examination
OBSTETRICS &
GYNAECOLOGY

examination
OBSTETRICS &
GYNAECOLOGY

4th edition

Judith Goh
AO, MBBS, FRANZCOG, PhD, CU
Urogynaecologist,
Greenslopes Private Hospital, Queensland
Professor, Griffith University, Gold Coast, Queensland

Michael Flynn
MBBS, FRANZCOG, FRCOG
Pindara Private Hospital, Gold Coast, Queensland

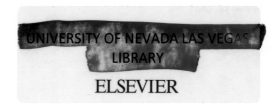

UNIVERSITY OF NEVADA LAS VEGAS
LIBRARY

ELSEVIER

ELSEVIER

Elsevier Australia. ACN 001 002 357
(a division of Reed International Books Australia Pty Ltd)
Tower 1, 475 Victoria Avenue, Chatswood, NSW 2067

Notice
This publication has been carefully reviewed and checked to ensure that the content is as accurate and current
as possible at time of publication. We would recommend, however, that the reader verify any procedures,
treatments, drug dosages or legal content described in this book. Neither the author, the contributors, nor the
publisher assume any liability for injury and/or damage to persons or property arising from any error in or
omission from this publication.

National Library of Australia Cataloguing-in-Publication Data

---

Goh, Judith, author.

Examination obstetrics and gynaecology / Judith Goh ; Michael Flynn.

4th edition

9780729542524 (paperback)

Obstetrics.
Gynecology.
Pregnancy.
Women–Medical examinations.

Flynn, Michael (Michael B.) author.

618

Content Strategist: Larissa Norrie
Content Development Specialist: Lauren Santos
Project Manager: Devendran Kannan
Edited by Leanne Poll
Proofread by Forsyth Publishing Services
Cover and internal design by Stan Lamond
Index by Innodata
Typeset by Toppan Best-set Premedia Limited
Printed in China by CTPS

Dedication

To my family and friends, for their endless support and encouragement.

JTWG

To Karen, who shared with me the wonder of childbirth. And to Molly, Daniel and Grace, who remind me daily!

MBF

Contents

Preface to the 4th edition

When writing the first edition of *Examination Obstetrics and Gynaecology* in 1996 we aimed to present a practical guide for medical students, junior medical staff, specialist trainees and general practitioners. The book not only became a checklist for those undergoing their undergraduate and specialist examinations, but also a handy point-form backup for daily clinical work.

The need has not changed over the second, third and now fourth editions for clear, concise explanations and management; however, obstetrics and gynaecology has. The specialty has evolved from an art to a practice with an evidence-based platform. This is a very positive change in our profession and reflecting this we have invited a number of contributors to this edition. Each in their own way has focused on their special area of obstetrics and gynaecology to impart a greater depth to the topic, but retain the note and checklist format. Many chapters have entirely changed to reflect this. Many references now also contain web addresses to long-term ongoing trials, reflecting the fluid nature of our specialty.

A clear focus of the book is passing exams and so sample Objective Structured Clinical Examination (OSCE) cases have been provided from examiners.

Our ultimate goal would be for the reader to not only pass an exam, but also to get the feel for the passion, enjoyment and great satisfaction of a truly wonderful specialty.

Michael Flynn
Judith Goh AO

Contributors

Based on their respective expertise, the following people have contributed content to chapters and we would like to extend our gratitude to them for dedicating their time, knowledge and input to ensure the success of this project.

Dr Helen L Barrett, FRACP
Obstetric Physician and Endocrinologist, Royal Women's Hospital
Brisbane, Queensland

Dr Clare Boothroyd, MBBS (Hons), MMed Sci, FRACP, FRANZCOG, CREI
IVF Med, Greenslopes Private Hospital
Brisbane, Queensland

Dr Thea Bowler, MBBS, MRANZCOG, BSc
Senior Registrar, Mater Hospital
Brisbane, Queensland

Dr Jackie Chua, MBBS, DRCOG (UK), FRANZCOG, DDU, COGU
Director, Queensland Ultrasound for Women
Senior Medical Officer, Mater Mothers Hospital
Associate Senior Lecturer, University of Queensland
Brisbane, Queensland

Dr Glenn Gardener, MBBS, DipRACOG, FRANZCOG, CMFM
Director, Mater Centre for Maternal Fetal Medicine
Brisbane, Queensland

Dr Peta Higgs, MBBS, FRANZCOG, CU
Urogynaecologist, The Sunshine Coast Private Hospital, Nambour Hospital
Sunshine Coast, Queensland

Dr Yasmin Jayasinghe, FRANZCOG, PhD
Senior Lecturer, Department of Obstetrics and Gynaecology, University of Melbourne
Consultant Gynaecologist, Royal Children's Hospital, Royal Women's Hospital Melbourne
Parkville, Victoria

Dr Hannah Krause, AO, MBBS, FRANZCOG, CU, MPhil
Urogynaecologist, Queen Elizabeth II Jubilee Hospital, Ramsay Specialist Centre, Greenslopes Private Hospital
Brisbane, Queensland

Associate Professor Karin Lust, FRACP
Interim Clinical Director, Obstetrics and Gynaecology, General and Obstetric Physician, Associate Professor, University of Queensland
Brisbane, Queensland

Dr Amy Mellor, MBBS, FRANZCOG (medal), IFEPAG
Arrivals Obstetric Centre, Eve Health, Mater Health Services
Brisbane, Queensland

Dr Justin Nasser, MBBS, FRANZCOG, DDU, MReprodMed
Senior Staff Specialist, Maternal Fetal Medicine Unit, Gold Coast University Hospital
Southport, Queensland

Dr Neroli Ngenda, MBBS, MRACOG, FRANZCOG
Visiting Medical Officer, Royal Brisbane and Women's Hospital and Sunnybank Private
Hospital
Brisbane, Queensland

Associate Professor Vivienne O'Connor, MEd, MBChB, MRCOG, FRCOG, FRANZCOG
Obstetrician and Gynaecologist, Director of the Simulated Patient Program, University of
Queensland
Brisbane, Queensland

Dr William Parsonage, BMedSci (Hons), BM, BS, DM, MRCP, FRACP
Royal Brisbane and Women's Hospital
Herston, Australia

Dr Gary Swift, MBBS, FRANZCOG, MReprodMed
Senior Visiting Medical Officer, Pindara Private Hospital, Gold Coast University Hospital and
Robina Hospital. Senior Specialist Queensland Fertility Group

Dr Amy Tang, MBBS, FRANZCOG, CGO
Gynaecological Oncologist, Queensland Centre for Gynaecological Cancer
Brisbane, Queensland

Dr Nikki Whelan, MBBS, FRANZCOG
Member of Queensland Maternal and Perinatal Quality Council, International Society for the
Study of Hypertension in Pregnancy, and International Association of Diabetes and Pregnancy
Study Groups
Clinical Tutor, The Wesley Clinical School
Auchenflower, Queensland

Associate Professor Anusch Yazdani, MBBS (Hons), FRANZCOG, CREI
Director of Research and Development, Queensland Fertility Group Research Foundation
Associate Professor of Gynaecology, University of Queensland
Brisbane, Queensland

Dr Susan Roberts, MBBS (Hons), FRANZCP
Perinatal and Consultation Liaison Psychiatrist, Gold Coast University Hospital
Gold Coast, Queensland

Reviewers

Dr Deborah Bateson, MA (Oxon), MSc, MBBS
Medical Director, Family Planning NSW
Clinical Associate Professor, Department of Obstetrics, Gynaecology and Neonatology, University of Sydney
Ashfield, New South Wales

Dr Anju Basu, MBBS, FRANZCOG
Gynaecologist, Southern Cross Hospital
Wellington, New Zealand

Dr Penelope M Sheehan, MBBS, GDEB, FRANZCOG,
Obstetrician, Head of Unit, Royal Women's Hospital
Lecturer in Obstetrics and Gynaecology, University of Melbourne
Parkville, Victoria

Dr Sebastian Hobson, MBBS, BMedSc, PGCSexHlth, MPH, FRANZCOG
Obstetrician and Maternal Fetal Medicine Fellow, Monash Health
Clayton, Victoria

Associate Professor Louis Izzo, MBBS, FRCOG, FRANZCOG
Associate Professor (Clinical) Obstetrics and Gynaecology, Head Department Obstetrics and Gynaecology, Canterbury Hospital
Canterbury, New South Wales

Gynaecology

Chapter 1

Gynaecological history and examination

Judith Goh

History

The gynaecological history and examination are a modification of standardised history taking designed for the efficient elucidation of the presenting problem, concluding with a provisional or differential diagnosis and a plan for further management. This guide to taking a gynaecological history may need to be modified, depending on the presenting complaint:

- name and age
- presenting complaint
- menstrual history
  - age of menarche/menopause
  - date of last menstrual period
  - length of menstruation and cycle
  - frequency/regularity of cycles
  - menstrual loss, presence of clots or flooding
  - duration of dysmenorrhoea and its relationship to periods
- abnormal bleeding
  - intermenstrual
  - postcoital
  - postmenopausal
- abnormal discharge
  - colour, pruritus, offensive odour
- cervical cytology
  - date of last examination and result
- sexual history
  - dyspareunia (superficial, deep), vaginal dryness
  - contraception
  - previous sexually transmitted infections
- hormonal therapy
  - oral/implant/injectable/intrauterine contraceptives
  - hormone replacement therapy

- menopausal symptoms
- pain
  - onset, duration, nature, site
  - relationship to menstrual cycles
- symptoms of prolapse
  - vaginal lump, dragging
- lower urinary tract
  - incontinence (stress or urge)
  - nocturia, frequency, urgency, dysuria, haematuria, pain
  - voiding symptoms: slow stream, hesitancy, sensation of incomplete emptying
- anorectal
  - constipation, obstructed defecation
  - peri-rectal (PR) bleeding
- other systems review
- past obstetric and gynaecological history
- past medical and surgical history
- social history
- cigarette smoking and alcohol intake
- medications, other drug use, allergies

Examination

Examination always begins with inspection, then palpation, followed by percussion and auscultation.

General
- appearance, colour
- blood pressure, pulse
- breast, thyroid examination
- presence of lymphadenopathy
- abdominal examination: scars, tenderness, masses

Genital examination
- inspection of the external genitalia, urethral meatus, perineal body
- evidence of oestrogen deficiency, prolapse, unusual masses, ulcers, bleeding/blood
- speculum: inspection of the vagina and cervix; checking for presence of a discharge/blood; taking specimens for cervical cancer screening and microbiological swabs; using Sims' speculum to assess uterovaginal prolapse
- assessing for urinary incontinence with coughing and prolapse reduced
- bimanual examination to assess: uterine size, shape, ante/retroversion, mobility, tenderness; cervical motion pain; adnexal tenderness, masses; pelvic masses and their relationship to the uterus (e.g. separate from uterus, moving with uterus); uterosacral ligament tenderness, presence of nodules; pouch of Douglas (presence of tumour nodules); rectovaginal septum

Conclusion

- summary of history and clinical findings
- provisional diagnosis, further investigations and management

Chapter 2

Amenorrhoea

Clare Boothroyd
Judith Goh

Puberty

Definition. Puberty is the physiological stage of development which results in becoming capable of reproduction (ovulation in the female and spermatogenesis in the male).

Endocrinology of puberty

In the fetus, the hypothalamic–pituitary axis responsible for pubertal development is able to function normally, but chronic inhibitory tone secondary to high levels of sex hormones from the fetoplacental unit inhibits fetal gonadotrophin release. After birth, increasing central nervous inhibition prevents gonadotrophin secretion. Puberty occurs when the gradual rise in gonadotrophin-releasing hormone (GnRH) secretion stimulates the pituitary to release gonadotrophins. With the lowering in central nervous system inhibition, there is an increase in hypothalamic generation of GnRH and increasing ovarian sensitivity to gonadotrophins.

Secondary sexual characteristics

MAJOR PHYSICAL CHANGES DURING PUBERTY

- development of secondary sexual characteristics
- changes in body mass and fat distribution
- rapid skeletal growth, with fusion of epiphyses

SECONDARY FEMALE CHARACTERISTICS

These include the enlargement of the ovaries, uterus, vagina, labia and breasts, and the growth of pubic hair.

- **Breast development** (thelarche) is classified into Tanner stages 1–5. Development normally starts between 8 and 13 years of age. It is often the first physical sign of puberty and is primarily controlled by ovarian oestrogens.
- **Pubic hair growth** is under the control of adrenal androgens. There is a high correlation between breast and pubic hair stages.

- **Growth in height** usually occurs, with the peak growth velocity coinciding with Tanner stages 2–3 (at about 12 years of age). In the year of maximum growth, 6–11 cm is added to the height.
- **Axillary hair growth** begins at about 12.5–13 years of age. It takes about 15 months from the first appearance of axillary hair to achieve adult distribution and is under control of adrenal androgens.
- **Menarche** occurs at the average age of 13 years (range 12.2–14.2 years). It occurs within 2 years of the onset of breast development, regardless of the age at which this occurs. Menarche occurs after the peak of the growth spurt in height but growth continues for a few months after menarche.
- **Skeletal age** corresponds better to maturity than chronological age.
- **Vaginal length** increases before the development of secondary sexual characteristics. There is also enlargement of the vulva.
- **Uterine growth** is mainly due to enlargement of the myometrium.

Primary amenorrhoea

Definition. Primary amenorrhoea is defined as no spontaneous uterine bleeding by age 16 years when normal growth and secondary sexual characteristics are present, or no sexual development by age 14.

The average age of menarche is 12.7 years. The requirements for having menses are:
- a functional outflow tract and uterus
- normal ovarian hormone production and follicular development
- anterior pituitary stimulation
- hypothalamic/central nervous system regulation

Management of primary amenorrhoea

WHEN TO INVESTIGATE
- no sexual development by age 14 years
- no spontaneous menstruation by age 16 years or within 2 years of onset of breast development
- Before evaluation, exclude:
- pregnancy
- chronic disease

HISTORY
- secondary sexual characteristics, sequence of events
- weight gain or loss
- excessive physical activity
- galactorrhoea
- medication and drugs
- past medical history
- family history, genetic anomalies
- anosmia, colour blindness

EXAMINATION
- height, weight, blood pressure
- webbed neck, inguinal hernia

- secondary sexual characteristics (feminising, masculinising, infantile)
- genitalia (avoid vaginal examination if the patient is not sexually active; instead, part the labia to observe, for example, an imperforate hymen)

INVESTIGATIONS

Investigations will depend on historical and clinical findings:
- ultrasound scan of the pelvis, magnetic resonance imaging (MRI)
- follicle-stimulating hormone (FSH), luteinising hormone (LH), prolactin, thyroid function tests
- karyotype
- androgens: testosterone, androstenedione, dehydroepiandrosterone sulfate (DHEAS), 17-hydroxyprogesterone
- endometrial cultures, such as tuberculosis and schistosomiasis where indicated

Classification of primary amenorrhoea

This classification is based on secondary sexual characteristics.

SEXUALLY INFANTILE

- short stature (Turner's syndrome, hypothalamic/pituitary causes, hypothyroidism)
- normal stature (true gonadal dysgenesis, hypogonadotrophic hypogonadism)

FEMINISING SECONDARY SEXUAL CHARACTERISTICS

- constitutional delay
- testicular feminisation
- müllerian anomalies

MASCULINISING SECONDARY SEXUAL CHARACTERISTICS

- polycystic ovarian syndrome
- congenital adrenal hyperplasia
- 5-alpha-reductase deficiency
- ovarian tumours
- true hermaphroditism

Causes of primary amenorrhoea

HYPOGONADOTROPHIC HYPOGONADISM

Causes of hypogonadotrophic hypogonadism include physiological delay, weight loss, anorexia and excessive exercise, GnRH deficiency with anosmia, and central nervous system defects/trauma.

Investigate with the GnRH test: administer GnRH; if the LH response is appropriate, this indicates hypothalamic failure; in the absence of LH response, pituitary failure is most likely.

The commonest cause of isolated hypogonadotrophic hypogonadism due to deficient GnRH secretion is Kallman's syndrome. This is an autosomal dominant condition, more common in males than females. There is associated anosmia secondary to defective development of the olfactory bulb and tract. Management is by ovulation induction with gonadotrophins or GnRH, and hormone replacement therapy.

HYPERGONADOTROPHIC HYPOGONADISM (GONADAL DYSGENESIS)

This is due to genetic or enzymatic abnormality, resulting in failure of gonadal development or abnormal functioning of the ovary.

Causes. Causes include: structural abnormalities of the X chromosome, 45XO; pure gonadal dysgenesis with 46XX, 46XY; 46XX with 17-hydroxylase deficiency (this enzyme is required for oestrogen synthesis); and other causes of premature ovarian failure (*see Ch 12*).

Investigations. Karyotyping is performed; as for premature ovarian failure (*see Ch 12*).

Management. The patient is usually infertile, and pregnancy is generally achieved with donor eggs though spontaneous conceptions have been reported and new techniques of ovarian cortex autotransplantation are developing. For breast development, use very low doses of oestrogen (e.g. 12.5 μg transdermal oestradiol or 1 mg oestradiol valerate every second day) for 6–12 months, then daily oestrogen for 6 months, and then introduce progestin. Transfer to the combined oral contraceptive pill can occur when contraception is required.

ANDROGEN INSENSITIVITY SYNDROME (TESTICULAR FEMINISATION)

Prevalence. Prevalence is 1 in 20 000 to 1 in 64 000.

Genetics. This is an X-linked inheritance condition, so a family history is important.

Endocrinology. To use testosterone, peripheral tissues need to convert testosterone to dihydrotestosterone via the enzyme 5-alpha-reductase. Testicular feminisation is associated with a variety of defects in androgen receptors (e.g. total absence of androgen receptors, abnormal binding of androgen to receptors and postreceptor binding abnormalities).

Presentation. Primary amenorrhoea; absent uterus and ovaries; sparse pubic/axillary hair; breast development is present; inguinal hernia, possibly with testes present at hernial orifice; vaginal pouch/pit is present; tall stature, absence of pimples or acne.

Investigations. The karyotype is male (XY); serum testosterone is above the normal female range and is in the male range.

Management. The patient is phenotypically female; remove gonads after pubertal development (age 18–20 years) because of a risk of malignant change in the gonads. Hormone replacement therapy is required with the use of oestrogen alone. The patient is infertile and generally families are created with donor oocytes and surrogate arrangements and/or adoption.

MÜLLERIAN ANOMALIES

Presentation is variable but can be primary amenorrhoea with secondary sexual characteristics present (*see Ch 14*).

OTHER CAUSES OF PRIMARY AMENORRHOEA

- hyperprolactinaemia (rare)
- polycystic ovarian disease
- agonadism
- 46XY with 17-hydroxylase deficiency
- premature ovarian failure

Constitutional delay in puberty

Definition. This is constitutional delay of growth occurring in an otherwise healthy adolescent. Height is below chronological age, but generally appropriate for bone age and stage of pubertal development, both of which are usually delayed. If the normal pattern of growth and puberty is lost, the delay in puberty is likely to be due to an endocrinological abnormality. There is delayed growth in patients with severe systemic disease (e.g. asthma, renal disease, coeliac disease, inflammatory bowel disease and long-term use of corticosteroids).

Principles of management of primary amenorrhoea

Prevent serious/life-threatening disease by:
- monitoring for gonadoblastoma and removing gonad if Y chromosome is present
- using hormone replacement therapy (initially unopposed oestrogen for 12 months, starting with low-dose oestrogen for breast development and to avoid premature epiphyseal closure)
- treating underlying disease (e.g. anorexia nervosa)

FERTILITY
- induction of ovulation, donor eggs
- adoption

PHYSICAL/EMOTIONAL DEVELOPMENT
- secondary sexual characteristics
- sexual function
- stature

Secondary amenorrhoea

Definition. Secondary amenorrhoea is defined as no menses for over 6 months in the absence of pregnancy, lactation, hysterectomy, endometrial ablation/resection or hormonal manipulation. The definition of oligomenorrhoea is a cycle length of over 35 days or fewer than or equal to eight periods per year.

Causes of secondary amenorrhoea

OESTROGEN DEFICIENCY
- gonadal failure
- hypothalamic causes (e.g. stress, exercise, anorexia)
- pituitary lesions
- hyperprolactinaemia

UNOPPOSED OESTROGEN
- polycystic ovarian syndrome/chronic anovulation
- follicular cysts
- androgen excess

OTHER CAUSES
- intrauterine synechiae (Asherman's syndrome)
- congenital adrenal hyperplasia (late-onset)
- other medical conditions (e.g. thyroid disease)

HISTORY
- menstrual history (Have all periods occurred while taking hormone therapy?)
- medication: oral contraceptive pill
- weight: anorexia, exercise

- stress: physical, emotional
- hirsutism, acne
- galactorrhoea, visual changes
- hot flushes, dry vagina
- past history of curettage

EXAMINATION

- general observations, weight, blood pressure
- sexual characteristics
- hirsutism
- galactorrhoea
- thyroid
- genital/vaginal examination

INVESTIGATIONS

- exclude pregnancy
- FSH with E_2, +/− LH
- thyroid function test, serum prolactin
- if hirsute, perform tests, including serum testosterone, DHEAS, 17-hydroxyprogesterone
- hysteroscopy/hysterosalpingogram

Management and further investigations of secondary amenorrhoea

PREMATURE OVARIAN FAILURE

(See Ch 12.)

- investigations: chromosomes, autoantibody tests
- management: hormone replacement therapy

HYPOTHALAMIC AMENORRHOEA

Investigations reveal normal serum prolactin levels, normal thyroid function tests, normal or low LH and FSH, and reduced oestrogen levels (inappropriately low gonadotrophin levels for low oestrogen).

Management depends on the cause of amenorrhoea (e.g. anorexia nervosa requires psychiatric referral).

POLYCYSTIC OVARIAN SYNDROME

(See Ch 5.)

ASHERMAN'S SYNDROME

- hysteroscopic division +/− resection of adhesion
- may use various means to reduce the risk of re-adherence of endometrial walls (e.g. oestrogen supplementation, intrauterine device)

MEDICAL PROBLEMS

- Treat and/or refer to other subspecialist as appropriate.
- Hyperprolactinaemia: treat with pharmacological agents or surgery.

TUMOURS

- Adrenals: these patients have greatly raised DHEAS and 17-hydroxyprogesterone.
- Ovarian tumours are associated with raised testosterone and androstenedione levels.

Further reading

Edmonds, D.K., 2003. Congenital malformations of the genital tract and their management. Best Pract. Res. Clin. Obstet. Gynaecol. 17, 19–40.

Lalwani, S., Reindollar, R.H., Davis, A.J., 2003. Normal onset of puberty: have definitions of onset changed? Obstet. Gynecol. Clin. North Am. 30, 279–286.

Timmreck, L.S., Reindollar, R.H., 2003. Contemporary issues in primary amenorrhoea. Obstet. Gynecol. Clin. North Am. 30, 287–302.

Chapter 3

Abnormal uterine bleeding

Anusch Yazdani

Terminology for disorders of menstruation

The terminology for describing the disorders of menstruation has been extensively revised with the eradication of non-descriptive terms with Latin or Greek roots, such as menorrhagia, dysfunctional bleeding or polymenorrhoea. Abnormal uterine bleeding (AUB) is the accepted term used to describe any deviation from the normal menstrual cycle. The key characteristics of an abnormal cycle (i.e. regularity, frequency, heaviness of flow and duration of flow) are now used descriptively.

Disturbances of regularity

Irregular menstrual bleeding. Cycle length variation of more than 20 days in individual cycles over a period of 1 year.

Absent menstrual bleeding (amenorrhea: this term has been retained). No bleeding in a 90-day period.

Disturbances of frequency

Infrequent menstrual bleeding. One to two episodes of bleeding in a 90-day period.

Frequent menstrual bleeding. More than four episodes of bleeding in a 90-day period.

Disturbances of flow

Heavy menstrual bleeding (HMB). Excessive menstrual blood loss that interferes with the woman's physical, emotional, social and material quality of life. It can occur alone or in combination with other symptoms. HMB is the most common presentation of AUB.

Disturbance of the duration of flow

Prolonged menstrual bleeding. Menstrual periods exceeding 8 days in duration on a regular basis.

Irregular non-menstrual bleeding

Irregular episodes of bleeding, often light and short, occurring between normal menstrual periods. Mostly associated with benign or malignant structural lesions. May occur during or following sexual intercourse.

Bleeding outside of the reproductive age

Postmenopausal bleeding (PMB). Bleeding occurring more than 1 year after the acknowledged menopause.

Precocious menstruation. Bleeding occurring before 9 years of age.

Acute AUB

An episode of bleeding in a woman of reproductive age, who is not pregnant, of sufficient quantity to require immediate intervention to prevent further blood loss.

Chronic AUB

Bleeding from the uterine corpus that is abnormal in duration, volume and/or frequency, and has been present for the majority of the last 6 months.

Causes of AUB: the PALM-COEIN classification system

In 2011 the FIGO PALM-COEIN classification of causes of AUB was introduced (see Table 3.1).

Any patient may have more than one potential cause contributing to AUB.

It is important to emphasise that women who present with AUB may have non-uterine causes of vaginal bleeding, including vulvar, urethral, vesical, vaginal, cervical and recto-anal disorders.

Anatomical and structural (PALM)

POLYPS (AUB-P)

AUB is the most common presenting symptom of endometrial or endocervical polyps. Diagnosed by ultrasound, saline infusion sonography, or hysteroscopy, it can be managed hysteroscopically.

Table 3.1 FIGO PALM-COEIN classification of causes of AUB		
PALM	**COEI**	**N**
visually objective structural	unrelated to structural anomalies	entities not yet classified
Polyps (AUB-P) **A**denomyosis (AUB-A) **L**eiomyoma (AUB-L) **M**alignancy (AUB-M)	**C**oagulopathy (AUB-C) **O**vulatory disorders (AUB-O) **E**ndometrial (AUB-E) **I**atrogenic (AUB-I)	**N**ot classified

Source: Adapted from Committee on Gynecologic Practice. Management of acute abnormal uterine bleeding in nonpregnant reproductive-aged women. Committee Opinion No. 557. American College of Obstetricians and Gynecologists. Obstet Gynecol 2013;121:891–6. Available from: http://www.acog.org/Resources-And-Publications/Committee-Opinions/Committee-on-Gynecologic-Practice/Management-of-Acute-Abnormal-Uterine-Bleeding-in-Nonpregnant-Reproductive-Aged-Women

ADENOMYOSIS (AUB-A)

In women with adenomyosis, 70% have AUB and 30% have menstrual pain. Putative diagnosis may be made by examination, ultrasound or magnetic resonance imaging (MRI), though the diagnosis is histological.

LEIOMYOMAS (AUB-Lsm OR AUB-Lo)

Fibroids or leiomyomas are the most common tumour of the genital tract. Submucosal and large intramural fibroids may be associated with AUB.

Malignancy (AUB-M)

This category includes malignancy and premalignant conditions, such as endometrial cancer and endometrial hyperplasia.

Unrelated to structural anomalies (COEI)

COAGULOPATHIES (AUB-C)

Disorders of hemostasis are an important cause of AUB that may be overlooked during the differential diagnosis.

Ovulatory dysfunction (AUB-O)

Patients with menses that are variable in timing and flow usually have ovulatory abnormalities associated with endocrinopathies, such as polycystic ovary syndrome (PCOS) or hypothyroidism. Investigations focus on the assessment of ovulatory dysfunction.

Endometrial causes (AUB-E)

Patients in this category may have regular cycles, normal ovulation and no other definable cause of AUB. This category includes idiopathic causes of AUB. Others may present with intermenstrual bleeding (IMB), which may be secondary to infection or inflammatory processes.

Iatrogenic (AUB-I)

Iatrogenic causes include intrauterine device (IUD) and other systemic drugs.

Not yet classified (AUB-N)

This is a mixed category that includes conditions such as arteriovenous malformations.

Assessment of AUB

History
- menstrual history
  - menarche
  - cycle, regularity, frequency
  - loss (clots, flooding)
  - pain
  - impact on life
- sexual and reproductive history including contraception
- medical history including iron deficiency, anaemia, thyroid disease, bleeding tendency
- pictorial chart of menstrual loss and number of pads/tampons used is of limited benefit other than for research purposes

Examination

- observations for evidence of haemodynamic compromise
- general examination for evidence of bleeding disorder or endocrinopathy
- abdominal examination, with evidence of masses, such as a large uterus or hepatosplenomegaly
- vaginal and speculum examination to assess the cervix and uterus, including cervical cancer screening

Investigations

- full blood count, iron studies
  - prolactin, thyroid function, follicle-stimulating hormone (FSH), luteinising hormone (LH), oestradiol and progesterone if abnormal cyclicity, human chorionic gonadotrophin (hCG)
- targeted screening for bleeding disorders (when indicated, based on history), including platelet function studies for platelet/coagulation disorders (which cause up to 20% of adolescent admissions for menorrhagia)
- cervical cytology
- ultrasound scan of pelvis as a first-line diagnostic tool to exclude structural anomalies
- hysteroscopy and endometrial sample
  - women > 45 years old
  - failure to respond to therapy
  - non-menstrual bleeding
  - patients with other risk factors such as PCOS, hereditary non-polyposis colorectal cancer (HNPCC)

Management of AUB: HMB

The general treatment for AUB depends on many factors, including the woman's choice, contraindications and future fertility needs.

1. correct any lifestyle factors: stop smoking
2. correct any primary disorders
3. manage the AUB

Prostaglandin inhibitors

- mefenamic acid
- naproxen or other non-steroidal anti-inflammatory drugs (can reduce menstrual loss by 20%–50%, which may be improved if used in conjunction with the oral contraceptive pill; also beneficial in women with dysmenorrhoea)

Antifibrinolytics and haemostatics

- tranexamic acid

Hormonal therapy

COMBINED ORAL CONTRACEPTIVE PILL

This reduces menstrual blood flow by inhibiting ovulation and decreasing endometrial thickness.

PROGESTERONE

- Routes of administration are oral, intramuscular, intrauterine and subcutaneous implants.
- It may cause irregular bleeding.
- Cyclical oral progesterone therapy:
  - This reduces menstrual loss, but is not as effective as tranexamic acid or Mirena device (Cochrane review).
  - Cyclical progesterone therapy may be more effective in women with ovulatory disorders.
  - High doses of norethisterone are commonly used to reduce or arrest bleeding in emergency treatment of dysfunctional uterine bleeding.
- The levonorgestrel-releasing intrauterine system has the added advantage of being an effective form of contraception and reducing progesterone systemic side effects. A common side effect is irregular bleeding for the first 6 months.

Surgical management of menorrhagia

Hysteroscopic removal of polyps and fibroids

- Hysteroscopy and endometrial sampling are essential diagnostic tools, but curettage has limited long-term benefit on HMB.
- Endometrial polyps and submucosal fibroids may be removed via the hysteroscope.

Endometrial ablation/resection

- an option for a woman who has completed her childbearing and has HMB
- produces amenorrhoea or an acceptable reduction in blood loss during periods in 80% of patients
- considered with normal uterus
- efficacy is reduced with large uteri, fibroids or adenomyosis

Hysterectomy

- has the advantage of no risk of menstrual loss following the procedure
- is the option when other treatment options have failed
- possible loss of ovarian function even if ovaries conserved

Uterine artery embolisation

This is an option for a woman who has a large fibroid and wishes uterine conservation.

Chapter 4

Endometriosis

Gary Swift

Definition. Endometriosis is defined as the presence of endometrial-like tissue outside the uterus, which induces a chronic inflammatory reaction and is associated with pain, subfertility and impaired quality of life.

Cyclical bleeding into deposits causes inflammation, scarring and adhesions, leading to pain, anatomical distortion and pelvic organ dysfunction. Dysmenorrhoea, dyspareunia, non-cyclical pelvic pain, dysuria, dyschezia and infertility result from the disease, though it may be asymptomatic in a minority. Symptoms in women subsequently found to have endometriosis may commence soon after menarche, with the disease varying widely in severity, symptomatology, and clinical and social impact. The disease ranges from relatively trivial superficial deposits causing few symptoms to severe deep infiltrating endometriosis (DIE) affecting the full thickness of the posterior vaginal fornix, muscularis of the bowel, bladder and/or the rectovaginal septum with associated quality of life implications.

Prevalence. An estimated 10% of reproductive-age women, in all social and ethnic groups, have endometriosis; up to 50% of women presenting with infertility will be found to have endometriosis; 50%–60% of women presenting with pelvic pain have endometriosis as an underlying cause. Endometriosis is an incidental finding in 1%–7% of laparoscopic procedures for sterilisation.

Risk factors

- higher risk with early menarche, short cycles and heavy menstrual flow (> 8 days' relative risk [RR] 2.4)
- increased risk with Müllerian anomalies and cervical or vaginal obstruction
- relative risk greatly increased with first-degree relative afflicted
- pregnancy has protective effect, reducing with time
- risk reduces with increasing parity and prolonged lactation
- reduced incidence with smoking (reduced oestrogen) and exercise (increased sex hormone-binding globulin [SHBG] and reduced luteal oestrogen levels)

- dietary factors: reduced risk with high fruit (odds ratio [OR] 0.6) and vegetable (OR 0.3) intake and fish oil (animal studies); increased risk with high red meat consumption (OR 2.0)
- increased risk with higher levels of vitamin D
- inverse association between endometriosis and body mass index (BMI)
- possible increased risk with alcohol, caffeine, and polychlorinated biphenyls (PCB) and dioxin exposure

Aetiology

The exact aetiology is still not known. The most widely accepted theory is related to viable endometrial cells reaching the peritoneal cavity through retrograde menstruation along the fallopian tubes (Sampson 1927). At least 90% of women with patent fallopian tubes will have evidence of retrograde menstruation; yet, in the majority, the menstrual debris is rapidly and efficiently cleared, by macrophages and natural killer (NK) cells leading to a suspicion of defective immune processing.

Alternative theories of 'coelomic metaplasia' and 'embryonic cell rests' are less favoured.

Increased susceptibility is possibly related to:
- increased exposure to menstrual debris
- abnormal eutopic endometrium
- altered peritoneal environment
- reduced immune surveillance
- increased angiogenic capacity

Genetics

Genes influence susceptibility to endometriosis, though exact genetic loci and the mechanisms of aberrant expression are still not elucidated.
- considered to be a complex heritable trait with many genes contributing to risk, with the contribution of any one individual gene likely to be small
- genomic linkages found on chromosomes 7, 10 and 20 so far
- relative increased risk with sibling affected: 2.34 to 15 times (higher risk in more severe forms of the disease)

Pathology

The lesions of endometriosis vary from superficial to deep and in appearance from clear to white to red to black in proportion to degree of inflammation, vascularity and haemosiderin deposition. Newly formed lesions tend to be clear to red, with older lesions more deeply pigmented, and with variable proportions of pale scarring and fibrosis. With increasing fibrosis, lesions become nodular. Lesions in postmenopausal or hormonally suppressed women will tend to be paler.

The inflammation and fibrosis leads to adhesions and anatomical distortion. Shortening and thickening of uterosacral ligaments reduces uterine mobility and causes fixed retroversion or lateral deviation. Shortening and thickening of ovarian ligaments displaces ovaries postero-medially. Pouch of Douglas obliteration follows involvement of rectal serosa and sometimes muscularis.

Endometriomas or 'chocolate cysts' are specific lesions that form in the ovaries. They are thought not to be true cysts but invaginations of the ovarian cortex lined by typical endometriotic tissue. The thick altered blood content resembles melted chocolate. These lesions have high recurrence rates if not excised completely. Endometriosis deposits are histologically similar to eutopic endometrium, but not identical. Plaques contain oestrogen, progesterone and androgen receptors, growing in the presence of oestrogen and atrophying with androgens.

Abnormal levels and function of growth factors, macrophages and proinflammatory cytokines have been observed in the peritoneal fluid and serum of women with endometriosis.

Pathogenesis

- Angiogenic processes are fundamental to the establishment of endometriosis.
- Polymorphisms in the vascular endothelial growth factor (VEGF) gene increase susceptibility to endometriosis in humans.
- There are current searches for endometriosis-specific angiogenic mechanisms.

Clinical presentation

Symptoms include the classic triad of dysmenorrhoea, dyspareunia and subfertility but may vary according to the anatomic site involved and may be asymptomatic. Symptom onset may be soon after menarche or delayed by interim menstrual suppression with the oral contraceptive pill, other hormonal contraceptives or child bearing.

Other symptoms include:

- chronic pelvic pain (cyclical and non-cyclical)
- ovulation pain (due to ovarian adhesions or endometriomas)
- cyclical rectal pain (dyschezia), bleeding or dysfunction (symptoms similar to irritable bowel syndrome)
- cyclical bladder pain or functional disturbance (dysuria, frequency, urgency)
- abnormal bleeding from the bladder (cyclical haematuria)
- infertility (as a result of direct anatomical or physiological impact)
- non-specific systemic symptoms such as low energy or chronic fatigue
- extrapelvic symptoms are rare but may include cyclical haemoptysis, migraine, right upper quadrant pain, umbilical discharge, perineal pain or discharge
- cyclical pain and tenderness in caesarean section scars (due to seeded deposits in the rectus abdominis muscles, sheath or subcutaneous tissues)

Diagnosis

There is no reliable non-surgical diagnostic test for endometriosis. Endometriosis may be suspected clinically with appropriate symptoms and examination findings (tenderness and nodularity in pouch of Douglas or uterosacral ligaments) or radiologic evidence of endometriomas.

Ultrasound, especially with 3D and dynamic assessment, can reliably diagnose endometriomas, many rectal nodules (including size and depth of muscularis involvement) and often adhesions between pelvic structures. The often-associated condition of adenomyosis may also be diagnosed by this modality.

Magnetic resonance imaging (MRI) may offer superior imaging quality for endometriosis involving deep tissue planes as well as endometriomas and adenomyosis, but is generally more expensive with less availability.

Although imaging may be highly suggestive, unless endometriotic 'blue dome cysts' are visible in the posterior vaginal fornix at speculum examination, direct visualisation at laparoscopy is required for definitive diagnosis, with preferably histological confirmation, and is regarded as the 'gold standard'.

Staging
- combination of clinical, radiological and surgical
- ideal system yet to be developed
- terminology includes minimal, mild, moderate and severe depending on number, size and depth of lesions
- American Fertility Society (AFS) staging is complex and detailed, but is most used in research settings

Treatments

Medical treatment
- primary therapy, postoperative, preventative
- no evidence that medical therapy is curative
- therapeutic goals: analgesia, menstrual suppression, disease suppression (primary and recurrent)

CONTRACEPTIVE
- hormonal medical therapies equally effective in symptom control, but vary in side effects and costs
- no evidence of improved fertility outcomes and may delay natural attempts at conception or the appropriate application of assisted reproductive technologies (ART)
- higher recurrence rates after medical treatment compared to surgical

Options
- progesterones: progesterone-only pill (POP), depot medroxyprogesterone acetate (DMPA), oral progestins (norethisterone, medroxyprogesterone acetate, dienogest), progesterone-containing intrauterine contraceptive devices (IUCDs)
- combined oral contraceptive pill (COCP)
- danazol (synthetic steroid, suppresses gonadotrophins + weak androgen)
- gestrinone (synthetic steroid progestogenic, anti-progestogenic and weak androgenic activity)
- gonadotrophin-releasing hormone (GnRH) agonists (goserelin, nafarelen, leuprolide)

Surgical treatment
Goals of surgical management to alter the natural course of disease:
- excision of all macroscopic disease
- pain relief
- restoration of function (menstrual, coital, bladder, bowel)
- fertility restoration or enhancement (primarily or as an adjunct to ART)

Laparoscopy is the 'gold standard' for diagnosis and therapeutic intervention. If endometriosis is present at laparoscopy, it is recommended that it is surgically removed at the same time as diagnosis, as it is an effective treatment for endometriosis-associated subfertility and pain. In cases of severe disease, diagnostic laparoscopy allows appropriate surgical planning for a subsequent procedure including counselling, consent and multi-disciplinary involvement (urology, colorectal surgery).

Excision of endometriotic deposits is more precise and potentially effective compared to in situ diathermy, with the additional benefit of histologic confirmation. Excision of ovarian endometriomas is superior to drainage and cautery with lower recurrence rates but with a potential to reduce ovarian reserve from collateral damage.

Segmental bowel resection may be required with muscularis involvement of the intestine at any level; discoid excision of deep localised disease is possible in the rectosigmoid.

The risks and potential complications with endometriosis surgery will vary with the stage of disease, anatomical distortion and visceral involvement. As such, complex cases require treatment where appropriate expertise exists and in dedicated units.

Alternative treatment

- acupuncture, Chinese medicine, naturopathy: potential positive effects on symptom control, but evidence based on randomised controlled trials is lacking

Prognosis

- natural history of early stage disease understanding is lacking
- tendency to progressive increase in number and size of deposits until excision, pregnancy, suppressive treatment or menopause
- optimal surgical resection of all macroscopic disease still associated with recurrence rates of at least 30%
- uncertain yet if early intervention in teenagers with surgical excision of all macroscopic disease will ultimately alter the underlying course of the disease, preserve future fertility or prevent chronic pain syndromes and analgesic dependence

Special areas

Endometriosis in adolescence

Endometriosis can be responsible for admissions with pain in the postmenarcheal 10–17-year-old age group. For adolescents with pelvic pain refractory to non-steroidal anti-inflammatory drugs (NSAIDs) and/or COCPs, it is estimated 50% will have underlying endometriosis. First-line medical treatment is appropriate, followed by laparoscopy and surgical management if unsuccessful.

Endometriosis and fertility

IMPACT ON FERTILITY

- spontaneous and assisted conception reduced in proportion to stage of disease and anatomical distortion
- quality of oocytes, ovarian reserve and implantation success reduced
- pain and menstrual disturbance have a negative impact on coital frequency

MEDICAL THERAPIES CONTRACEPTIVE

Surgical management is proven to improve mild and moderate disease stages, with severe forms difficult to evaluate due to variables, but trends to improved fertility, natural and assisted, with optimal surgical management.

IMPACT ON AND ROLE OF ASSISTED REPRODUCTIVE TECHNOLOGY (ART)

Endometriomas may be associated with reduced follicle numbers and ovarian responsiveness to gonadotrophin stimulation, especially with increasing volume. Currently, there is debate on excision prior to in vitro fertilisation (IVF). Surgical excision is not proven to improve outcomes with IVF and may reduce ovarian reserve further. Generally, excision is recommended if ≥ 4 cm, there is pain or access to follicles is affected.

There is an increased risk of ovarian abscess at oocyte retrieval if an endometrioma is entered (deliberately to drain or inadvertently).

Deep infiltrating endometriosis

- defined as deposits invading over 5 mm in depth
- severe form of endometriotic disease forming a subset with infiltrating deposits in bowel and/or bladder muscularis and rectovaginal septum
- management is complex with advanced surgical techniques required
- referral to centre with necessary expertise strongly recommended

Extrapelvic disease

This is rare, but it can affect any organ. Deposits have been documented in the umbilicus, lungs and central nervous system. It should be considered in any symptoms with a cyclical pattern, especially if it is associated with pain and/or bleeding.

References and further reading

American Society of Reproductive Medicine (ASRM) Guidelines. Available at: <www.asrm.org>.

D'Hooghe, T.M., Debrock, S., 2003. Future directions in endometriosis research. Obstet. Gynecol. Clin. North Am. 30, 221–244.

Eskenazi, B., Warner, M.L., 1997. Epidemiology of endometriosis. Obstet. Gynecol. Clin. North Am. 24, 235–238.

European Society of Human Reproduction and Embryology (ESHRE) Guidelines. Available at: <www.eshre.eu>.

Garcia-Velasco, J.A., Somigliana, E., 2009. Management of endometriomas in women requiring IVF: to touch or not to touch. Hum. Reprod. 24, 496–501.

Hull, M.L., Charnock-Jones, D.S., Chan, C.L.K., et al., 2003. Antiangiogenic agents are effective inhibitors of endometriosis. J. Clin. Endocrinol. Metab. 86, 2889–2899.

Kennedy, S., 1998. The genetics of endometriosis. J. Reprod. Med. 43 (Suppl. 3), S263–S268.

Kennedy, S., Bergqvist, A., Chapron, C., et al., 2005. on behalf of the ESHRE Special Interest Group for Endometriosis and Endometrium Guideline Development Group. ESHRE Guideline for the diagnosis and treatment of endometriosis. Hum. Reprod. 20, 2698–2704.

Parazzini, F., Chiaffarino, F., Surace, M., et al., 2004. Selected food intake and risk of endometriosis. Hum. Reprod. 19, 1755–1759.

Rogers, M.S., D'Amato, R.J., 2006. The effect of genetic diversity on angiogenesis. Exp. Cell Res. 312, 516–574.

Sampson, J.A., 1927. Peritoneal endometriosis due to the menstrual dissemination of endometrial tissue to the peritoneal cavity. Am. J. Obstet. Gynecol. 14, 422–469.

Treloar, S.A., Wicks, J., Nyholt, D.R., et al., 2005. Genome-wide linkage study in 1176 affected sister pair families identifies a significant susceptibility locus for endometriosis on chromosome 10q26. Am. J. Hum. Genet. 77 (3), 356–376.

Zondervan, K.T., Treloar, S.A., Lin, J., et al., 2007. Significant evidence of one or more susceptibility loci for endometriosis with near-Mendelian autosomal inheritance on chromosome 7p13–15. Hum. Reprod. 22, 717–728.

Chapter 5

Polycystic ovarian syndrome

Clare Boothroyd

Definition. The definition of polycystic ovarian syndrome (PCOS) was revised in 2003 (Rotterdam Consensus criteria). The diagnosis is based on two out of three of the following criteria:

- oligomenorrhoea (8 menses or less per year, or menstrual cycles > 35 days in length) or anovulation
- clinical and/or biochemical signs of hyperandrogenism
- polycystic ovaries, defined as at least one of the following:
  - 12 or more follicles measuring 2–9 mm in diameter; this was recommended to be revised to 25 follicles per ovary by the Taskforce in November 2014 because of the improved resolution with ultrasound probes (e.g. 8 mHz)
  - increased ovarian volume (> 10 cm^3)

If there is evidence of a dominant follicle (> 10 mm) or a corpus luteum, the scan should be repeated during the next cycle. Only one ovary fitting this definition or a single occurrence of one of the above criteria is sufficient to define the PCOS. It does not apply to women taking the oral contraceptive pill. Regularly menstruating women should be scanned in the early follicular phase (days 3–5). Oligomenorrhoeic and amenorrhoeic women should be scanned either at random or between days 3 and 5 after a progestogen-induced bleed *and* the exclusion of other aetiologies (congenital adrenal hyperplasia, androgen-secreting tumours, Cushing's syndrome).

The use of measurement of serum anti-müllerian hormone (AMH) as a diagnostic test is likely in the future but currently remains a research tool.

Prevalence. Prevalence is 5%–7% overall, 85% of oligomenorrhoeic females, 90% of women with hirsutism and 30% of infertile women.

Clinical presentation

- menstrual irregularities
  - amenorrhoea or oligomenorrhoea; particularly oligomenorrhoea soon after menarche
  - variable menstrual loss

- infertility
- androgen excess, such as hirsutism or acne

Aetiology

- Aetiology is multifactorial.
- About 50% of women with PCOS have affected sisters.
- Multiple candidate genes have been identified, but it is likely that a number of different pathways, both genetic and environmental, contribute to the same phenotype.

Pathophysiology

PCOS is characterised by ovarian, hypothalamic–pituitary, peripheral and adrenal dysfunction. The phenotype develops through chronic anovulation of any aetiology and a clear sequence of events is therefore not identifiable.

Ovaries

- High luteinising hormone (LH) levels drive ovarian androgen production.
- High intraovarian androgen concentrations inhibit follicular maturation and lead to inactive granulosa cells with minimal aromatase activity.
- The large number of ovarian follicles produces a high inhibin B, which inhibits follicle-stimulating hormone (FSH).

Hypothalamus–pituitary

- Hypothalamic dysfunction is associated with increased gonadotropin-releasing hormone agonist (GnRH) frequency and tonic (i.e. non-cyclic) LH release, elevating the LH/FSH ratio. The increase in LH is more pronounced in lean patients.
- The large number of ovarian follicles produces a high inhibin B, which inhibits FSH; however, as FSH is not fully suppressed, continuous follicular recruitment and stimulation proceeds but not to the level of full maturation and ovulation.
- Increased oestrogen production stimulates an increase in prolactin.

Peripheral compartment

- Reduced sex hormone-binding globulin (SHBG) concentrations perpetuate hyperandrogenaemia:
  - hyperinsulinaemia
  - obesity
  - hepatic dysfunction
- Peripheral alteration in insulin-like growth factor (IGF-1), androgen and oestrogen levels perpetuate hypothalamic dysfunction.
- Obesity reduces SHBG and increases peripheral aromatisation of androgens (androstenedione), which produces a chronic hyperoestrogenic state with reversal of the oestrone : oestradiol ratio.

Adrenal compartment

- dysregulation of cytochrome p-450c17 (as in the ovaries), but dehydroepiandrosterone sulfate (DHEAS) (of adrenal origin) is only increased in 50% of PCOS
- exaggerated adrenarchal response

Consequences of PCOS

Consequences are worsened by weight gain.

Reproductive consequences

- anovulation/oligo-ovulation leading to:
  - menstrual disturbances
  - infertility
  - reproductive failure
- abortion
  - controversial
  - may be related to hyperinsulinaemia

Metabolic consequences

- obesity
  - at least 50% of women with PCOS are obese
  - most are also hyperinsulinaemic and insulin resistant, independent of obesity
- metabolic syndrome: present in up to 40% of PCOS patients
- hyperinsulinaemia/diabetes
  - hyperinsulinaemia: 80% of obese PCOS; 30% of lean PCOS
  - diabetes
    — increased prevalence of impaired glucose tolerance (IGT) (35%) and type 2 diabetes (10%) in women with PCOS compared with age-matched and weight-matched populations of women without PCOS (Legro 2006)
    — a 5–10 time increased risk of type 2 diabetes
    — 10%–30% of women will develop type 2 diabetes within 3 years
    — conversion from IGT to type 2 diabetes is accelerated in PCOS
    — risk is increased further if positive family history
  - gestational diabetes: increased risk of gestational diabetes, regardless of body mass index (BMI)
- hyperlipidaemia: conflicting data

Neoplasia

- increased endometrial hyperplasia and perhaps carcinoma
  - hyperplasia: women with anovulatory infertility are at increased risk of endometrial hyperplasia
- carcinoma
  - reported three times increased risk of endometrial carcinoma
  - the evidence for an increased risk of endometrial carcinoma in PCOS is incomplete and contradictory
- increased breast cancer: data inconclusive

Cardiovascular disease

- poor data
- limited epidemiological data to support increased coronary heart disease

Other

- increased sleep apnoea
- non-alcoholic steatohepatitis

Differential diagnosis

- constitutional obesity
- idiopathic hirsutism
- Cushing's syndrome
- congenital adrenal hyperplasia
- hypothyroidism
- androgen producing tumours

Assessment

Assessment is based on clinical presentation and investigations to validate the diagnostic criteria, and exclude other endocrinopathies and sequelae.

History

- menstrual history
- reproductive history
- weight gain
- hirsutism, acne
- galactorrhoea, headaches

Examination

- hirsutism
- evidence of virilisation
- evidence of Cushing's syndrome (red striae, dermal wasting, facial plethora, hypertension), thyroid disorders
- acanthosis nigricans (a marker of insulin resistance)

Investigations

- FSH, oestradiol (LH/FSH ratio is not a diagnostic criterion)
- thyroid function test
- prolactin
- fasting glucose, insulin, lipids
- testosterone levels: if above 6 nmol/L, further investigations are required to check for adrenal or virilising tumours
- DHEAS: levels above 18 nmol/L necessitate exclusion of Cushing's syndrome
- 17-hydroxyprogesterone: if the morning level is <5.5 nmol/L, no further investigations are needed; if the levels are raised, check for congenital adrenal hyperplasia by a Synacthen stimulation test
- endometrial sampling, especially if history or prolonged amenorrhoea followed by heavy and/or irregular menses
- ultrasound scan of the pelvis
  - more than 80% of women with PCOS have a classic ultrasound appearance
  - morphologic changes have been found in different studies in different settings:
    — in 90% of women with hirsutism
    — in 90% of women with oligomenorrhoea
    — in 40% of women with a history of gestational diabetes
    — in 25% of women who considered themselves normal and reported regular menstrual cycles; this is called polycystic ovaries (PCO) or polycystic ovarian morphology (PCOM)
    — in 15% of women on a combined oral contraceptive pill (COCP)

Management

Management is dictated by the clinical presentation (e.g. menstrual changes, hirsutism and/or infertility).

Supportive

- lifestyle changes: the most important intervention
- weight reduction: 5%–10% of body weight over 6 months is sufficient to re-establish ovarian function in more than 50% of patients
- hirsutism: see management of hirsutism (*Ch 6*)

Not wanting to conceive

COCP

- protects endometrium by progestational changes
- oestrogen increases SHBG, resulting in reduced free testosterone and suppresses ovarian androgen production
- progestins inhibit 5-alpha-reductase in the skin, resulting in decreased hirsutism
- progestins suppress LH, resulting in decreased androgen production

PROGESTERONE (CYCLICAL ORAL OR DEPOT MEDROXYPROGESTERONE ACETATE, DMPA)

- negative feedback decreases GnRH production, resulting in decreased oestrogen and androgen
- protects endometrium
- not recommended in those planning or potentially planning a family because of the delay in return of ovulatory function

INSULIN-SENSITISING DRUGS

- thiazolidinediones (TZDs)
  - insulin sensitisers
  - specifically contraindicated for conception and associated with an increased risk of weight gain; unlikely to become a major component of PCOS management
- metformin (anecdotal evidence that standard-release preparation is more effective than extended-release preparation)
  - no change in BMI, waist : hip ratio
  - no effect on clinical hyperandrogenaemia (e.g. hirsutism)
  - reduced fasting glucose (statistically but not clinically significant)
  - reduced fasting insulin; also reduces conversion to diabetes mellitus in those with impaired glucose tolerance
  - reduced biochemical androgens
  - altered lipids
  - increased nausea and gastrointestinal side effects: dose related and should be reduced by slow introduction
- oral contraceptive pill (OCP) and metformin
  - OCP is more effective than metformin in improving menstrual pattern and reducing serum androgen levels
  - limited evidence demonstrating that the addition of metformin to the OCP is more effective than the OCP alone in improving hirsutism score and increasing serum SHBG levels

- insufficient evidence to demonstrate any benefit to adding metformin to the OCP in terms of reducing body weight, reducing serum androgen levels, and reducing fasting serum levels of metabolic parameters such as insulin, glucose or lipids

Wanting to conceive
See Fig. 5.1.

MEDICAL
- letrozole (not approved for ovulation induction in Australia): aromatase inhibitor, effective, reduced twinning
  - mechanism is selective reversible inhibition of aromatase (a product of CYP19 gene, part of the cytochrome P450 complex), which catalyses the rate-limiting step in the production of oestrogens
  - supposed benefit over clomiphene is reduced negative effects on target tissues such as endometrium and cervix
- clomiphene
- selective oestrogen receptor modulator
- central oestrogen receptor antagonism leads to reflex elevation in FSH and thereby ovulation
- commence on low dose
- 85% ovulation
- 50% conception: possibly due to negative effect of clomiphene on endometrium/ mucus
- 7% multiple pregnancy

METFORMIN
- metformin: increased ovulation rate but not clinical pregnancy rate
- clomiphene and metformin
  - increased live-birth rate: effective also in clomiphene resistance
  - increased ovulation rate
- metformin and gonadotrophin treatment: does not increase pregnancy rate, but reduces total FSH requirement and risk of ovarian hyperstimulation syndrome (OHSS)

OTHER MEDICAL TREATMENT
- increased benefit from addition of dexamethasone to clomiphene: resulted in a significant improvement in the pregnancy rate
- pulsatile GnRH (Cochrane): insufficient evidence from trials to show the effectiveness of pulsatile GnRH in PCOS
- FSH: chronic low-dose stimulation protocol has lower OHSS and multiple pregnancy rate
- in vitro fertilisation (IVF)
  - 7% of PCOS patients need IVF
  - high risk of OHSS (20%)
- surgical
  - wedge resection: high incidence of adnexal adhesions
  - laparoscopic golf balling/pepper potting/ovarian drilling (LOD) (see Table 5.1)
  - high incidence of adnexal adhesions
  - unknown long-term effect on ovarian function
  - effect may be permanent
  - consider in failed ovulation induction

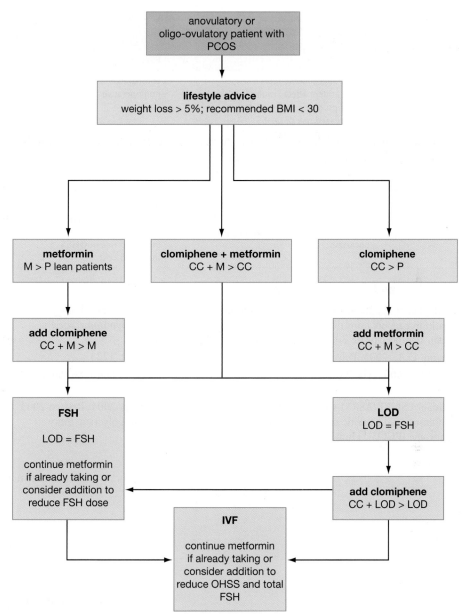

Notes: BMI = body mass index, CC = clomid, FSH = follicle-stimulating hormone,
IVF = in vitro fertilisation, LOD = laparoscopic ovarian drilling, M = metformin,
OHSS = ovarian hyperstimulation syndrome, P = placebo,
PCOS = polycystic ovarian syndrome

Figure 5.1 **Patients with a diagnosis of PCOS wishing to conceive**

Table 5.1 Comparison of laparoscopic ovarian drilling and FSH stimulation in fertility management in patients with PCOS

	LAPAROSCOPY	FSH
Benefits	comparable success rates one treatment affects multiple cycles usually produces mono-ovulation no increased risk of OHSS may lower miscarriage rate no medications required no intensive monitoring required lower cost	comparable success rate non-operative
Problems	surgical risks adhesion ovarian atrophy long-term effect on ovarian function uncertain	multiple cycles required intensive monitoring required increased risk of multiple pregnancy increased risk of OHSS increased cost

References and further reading

Deqailly, D., et al., 2014. Definition and significance of polycystic ovarian morphology: a taskforce report from the Androgen Excess and Polycystic Ovarian Syndrome Society. Hum. Reprod Update 20, 334.

Ehrmann, D.A., 2005. Polycystic ovary syndrome. N. Engl. J. Med. 352, 1223.

Legro, R.S., 2006. Type 2 diabetes and polycystic ovary syndrome. Fertil. Steril. 86 (Suppl. 1), S16–S17.

Rotterdam ESHRE/ASRM-sponsored PCOS consensus workshop group, 2004. Revised 2003 consensus on diagnostic criteria and long-term health risks related to polycystic ovary syndrome (PCOS). Hum. Reprod 19 (1), 41–47.

Chapter 6

Hirsutism

Anusch Yazdani
Judith Goh

Definition. *Hirsutism* is the growth of coarse/terminal hair in amounts that are socially unacceptable to a woman. For the woman, this is typically in a male pattern (sexual hair), with a Ferriman–Gallwey (see below) hirsutism score over 8. Under 5% of women (various ethnic origin) in the reproductive age group have scores over 7. *Hypertrichosis* is generalised excess hair growth that may be hereditary. This is in a non-sexual pattern and is not related to, but may be aggravated by, excess androgens. *Virilism* is a condition usually secondary to hyperandrogenism and is associated with one or more of clitoral hypertrophy, breast atrophy, male baldness and deepening of the voice.

    Prevalence. About 15% of women normally have terminal hair on their faces, and this tends to increase with age. Up to 4% of women seek treatment for hirsutism.

Physiology of hair growth

There are three major groups:
1. lanugo: fine, lightly pigmented hair
2. vellus hair: short, fine, unpigmented
3. terminal hair: longer, thicker and pigmented

    Non-sexual hair is present on the scalp, eyebrow and distal extremities. Its growth is not affected by androgens. **Ambisexual hair** is present in both sexes on the axilla and lower pubic triangle. Small amounts of androgens are required for its growth. **Sexual hair** is present on the upper pubic triangle, face, chest, ear and nose. It is induced and maintained by androgens.

Hair growth and hirsutism

In the skin, plasma testosterone is converted by 5-alpha-reductase to dihydrotestosterone, which is required for the local stimulation of vellus hair follicles to produce terminal hair. Sensitivity of hair follicles is affected by local metabolism of androgens. Once the hair follicle has been stimulated by androgens to produce terminal hair, the changes persist even in the absence of androgen excess.

Causes of hirsutism

Common
- idiopathic
  - diagnosis based on:
    — hirsutism
    — normal serum androgen concentrations
    — no menstrual irregularity
    — exclusion of other factors
  - may be a steroidogenic abnormality despite the apparently normal serum androgen levels
  - distinction between idiopathic disease and the PCOS may be one of degree
  - increased 5-alpha-reductase in the skin
- PCOS

Uncommon

NON-ANDROGENIC
- genetic
  - hirsutism is more prevalent in certain races and may be familial
- menopause
- endocrinopathies
  - hypothyroidism
  - acromegaly
  - hyperinsulinaemia
    — 5-alpha-reductase is stimulated by IGF-1
  - hyperprolactinaemia
    — uncertain whether hyperprolactinaemia per se contributes to hyperandrogenism
- drugs
  - phenytoin
  - diazoxide
  - minoxidil
  - glucocorticoids

ANDROGENIC
Adrenals
- congenital adrenal hyperplasia
  - prevalence of late-onset congenital adrenal hyperplasia among hirsute women has varied from 1% to 15%
- Cushing's disease
- adrenal tumours
  - rare cause of androgen excess
  - minority: adenoma → produce mainly testosterone
  - majority: carcinoma → often secrete not only androgens (DHEA and DHEAS) but also cortisol, therefore androgen excess and Cushing's syndrome

- elevated serum DHEA-S suggestive of adrenal carcinoma
  — some carcinomas may lose the ability to sulfate DHEA

Ovarian

- hyperthecosis
  - non-malignant ovarian disorder
  - increased production of testosterone by luteinised thecal cells in the stroma, leading to increased serum testosterone concentrations
  - clinical features of hyperthecosis are similar to those of PCOS but:
    — more hirsutism
    — much more likely to be virilised
    — more likely to be obese
    — can occur in postmenopausal women; severe hirsutism and virilisation in post-menopausal women are more often due to ovarian hyperthecosis rather than virilising ovarian tumours
- luteoma
  - exaggerated response to pregnancy
  - unilateral in 45%
  - multifocal in 50%
  - more common in multiparous black women in third and fourth decades
  - solid mass; may be up to 20 cm (median 6 cm)
  - associated with normal pregnancy
  - produces:
    — maternal virilisation in 35%
    — fetal effects
      – masculinisation in 80% of female fetus; exposure to high androgens has to occur early in pregnancy (before 9–14 weeks gestation)
      – virilisation will occur if exposure after 9–14 weeks gestation
  - regress spontaneously postpartum
- theca-lutein cysts
  - related to high hCG
    — trophoblastic disease
    — multiple pregnancy
  - usually bilateral
  - produces:
    — 30% maternal virilisation
    — no risk of masculinisation of female fetus
- ovarian tumours
  - hormonally active tumours
    — Sertoli-Leydig tumours
    — granulosa-theca cells tumours
    — hilus cell tumours
  - occur later in life and more rapid course than PCOS

Drugs

- androgens
- androgenic progestogen
- danazol
- anabolic steroids

Investigation and diagnosis

History
- onset, duration, pattern of growth
- weight gain, acne, change in voice
- menstrual changes
- diabetes, Cushing's syndrome, thyroid disease
- medication, family history

Examination
- general, blood pressure, weight, acne
- Ferriman–Gallwey score for hirsutism
- signs of virilisation
- abdominal and pelvic examination

  The diagnosis is a clinical one and the hirsutism score does not necessarily correlate to androgen levels. This is thought to be due to the variable response of follicles to androgen.

Investigations
The aim is to exclude serious disease and establish the source of androgens.
- pregnancy test
- early follicular phase tests of serum LH, FSH, oestradiol, progesterone
- thyroid function and prolactin
- fasting insulin and glucose
- serum levels of testosterone, DHEAS, androstenedione and 17-hydroxyprogesterone
- ultrasound scan of ovaries for polycystic ovaries or tumour
- there is a significant overlap of PCOS with early Cushing's
  - hypertension is the greatest clinical differentiator
  - if Cushing's is suspected, an adrenal disorder must be excluded

Management

Exclude or treat causes (see above).

Principles
- androgen suppression
- peripheral androgen suppression
- removal of unwanted hair
- weight control

Counselling
- reassurance that it is a common condition
- weight loss
- fertility not excluded

Hair therapy
- bleaching to mask hairs
- temporary removal of hair
- epilation, such as plucking or waxing

- depilation, such as shaving, is the removal of hair shaft from the skin surface
- chemicals may be used to dissolve the hair

PERMANENT HAIR REDUCTION

- electrolysis by thermal or chemical methods: causes destruction of hair follicle
- photoepilation using lasers or non-laser light sources: destroys hair follicles

TOPICAL TREATMENT

- eflornithine: an irreversible inhibitor of ornithine decarboxylase, an enzyme necessary for hair growth; reduces hair growth rate but does not remove hair

Pharmacological

ORAL CONTRACEPTIVES

- Due to teratogenic potential of antiandrogens (see below), contraception should be used.
- Oral contraceptives also reduce hyperandrogenism by reducing gonadotropin drive (which reduces ovarian androgens) and increasing SHBG (which reduces free serum androgen). Some progesterones (e.g. cyproterone acetate) also act as androgen receptor antagonists.

SPIRONOLACTONE

- an aldosterone antagonist with dose-dependent inhibition of androgen receptor
- inhibition of 5-alpha-reductase activity
- dose: spironolactone 100–200 mg daily
- contraception required: spironolactone may feminise a male fetus

CYPROTERONE ACETATE

- a potent androgen receptor antagonist
- inhibits androgen receptor and inhibits 5-alpha-reductase in the skin
- a potent progesterone that inhibits gonadotrophin and androgen levels
- dose: combined ethinyloestradiol 20–50 µg with cyproterone acetate 50–100 mg
- available as oral contraceptive pill with smaller dose of cyproterone acetate
- side effects include fatigue, reduced libido, weight gain

FINASTERIDE

- inhibition of type 2, 5-alpha reductase activity (types 1 and 2 5-alpha-reductase is involved in hirsutism)
- mixed reports of efficacy compared to spironolactone, with finasteride having either equal or reduced efficacy

FLUTAMIDE

- an antiandrogen, inhibiting androgen receptors
- small studies show similar efficacy to spironolactone
- major risk is hepatic toxicity with reported liver failure

INSULIN-LOWERING MEDICATIONS

- metformin in women without menstrual or metabolic dysfunction is controversial
- trials have shown reduced efficacy in treating hirsutism compared to spironolactone

GLUCOCORTICOIDS

- in small doses, reduce adrenal androgens
- dose is dexamethasone 0.25–0.5 mg/day
- with antiandrogens, the male fetus may be feminised
- side effects include hypertension, weight gain, skin striae, decrease in bone density

GONADOTROPIN-RELEASING HORMONE AGONIST (GNRH) AGONIST

- GnRH analogues are now rarely used
- rationale: reduce LH and FSH and thus reduce ovarian androgens

Chapter 7

Contraception

Thea Bowler
Michael Flynn

The chance of pregnancy when no contraception is used is approximately 20% per cycle.

A standard measure of contraceptive effectiveness is the Pearl index—the number of pregnancies per 100 woman-years in those at risk of pregnancy. One woman-year equals 12 menstrual cycles.

Natural methods

Natural methods are based on avoiding sexual activity that might lead to conception at the time when the ovum can be fertilised. It is necessary to predict the time of ovulation (generally by observing changes in body temperature) and to allow for the time that the sperm can survive with fertilising potential in the female genital tract. Intercourse is prohibited until 72 hours after the rise in basal body temperature. The Pearl index is 25/100 woman-years; with coitus interruptus, it is 18/100.

Barrier methods

Diaphragm

The diaphragm lies diagonally across the cervix, vaginal vault and anterior vaginal wall (extends from posterior vaginal fornix to behind pubic bone). Types of design are arcing, coil or flat; it is manufactured from natural rubber, latex or silicone.

FUNCTION
- acts as retainer of spermicide
- keeps sperm away from alkaline cervical mucus, as sperm die in the acidic pH of the vagina
- prevents physical aspiration of sperm into the cervix and uterus

- with perfect use, Pearl index 6/100 (normally increased by 3–7 times)
- may be protective against some sexually transmitted diseases, but not human immunodeficiency virus (HIV)
- not suitable for women with anatomical abnormalities of the genital tract and those with large cystoceles, rectoceles or uterine prolapse

Cervical/vault caps
- three types: cervical, vault, vimule (both cervix and vault); manufactured from latex, silicone
- function: to occlude the cervix
- spermicides recommended with use
- Pearl index 7/100

ADVANTAGES
- can be used in the presence of genital prolapse
- no rim; therefore, not felt by partner
- fitting not changed by changes in the size of the vagina

Sponge
- function: release spermicide; absorb the ejaculate; block the cervix
- Pearl index 17/100

Condoms
- reduce transmission of sexually transmitted diseases, including HIV
- non-latex condoms (polyurethane) available
- Pearl index, with perfect use, 2/100

FEMALE CONDOMS
- cover the vulva and may protect against infections such as herpes simplex and human papillomavirus

Spermicides
- most commonly used is nonoxynol-9; newer agents: octoxynol, benzalkonium chloride
- act by disrupting sperm cell membrane, causing rupture of spermatozoa
- available in gels, foams, creams, pessaries and capsules
- variable efficacy depending on doses, formulations and compliance
- may protect against sexually transmitted disease, and have in vitro anti-HIV properties

Intrauterine contraceptive devices

Types
- copper, to increase effectiveness and reduce the surface area (e.g. Multiload 375, Slimline TT380)
- progestogen-containing device (e.g. levonorgestrel-releasing intrauterine device [LNG IUD]); releases 20 µg levonorgestrel per day over 5 years

Mechanisms of action

- both types: prevent fertilisation of the ovum
- both types: foreign body response in myometrium interferes with implantation of the blastocyst
- both types: interfere with sperm transport
- LNG IUD only: causes endometrial atrophy, thickening of cervical mucus, prevents or delays ovulation in some women; oligomenorrhoea or amenorrhoea a normal side effect

Effectiveness

- Copper devices have a Pearl index in the first year of 2–3/100, later falling to lower than 1/100. The failure rate is 0.8%.
- They can be used as a postcoital contraceptive.
- Progesterone devices have a failure rate of 0.2%.

Counselling

- Take a past medical, surgical and social history.
- Discuss risks.
- The ideal patient for the intrauterine contraceptive device is a multiparous, monogamous woman with regular, normal periods.

Before insertion

- Explain procedure and risks, and acquire consent.
- Conduct a general physical examination.
- Perform a vaginal/pelvic examination.
- Obtain bacteriological, *Chlamydia* swabs, and cervical cytology if indicated.

Insertion

- Preferably insert at menses or up to day 10 of the cycle.
- For postcoital contraception, it may be effective up to 5 days postcoitus.
- For postpartum contraception, insert at 6 weeks after delivery.
- Training in insertion procedure is essential.

Change of the contraceptive device

- Multiload 375 devices require a change every 5 years.
- Progesterone (LNG IUD) is effective for 5 years.

Risks

- increased menstrual blood loss and dysmenorrhoea in copper devices
- incidence of uterine perforation (usually at time of insertion) 1 in 1000
- infection: for pelvic inflammatory disease, relative risk in the first 6 months 1.6; *Actinomycosis israelii* is usually an incidental finding at cervical cytological examination; may be associated with use of an intrauterine contraceptive device (*see Ch 11*)
- no protection against sexually transmitted infections
- increased risk of abortion, premature labour and delivery if a pregnancy occurs while the device is present
- ectopic pregnancy more frequent than in women not using an intrauterine contraceptive device (as device does not prevent ectopic)
- no reduction in fertility after using an intrauterine contraceptive device

Oral contraceptives

Combined oral contraceptive pill (COCP)

TWO FORMULATIONS

- monophasic: contain same oestrogen/progestogen throughout 21 or 24 days of course
- triphasic: variations in oestrogen/progestogen content to reduce side effects

MECHANISMS OF ACTION

- prevention of ovulation by inhibiting the oestrogen-mediated positive feedback that is required for the mid-cycle luteinising hormone (LH) surge
- inhibit follicle-stimulating hormone (FSH) release, thus preventing follicular maturation
- produce a change in cervical mucus
- reduce endometrial receptivity to the blastocyst

EFFECTIVENESS

- efficacy 99.7% with perfect use and 91% with typical use

ASSESSMENT BEFORE COMMENCING COCP

- Assess for and advise/manage risk factors such as hypertension, cigarette smoking and abnormal bleeding, and risk factors for thrombosis.
- Perform cervical cytology and breast examination.
- Contraindications include the presence of an oestrogen-dependent tumour, unexplained vaginal bleeding, pregnancy, breastfeeding, previous thromboembolism or cerebrovascular accident, known thrombophilia, hepatic dysfunction, severe migraine, > 15 cigarettes daily in women > 35 years, type 2 diabetes with complications, body mass index (BMI) > 40.
- The woman must understand the method and solutions to problems (see below).

SIDE EFFECTS AND RISKS

- deep venous thrombosis
  - increased risk of thromboembolism 2–3 times background rate
  - lowest risk with pills containing < 35 µg ethinyloestradiol and levonorgestrel or norethisterone
  - hypercoagulation: may occur, but will reverse within 1 week of cessation of the oestrogen
- ischaemic stroke
  - risk is increased with COCP use in women suffering migraine with aura
- cardiovascular disease
  - no statistically significant increased risk of hypertension in non-smokers
  - increased risk of myocardial infarction especially in women who smoke, are > 35 years, have hypertension or hyperlipidaemia
- malignancy: reduced relative risk of endometrial and ovarian cancer, which may continue for some time after cessation of use
- decrease in functional ovarian cysts; useful in managing polycystic ovarian syndrome (PCOS)
- carbohydrate metabolism: ethinyloestradiol doses lower than 40 µg little or no effect
- decreased menstrual loss and dysmenorrhoea
- improvement in acne

MISSED PILLS

The high-risk time to miss pills, in terms of risk of pregnancy, is at the end of a packet or at the start of a new packet. Manage by continuing oral contraception and use other forms of contraception for 7 days. If these 7 days continue beyond the current 21-day packet, then start the next packet without a normal break (i.e. do not take the inactive pills).

PROBLEMS AND SOLUTIONS

- androgenic side effects: use nomegestrol, desogestrel, gestodene, drospirenone, etonogestrel, dienogest, cyproterone acetate; increase oestrogen content
- anticonvulsant therapy: use monophasic 50 μg ethinyloestradiol
- breakthrough bleeding, amenorrhoea, dry vagina: increase oestrogen content
- breast tenderness: increase progestogen, reduce oestrogen
- hormone withdrawal symptoms (e.g. pelvic pain, headache): newer COCP formulations with shortened placebo break (e.g. 24/4 or 26/2 regimens); these may also reduce menstrual loss and provide higher contraception effectiveness
- antibiotics: little effect on contraceptive efficacy except for rifampicin; when using antibiotics, continue oral contraception and use other methods during and for 7 days after treatment; hormone-free interval should be omitted if < 7 active pills remain in packet (i.e. continue directly with active pills in next packet)
- lactation: combined oral contraceptives may interfere

Progestogen-only pills

These pills contain progestogen only (levonorgestrel or norethisterone). All pills are active, and are taken continuously with no breaks. The mechanism of action is thickening of the cervical mucus, preventing sperm transport, rather than inhibiting ovulation (also possible interference with tubal motility and implantation). The pill should be taken at the same time each day, as efficacy is less than COCP (99.7% with perfect use and 91% with typical use). It is useful in breastfeeding women and those with certain medical contraindications to COCP.

Contraceptive implants

Depot medroxyprogesterone acetate (DMPA)

- dose: 150 mg by intramuscular injection every 12 weeks
- start first injection within 3 days of menstrual period
- Pearl index below 1/100 (i.e. as effective as COCP)

MECHANISMS OF ACTION

- inhibits ovulation
- atrophies endometrium
- increases viscosity of cervical mucus
- reduces motility of fallopian tubes

SIDE EFFECTS

- irregular vaginal bleeding, especially in first 3 months
- amenorrhoea in 50% of women by 12 months
- restoration of ovulation taking up to 18 months
- causes reversible reduction in bone density, therefore avoid as first-line therapy in women under 18 years and over 45 years

Subcutaneous progestogen implants

Etonogestrel's mechanisms of action are similar to those of DMPA. It represents a rapidly reversible contraception method. The implant requires a small procedure for insertion and is effective for 3 years. Training in insertion and removal procedures is essential. Effectiveness is 99.9%.

Combined vaginal ring

This is a combined hormonal contraceptive ring inserted vaginally by the woman, left in place for 3 weeks and removed for a 7-day interval, as with placebo pills in COCP packs (e.g. NuvaRing). It inhibits ovulation, thickens the cervical mucus preventing sperm migration, and may interfere with implantation. It is a rapidly reversible method of contraception. Efficacy is equivalent to COCP.

ASSESSMENT

- as for COCP
- useful for women having difficulty with daily pill taking and women with inflammatory bowel disease
- contraindicated in immediate postpartum period
- the woman must understand method and how to insert ring

SIDE EFFECTS AND RISKS

- may be accidentally expelled (e.g. in presence of prolapse, chronic constipation)
- possible increased vaginal discharge, vaginal infections
- decrease in menstrual loss and dysmenorrhoea
- contraindicated for first 6 months of breastfeeding
- late removal or late reinsertion of ring: cover insertion of new ring with condoms or other methods for 7 days

Pregnancy interception (emergency contraception)

Hormonal methods

- effectiveness dependent on time interval from unprotected intercourse to administration of medication; more effective when taken earlier
- mechanism of action: prevent or delay ovulation, therefore effective pre-ovulation; probably ineffective post-ovulation
- progestogen only
  - levonorgestrel 750 µg immediately
  - repeat dose in 12 hours, or 1.5 mg single dose
  - available over the counter in Australia
  - efficacy 85%
- Yuzpe regimen
  - oral ethinyloestradiol 100 µg and levonorgestrel 500 µg with an antiemetic
  - repeat dose in 12 hours
  - take within 72 hours of coitus
  - efficacy 57%–74%
- hormonal methods require follow-up for failure of method, future contraception, risk of ectopic pregnancy and risk of sexually transmitted infections
- anti-progesterone: mifepristone

Non-hormonal methods

- intrauterine contraceptive device (copper)
  - effective up to 5–8 days after coitus
  - works by inhibiting fertilisation and preventing implantation of fertilised ovum
  - efficacy 99%

Male contraception

Gonadotropin-releasing hormone (GnRH) analogues

- reduce testosterone levels and libido
- GnRH with testosterone may block spermatogenesis

Steroids

- androgens cause a negative feedback that results in a fall in gonadotrophins
- progesterone and testosterone result in oligospermia

Antiandrogen (cyproterone acetate)

- inhibits spermatogenesis
- reduces potency and libido

Gossypol

- interferes with the acrosome

Sterilisation

Female sterilisation

ABDOMINAL/LAPAROSCOPIC

- Methods include fimbriectomy, diathermy, Pomeroy technique, Falope rings, Hulka or Filchie clips.
- Failure rate of 2–4/1000 may rise if performed at caesarean section or immediately postpartum.

HYSTEROSCOPIC

- Block fallopian tubes by inserting titanium microinserts via tubal ostia.

Male sterilisation

- Vasectomy is not associated with changes in the endocrine function.
- Pearl index is 0.2/100.

Further reading

Sexual Health and Family Planning Australia, 2013. Contraception: An Australian Clinical Practice Handbook. SH&FP, Canberra.

Chapter 8

Miscarriage and abortion

Michael Flynn

Definition. Termination of pregnancy at less than 20 weeks gestation or with the fetus weighing less than 400 g (exact definitions depend on the jurisdiction). 'Miscarriage' is usually taken to mean spontaneous abortion. 'Abortion' or 'termination of pregnancy' (TOP) usually refers to induced abortion (by surgical or medical means).

- threatened miscarriage: presentation of bleeding in pregnancy less than 20 weeks with closed cervical os and viable fetus
- inevitable miscarriage: presentation of bleeding in pregnancy less than 20 weeks with open cervical os and miscarriage cannot be avoided

Incidence. About 15% of all pregnancies spontaneously abort (miscarry) at 6–13 weeks gestation. Up to 80% of spontaneous abortions are diagnosed at 8–12 weeks gestation. The miscarriage rate increases with age.

Aetiology of spontaneous miscarriage

- genetic: chromosomal abnormalities present in up to 50% of first-trimester pregnancy loss (e.g. trisomy, monosomy, triploidy)
- fetal malformations (e.g. neural tube defects)
- immunological disorders
- uterine abnormalities
- cervical incompetence
- endocrine disorders (e.g. luteal phase dysfunction, diabetes mellitus)
- infections: listeria, mycoplasma, ureaplasma
- trauma: surgery, amniocentesis, chorionic villus sampling

Risk factors associated with miscarriage include:
- age
- smoking
- previous miscarriage
- trauma
- alcohol
- fever in early pregnancy
- other causes including medications, environmental chemicals

Presentation and management

Presentation (spontaneous miscarriage)
- a period of amenorrhoea, followed by vaginal bleeding and cramping lower abdominal pain
- human chorionic gonadotrophin (hCG) positive

Examination
- general examination: colour, blood pressure, pulse
- abdominal examination
- vaginal examination
  - bleeding through the cervical os
  - bulky uterus
- cervical os may be open, with products of conception at the os or in the vagina

Investigations
- Full blood count, blood group.
- Ultrasound scan of the pelvis (in early first trimester, this is preferable via transvaginal scan).
- Protocol for ultrasound assessment of diagnosis of miscarriage:
  - First identify if fetal heartbeat present and the gestational sac is intrauterine.
  - If there is no fetal heartbeat present, measure the crown–rump length of the fetal pole.
    — If crown–rump length is less than 7 mm, correspond with history and first positive pregnancy test. If not clear, repeat scan not less than 7 days.
    — If crown–rump length is greater than 7 mm and corresponds with clinical history and time of first positive pregnancy test, a diagnosis of miscarriage is made.
- Consideration of clinical history with last menstrual period, combined with the time of positive pregnancy test, appropriate doubling times of quantitative hCG and ultrasound assessment, will give an accurate diagnosis of miscarriage.

Management
- threatened miscarriage
  - commonly, management is conservative with repeat scan 14 days or earlier if bleeding increases
- confirmed miscarriage:
  - if bleeding not heavy and patient agrees, can 'wait and see' (expectant management); complete abortion process may occur naturally
  - uterine curettage if incomplete abortion, non-viable pregnancy on ultrasound or patient request
  - misoprostol 800 µg vaginally may assist with expulsion of retained products
  - anti-D immunoglobulin if patient Rh-negative

Recurrent pregnancy loss

Definition. 'Recurrent pregnancy loss' is defined as three or more consecutive spontaneous abortions to the same partner.
Prevalence. Prevalence is 1%–2%.

Risk of miscarriage

- After one miscarriage, the risk of another abortion at the next pregnancy is 20%–25%.
- After two miscarriages, the risk rises to 25%.
- After three, the risk is 30%.
- After four, the risk is 35%.
- Despite the many listed causes, most women have no obvious aetiology.

Investigations for recurrent pregnancy loss

- depends on history and time of miscarriage, with differing aetiologies presenting at different times
- abnormal parental (both maternal and paternal) karyotype and fetal karyotype; accounts for up to 5% recurrent pregnancy loss and is usually early loss
- assessment of uterine cavity via hysteroscopy or ultrasound
- thyroid function tests
- anticardiolipin and lupus anticoagulant testing
- inheritable thrombophilias (protein C resistance, protein S deficiency, factor V Leiden mutation)

Management of recurrent pregnancy loss

- immunosuppressive therapy (prednisone) indications unclear and not supported by trials
- anticoagulation therapy (such as aspirin and/or clexane) is beneficial for anti-phospholipid syndrome: treatment with low-molecular-weight heparin indicated in disorders of inherited thrombophilias

ABORTIONS DUE TO UTERINE ABNORMALITIES

- surgery such as hysteroscopic resection of intrauterine adhesions

ABORTIONS DUE TO ENDOCRINE ABNORMALITIES

Treat the cause (e.g. maintain good blood sugar control, and appropriate thyroid replacement).

SUPPORT AND COUNSELLING

Women experiencing spontaneous abortion of a wanted pregnancy, especially those with recurrent abortions, may need effective psychological support and counselling.

Induced abortion

Surgical abortion

- carried out up to 12–13 weeks gestation
- suction curettage, increasingly preceded by misoprostol 400–800 μg 2–4 hours pre-operatively to soften and dilate cervix
- cover with antibiotics or take swabs preoperatively and treat infection
- anti-D for Rh-negative women

Medical abortion

- mifepristone plus misoprostol or misoprostol alone used for late abortion (usually for fetal abnormality or serious maternal conditions) in hospital setting

- misoprostol very effective, but process greatly shortened by the addition of mifepristone
- side effects: nausea, vomiting, diarrhoea from misoprostol; vaginal bleeding and pain from uterine contractions part of abortion process (analgesics should be given)
- anti-D for Rh-negative women

Support and counselling

- All women undergoing induced abortion need appropriate counselling prior to the procedure, and follow-up, including advice about contraception and safe sex as indicated.
- All women experiencing abortion, whether spontaneous or induced, should be told to report promptly following procedure if pain, fever or offensive discharge occurs. Septic abortion can lead to pelvic inflammatory disease and subsequent infertility.

References

Adelberg, A.M., 2002. Thrombophilias and recurrent miscarriage. Obstet. Gynecol. Surv. 57, 703–710.

Crenin, M.D., Potter, C., Holovanisin, M., et al., 2003. Mifepristone and misoprostol and methotrexate/misoprostol in clinical practice for abortion. Am. J. Obstet. Gynecol. 188 (3), 664–669.

Royal College of Obstetricians and Gynaecologists, 2011. Recurrent miscarriage, investigation and treatment of couples. Green-top Guideline No. 17, April. RCOG, London.

National Institute for Health and Care Excellence, 2012. Clinical Guidelines No. 154, December. NICE, London. Available at: <www.nice.org.uk/guidance/cg154>.

Chapter 9

Ectopic pregnancy

Michael Flynn

Definition. An ectopic pregnancy is implantation of a pregnancy outside the uterine cavity.

Incidence. Incidence varies with geographical location, from 1 in 28 to 1 in 300 pregnancies; 65% occur in the age group 25–34 years. In developed countries, incidence remains static at approximately 11 in 1000 pregnancies. Heterotrophic pregnancy (coexisting intrauterine and ectopic pregnancies) occurs in 1 in 30 000 spontaneous conceptions and in at least 1% of technically assisted conceptions. The mortality rate in developed countries is approximately 0.2 per 1000 estimated ectopic pregnancies

Site. The site of 97% of ectopic pregnancies is the fallopian tubes; the remainder are abdominal, ovarian or cervical.

Tubal ectopic pregnancy

Aetiology and risk factors
- pelvic inflammatory disease: associated with a seven-fold increased incidence of ectopic pregnancy
- tubal surgery
- past history of ectopic pregnancy: a 10%–15% chance of recurrence, rising to 50% if the contralateral tube is abnormal
- contraception associated with a risk of ectopic pregnancy
  - progesterone-only pill
  - postcoital pill
  - intrauterine contraceptive device (users who fall pregnant have a higher risk of ectopic pregnancy than oral contraceptive users)
- assisted reproductive techniques
- endometriosis
- abnormal embryo

Presentation

- amenorrhoea
- small amount of vaginal bleeding, often after the onset of pain
- lower abdominal pain, shoulder-tip pain
- cervical motion tenderness, adnexal tenderness/mass
- breast tenderness

Note that ectopic pregnancy often has an atypical presentation.

Investigations

QUANTITATIVE SERUM HUMAN CHORIONIC GONADOTROPHIN (HCG)

From 10 days post-fertilisation, the hCG level increases at least 63% every 48 hours. If there is an apparently inadequate rise in hCG levels, often associated with below-expected serum progesterone, suspect a failed pregnancy or ectopic pregnancy. Up to 1% of ectopic pregnancies have hCG levels < 25 IU/L.

ULTRASOUND

Intrauterine pregnancy can be identified by 6 weeks gestation via transabdominal ultrasound scan and by 5 weeks gestation when using transvaginal scans. Abdominal ultrasound scans should identify an intrauterine sac with hCG levels > 2000 IU/L; with transvaginal scans, the intrauterine sac may be seen with hCG > 1000 IU/L. If no intrauterine sac is present with these levels, ectopic pregnancy is suspected.

The diagnosis is pregnancy of unknown location until ectopic location is determined.

LAPAROSCOPY

This is the gold standard in investigation and diagnosis; 3%–4% of very early tubal pregnancies can be missed.

Management

SURGICAL

A laparoscopic approach is the preferred option in surgical management. This is particularly so in haemodynamic compromise.

It should be first-line management if:

- associated significant pain
- an adnexal mass of 35 mm or larger
- an ultrasound with visible heartbeat outside the endometrial cavity
- a hCG of 5000 IU or more
- no availability for follow-up of medical management

Salpingectomy and salpingostomy

Salpingectomy is the optimal treatment unless there are other risk factors for infertility.

- In those managed by removal of the ectopic tissue only, follow-up with weekly quantitative hCG test is required. At least 5% of these cases will have evidence of continuing trophoblastic activity (i.e. persistent ectopic pregnancy). Advise 1 in 5 may require further treatment.
- There is no randomised control trial evidence specifically comparing salpingectomy and salpingostomy. Cohort studies suggest no difference in subsequent intrauterine

pregnancy rates between either procedure, but a tendency towards higher subsequent ectopic pregnancies in the salpingostomy group.

Local injection of ectopic pregnancy
- methotrexate, potassium chloride, prostaglandins
- requires follow-up because of risk of persisting ectopic pregnancy

MEDICAL
Systemic methotrexate
Single-dose methotrexate is successful in over 90% of cases. The dose is calculated on body surface area at 50 mg/m^2. Criteria for use include:
- haemodynamic stability
- no fetal cardiac activity
- hCG level < 1500 IU/L
- ectopic mass ≤ 3.5 cm

About 15% will require a second dose if hCG levels have failed to fall more than 15% in 4–7 days. The outcome is comparable to that of surgery for unruptured ectopic pregnancy. It is useful for early cervical pregnancy, and has been used in continuing hCG activity after incomplete removal of an ectopic trophoblast.

Expectant management
This has been reported in the woman who does not have abdominal pain and who has falling hCG levels of < 1000 IU/L. However, there have been cases of ruptured ectopic pregnancy with low and declining levels of hCG.

Anti-D
Rh-negative women with confirmed ectopic pregnancy should be given 250 IU of anti-D.

CONTRACEPTION AND FUTURE PREGNANCIES
Because of the heightened risk of future ectopic pregnancies, the woman requires advice for subsequent pregnancies, such as an early hCG test and ultrasound scan.

Avoid contraception, which can increase the risk of ectopic pregnancies (e.g. progesterone-only pill, intrauterine contraceptive device).

Abdominal pregnancy

Incidence. Incidence is up to 1 in 10 000 live births. There is a higher incidence with low socioeconomic status and in developing countries.

Maternal mortality. Maternal mortality of 2%–10% of abdominal pregnancies (i.e. seven to eight times the risk compared with tubal ectopic pregnancies and 90 times the risk of intrauterine pregnancy).

Management
- If the fetus dies and a lithopedion develops, no treatment is required.
- If the fetus dies, wait 3–8 weeks to allow it to atrophy. However, coagulation disorders may develop.
- If the fetus is alive, intervene early because of the risk of maternal morbidity/ mortality.

- Management of the placenta is debatable:
  - if an attempt is made to remove it, there is a risk of bleeding
  - if the placenta is left in situ, there is a risk of infection and abscess formation
  - treat with methotrexate

Reference

National Institute for Health and Care Excellence, 2012. Clinical Guidelines No. 154, December. NICE, London. Available at: <www.nice.org.uk/guidance/cg154>.

Chapter 10

Infertility

Anusch Yazdani

Definitions. *Infertility* is the failure to conceive after 12 months of unprotected intercourse. *Primary infertility* defines no previous conception, regardless of the outcome, whereas *secondary infertility* means that there has been a previous pregnancy, regardless of the outcome. *Fecundability* is the probability of achieving a pregnancy per menstrual cycle. *Fecundity* is the probability of achieving a live birth per menstrual cycle.

Incidence. The overall incidence of primary infertility is 10%–15% of couples. Female fertility declines with age and the incidence of infertility increases: 5% under the age of 25; 10% under the age of 30; 15% under the age of 35; 30% under the age of 40; and 60% over the age of 40.

Conception

Conception requires:
- sperm*
  - adequate (quantity, quality)
  - deposition (in vicinity of cervix, prior to/at ovulation, permeable cervical mucus)
- egg*
  - adequate (quantity, quality)
  - ovulation
- reproductive environment
  - at least one patent fallopian tube to allow fertilisation*
  - transport to endometrial cavity
  - implantation

Probability of conception
The probability of conception is time dependent:
- after 3 months: 60%
- after 6 months: 75%

---

*denotes common problem.

- after 12 months: 85%
- after 24 months: 95%

Therefore, the majority of couples who have not conceived after 1 year are likely to conceive in the subsequent year.

Aetiology

The requirements for conception determine the aetiological factors that contribute to infertility:

- male factor: 40%
  - pretesticular factors: hypothalamic–pituitary abnormalities
  - testicular factors: primary testicular abnormalities, varicocele, torsion, trauma, orchiditis, cytotoxic drug treatment, radiotherapy, undescended testes
  - post-testicular factors: genital tract obstruction, may be congenital (congenital absence of vas deferens), inflammatory, Young's syndrome, postvasectomy, vasectomy
- female factor: 50%
  - tubal and pelvic pathology: 40%
    — endometriosis, adhesions, hydrosalpinges, pelvic inflammatory disease, fibroids, congenital abnormalities
  - ovulatory dysfunction: 40%
    — primary ovarian abnormalities, polycystic ovary syndrome, obesity, age
    — hypothalamic–pituitary disorders
- other: 20%
- unexplained: 10%

History

Female

- history of infertility
  - primary or secondary infertility
    — previous pregnancies: same or different partner, time to conception, outcome of pregnancy
  - duration of infertility
- sexual history
  - history of contraception
  - sexual function
    — dyspareunia
    — coital frequency, timing during cycle
- menstrual history
  - regularity, frequency of cycles, evidence of ovulation (such as mucus changes)
  - dysmenorrhoea
- evidence of endocrine disorder
  - galactorrhoea, hirsutism, acne
  - weight gain
- past medical history
  - obesity
  - hypertension, renal disease, gastrointestinal disease
  - thyroid disease

- pelvic inflammatory disease
- peritonitis, appendicitis, ovarian or pelvic surgery
- endometriosis
- medications
- social history, including smoking, alcohol or other substance abuse
- family history, including birth defects, mental retardation or reproductive failure

Male
- history of infertility
  - pregnancies to other partners
- sexual function
  - erectile or ejaculatory dysfunction
- past medical history
  - varicocele, undescended testicle, mumps
  - orchidopexy, inguinal hernia repair
  - urinary tract infection, sexually transmitted disease
  - testicular injury or infections
- medications
- social history, including smoking, alcohol or other substance abuse
- family history, including birth defects, mental retardation or reproductive failure

Examination

Female
- general
  - pulse rate, blood pressure, body mass index (BMI)
  - dysmorphic features, secondary sexual characteristics
- endocrine
  - breast and thyroid, hirsutism, acne, galactorrhoea, striae, acanthosis
- reproductive
  - vaginal examination
    — cervical cytology, microbiological studies, including *Chlamydia*
    — pelvic assessment (e.g. fixed retroversion of the uterus)

Male
- general
  - pulse rate, blood pressure, BMI
  - dysmorphic features, secondary sexual characteristics
- endocrine
  - gynaecomastia, hair distribution
- reproductive
  - phallus
  - spermatic cord: presence of vas, varicocele
  - testicular size and consistency

Investigations

Initial investigations
Initial investigations focus on the three main factors causing infertility (ovulatory, pelvic and male factors) and assess the suitability for pregnancy (antenatal screening).

- ovulatory factor assessment
  - a regular cycle with symptoms of ovulation is evidence of ovulation
  - basal body temperature (BBT) chart
    — progesterone is thermogenic and raises BBT after ovulation, which is maintained during the luteal phase
    — 20% of ovulatory women have a monophasic BBT
  - serum progesterone
    — tested in the luteal phase on day 21 of an ideal 28-day cycle or 7 days prior to menses
    — raised progesterone in the luteal range is evidence of ovulation in that cycle
- anti-müllerian hormone (AMH)
  - AMH levels correlate with the pool of antral follicles and, by association, the total pool of primordial follicles; AMH levels correlate with the total antral follicle count (AFC), an ultrasound assessment of the number of specific antral follicles in the early follicular phase of the ovarian cycle (these two tests have largely surpassed other tests of ovarian reserve, such as early follicular phase estimations of oestradiol or FSH)
  - in general, reduced ovarian reserve has been variably associated with a limited reproductive life span (time to conception), reproductive performance (ovarian response) and reproductive success (as defined by fertilisation or clinical pregnancy rates), as well as early menopause
- pelvic factor assessment
  - ultrasound scan of pelvis: ovarian morphology, antral follicle count, evidence of pelvic disease, such as fibroids
- preconception screening tests
  - all the tests performed as part of antenatal screening, including cervical screening, rubella serology
  - preconception screening also offers the opportunity for screening for genetic diseases, such as cystic fibrosis, or other genetic diseases in high-risk groups
- male factor assessment
  - semen analysis
    — 5th edn (2010) now uses a reference range (not normal values) where the quoted reference denotes 5% lower reference limit drawn from a sample of fertile males: *WHO laboratory manual for the examination and processing of human semen*
    — requires a minimum of 2 days and a maximum of 7 days of no ejaculation before collection
    — volume 1.5 mL
    — concentration 15 million sperm/mL
    — motility 40%
    — morphology 4% normal

Extended investigations

Extended investigations are performed when the initial investigations have not identified a cause or when further elucidation is required.

- ovulatory factor assessment
  - follicle-stimulating hormone (FSH), luteinising hormone (LH) and oestradiol in the follicular phase in those menstruating, or randomly when cycles are irregular or absent
  - serum prolactin, thyroid function tests

- endometrial biopsy in secretory phase
- if hirsutism is present, serum testosterone, androstenedione, dehydroepiandroster-one sulfate (DHEAS), sex hormone binding globulin and 17-hydroxyprogesterone
- pelvic factor assessment
  - assessment of tubal function
    — provides information regarding uterine cavity and tubes but no extratubal view: hysterosalpingogram, hysterosonography (HyCoSy)
  - laparoscopy, hysteroscopy, dye perturbation
    — detailed survey of the reproductive organs, hydrotubation to assess (and treat) tubal patency, pelvic adhesions, endometriosis
- male factor assessment
  - semen analysis: if the initial test is abnormal, repeat in 2–3 months (long develop-ment cycle of sperm may be affected by, for example, fever)
  - antisperm antibodies: immunobead test, mixed antiglobulin reaction test
  - endocrine tests
    — FSH/LH/total testosterone: to distinguish between obstructive disorders and primary testicular failure
    — inhibin, prolactin, thyroid-stimulating hormone (TSH)
  - chromosomal analysis
    — indications: azoospermia, raised FSH, reduced testicular volume, prolonged unexplained infertility, congenital abnormalities
    — in infertility clinics, 2% of males are chromosomally abnormal, rising to 15% in the azoospermic male
  - testicular biopsy
    — indication: obstructive azoospermia, diagnostic uncertainty

Management

Management of infertility is directed by the assessment of the three main factors (ovula-tory, pelvic and male) as above.

Principles
- optimise conception
  - lifestyle modification if required
  - folic acid supplementation in line with National Health and Medical Research Council (NHMRC) requirements
  - appropriate coital timing
- correct any primary pathology
  - treatment of endocrine disorders
- manage any non-correctible factors

Ovulatory factor infertility
Management options include:
- ovulation induction: induce ovulation in anovulatory or oligoovulatory females
- superovulation: induce the formation of two or three mature follicles in women who are ovulating
- controlled ovarian hyperstimulation: induce the formation of multiple mature fol-licles for the purposes of in vitro fertilisation (IVF)

CLOMIPHENE
- description
  - a non-steroidal agent distantly related to diethylstilbestrol
  - the principally antagonistic effect at the level of the hypothalamus activates the oestrogen–gonadotrophin feedback to the pituitary, causing a rise in FSH and LH (but especially FSH), which leads to induction of ovulation
- dose
  - 50–150 mg/day for 5 days on days 5–9 or days 2–6 of the menstrual cycle
  - a lower dose is often required in polycystic ovarian syndrome
  - a rise in luteal serum progesterone on day 21 confirms ovulation
- adverse reactions
  - vasomotor symptoms, breast and abdominal discomfort, visual changes, alopecia, multiple pregnancies (8%)

FOLLICLE-STIMULATING HORMONE (FSH)
- description
  - FSH in stimulation regimen may be derived from two sources:
    — synthetic FSH, a manufactured recombinant glycoprotein
    — purified urinary menopausal gonadotrophins, containing both FSH and LH, though the latter has minimal clinical efficacy
- dose
  - 50–450 IU/day self-administered from days 2–5 of the menstrual cycle
  - dosing determines whether one or multiple follicles are developed
  - response is monitored by ultrasound scanning and oestrogen-level measurement
- adverse reactions
  - breast and abdominal discomfort, multiple pregnancies (25%), ovarian hyper-stimulation syndrome

GONADOTROPIN-RELEASING HORMONE (GNRH) AGONIST/ANTAGONISTS
- Unless the pituitary is suppressed, the rising oestrogen levels will cause spontaneous LH surge and ovulation prior to follicles reaching the correct size for an egg pick-up.
- GnRH agonists administered in a non-pulsatile fashion (either as injections or nasal sprays) will cause GnRH receptor down-regulation and suppress the midcycle LH surge and ovulation; this effect requires 7–10 days.
- GnRH antagonists act as competitive inhibitors and can therefore be administered only at the time suppression is required.

HUMAN CHORIONIC GONADOTROPHIN (HCG)
- Purified urinary or recombinant hCG may be used to induce final oocyte maturation (analogous to the LH surge in a natural cycle).
- It is a cheaper alternative to LH.
- In ovulation induction or superovulation, ovulation is induced for IVF.
- In IVF, a transvaginal egg pick-up is performed prior to ovulation.

Pelvic factor infertility

TUBAL FACTORS
- success of repair depends on the site, nature and severity of the tubal damage
  - interstitial tubal obstruction
    — tubal reimplantation has a poor prognosis and is an indication for IVF

- proximal tubal obstruction
  — has an excellent prognosis, particularly if resulting from sterilisation
  — tubal reanastomosis requires at least one tube of over 4 cm in length with a healthy ampulla and fimbria
  — best results are with isthmo-isthmic anastomosis
  — pregnancy rate > 60%; 10% ectopic
- distal tubal obstruction
  — has a poor prognosis, as it is most often associated with severe tubal damage
  — neosalpingostomy 25% intrauterine pregnancy and 30% ectopic pregnancy rate
- success rates of tubal surgery must be compared to assisted reproductive techniques
- hydrosalpinges should be corrected or removed prior to any assisted reproduction

ADHESIONS

Removal of adhesions around the ovary and fimbriae, if the tube is otherwise normal, provide a 50% chance of a live birth and a 10% risk of ectopic pregnancy.

ENDOMETRIOSIS

(*See Ch 4.*)

FIBROIDS

(*See Ch 19.*)

Male factor infertility

PRETESTICULAR FACTORS

- gonadotrophin deficiency: gonadotrophin therapy
- note that testosterone supplementation results in a feedback suppression of gonadotrophins and cessation of spermatogenesis

TESTICULAR FACTORS

- most testicular factors are not correctible
  - if spermatogenesis persists, sperm may be used for insemination, IVF or intracytoplasmic sperm injection (ICSI)
  - in the absence of spermatogenesis, donor sperm will be required
- varicocele (with abnormal seminal analysis) may be repaired
- sperm auto-antibodies: corticosteroids are rarely useful; IVF–ICSI is now considered the primary treatment of choice

POST-TESTICULAR FACTORS

- surgical correction of obstruction may be considered depending upon the level of obstruction
- alternatively, testicular or epididymal sperm retrieval for IVF–ICSI has a high success rate

COITAL DISORDERS

- correction of primary pathology
- pharmacotherapy for erectile dysfunction
- psychosexual counselling

Assisted reproduction

Definitions. IVF: in vitro fertilisation; ICSI: intracytoplasmic sperm injection.

Success rates. IVF—fresh embryo transfer: 35%–60%; frozen embryo transfer: 25%–40%. Rates are dependent on the age of the female at the time of egg collection.

Steps in assisted reproduction

The aim of assisted reproduction is to induce the development of multiple mature ovarian follicles. There are five steps.

STEP 1: CONTROLLED OVARIAN HYPERSTIMULATION

- administration of FSH, commencing on day 3–5 of the cycle
- prevention of a premature LH surge and ovulation by either:
  - GnRH antagonist after day 5 of stimulation, or
  - pituitary down-regulation with a GnRH agonist
- ovarian response is carefully monitored by oestradiol assays and/or transvaginal ultrasound scans over a period of 9–12 days
- ovarian follicles grow at a predictable rate of approximately 2 mm/day
- once follicles have reached maturity (> 18 mm in diameter), an injection of hCG is given to initiate the final process of egg maturation

STEP 2: EGG COLLECTION

- performed under a local or general anaesthetic using a vaginal ultrasound probe at 36–38 hours following the hCG
- needle is guided through the vaginal fornix into the ovary and each follicle is aspirated
- follicular fluid is assessed by a scientist for the presence of an egg

STEP 3: FERTILISATION AND EMBRYO CULTURE

- semen sample (collected by masturbation) or surgically retrieved sperm is prepared in the laboratory
- oocyte is prepared
  - IVF: prepared oocytes are cultured with prepared sperm
  - ICSI: prepared oocytes are directly injected with a single sperm
- fertilisation is completed the following day and the embryo develops in culture
- 2–3 days after egg collection, the embryos have reached the 2–8 cell stage (cleavage)
- 5 or more days after egg collection, the embryos have reached several hundred cells (blastocyst); the full embryonic genome only switches on after the cleavage stage

STEP 4: EMBRYO TRANSFER

- performed in day theatres without anaesthetic or sedation
- embryos are transferred on day 3 (cleavage) or day 5 (blastocyst) stage, depending on the number and quality of embryos
- with the current high pregnancy rates, units perform single embryo transfers to minimise the risk of multiple pregnancy
- luteal support in the form progesterone pessaries or injections may be required after the embryo transfer to support the uterine lining

- spare embryos may be frozen and stored for future use
- in subsequent cycles, an embryo is thawed and transferred in synchrony with a natural or a hormonally optimised cycle

Ovarian hyperstimulation syndrome

Ovarian hyperstimulation syndrome (OHSS) is an exaggerated response to ovulation/ovulation triggers characterised by increased vascular permeability, intravascular depletion and third space fluid sequestration. It is usually an iatrogenic, self-limiting disorder associated with ovulation induction/ovarian stimulation. It may be:
- early onset: related to hCG trigger
- late onset: related to ensuing pregnancy, especially multiple

Incidence. Severe OHSS occurs in 0.5% episodes of assisted reproduction, but is increasingly rare with modern stimulation regimen.

Pathophysiology. OHSS occurs in response to exogenous hCG (more rarely, endogenous LH), resulting in increased vascular permeability, arterial dilation, fluid shift from vascular to third space, intravascular depletion and circulatory dysfunction.

RISK FACTORS
Patient factors
- young age
- low body weight
- history of OHSS
- polycystic ovaries

Cycle factors
- agonist down-regulated cycles are more likely to result in OHSS
- GnRH antagonists reduce incidence of severe OHSS
- high doses of exogenous gonadotrophins
- high absolute or rapidly rising oestradiol (E2)
- large number of developing follicles or oocytes retrieved (> 20)
- high-dose hCG ovulation trigger
  - hCG luteal support

MANAGEMENT
Outpatient
Mild forms may be managed as an outpatient.
- simple analgesia
- simple antiemetics
- maintain oral intake
- encourage mobilisation

Inpatient
Moderate to severe forms require admission.

Indications
- pain
- intractable nausea/vomiting/diarrhoea
- haemodynamic compromise
- respiratory compromise

Investigations
- haematocrit > 45 L/L
- white cell count > 15×10^9/L
- hyponatraemia
- hyperkalaemia
- abnormal liver function test
- renal impairment (creatinine > 0.12 μmol/L; creatinine clearance < 50 mL/minute)

Assessment
- regular assessment of vital signs (every 2–8 hours)
- daily weight
- daily abdominal circumference
- fluid balance sheet
- pulse oximetry
- ward test of urine

Investigations
- full blood examination
- electrolytes and liver function tests
- coagulation profile
- pelvic ultrasound scan
- chest X-ray if respiratory compromise
- echocardiogram if respiratory or cardiovascular compromise

Management
- bed rest
- analgesia
- antiemetic
- thromboprophylaxis
- fluid management
  - oral
  - intravenous fluids
- paracentesis

Intensive care unit admission
Indications are:
- haemodynamic compromise requiring invasive monitoring
- renal compromise requiring invasive monitoring (central venous pressure monitoring), dopamine agonist therapy or dialysis
- respiratory compromise requiring ventilation/positive end-expiratory pressure (PEEP)/oxygen

Reference

World Health Organization (WHO), 2010. WHO Laboratory Manual for the Examination and Processing of Human Semen, 5th ed. WHO, Geneva.

Chapter 11

Pelvic infections

Yasmin Jayasinghe

Pelvic inflammatory disease

Pelvic inflammatory disease (PID) is an upper genital tract infection. This includes any combination of cervicitis, endometritis, salpingitis, tubo-ovarian abscess and pelvic peritonitis.

Epidemiology
- no national surveillance data as non-notifiable
- in Australia, it is estimated that 10000 women treated in hospital annually and 10–30 times that are treated as outpatients

Pathogenesis
- ascending infection from the lower genital tract
- sexually transmitted infection (STI) may cause epithelial damage and allow ascent of vaginal bacteria
- infection risk could be associated with bacterial vaginosis or changes in the vaginal microbiome with degradation of cervical mucus and antimicrobial peptides
- fibrinous suppurative epithelial damage and adhesions
- genetic susceptibility factors may play a role in development of PID and tubal infertility
- postgynaecological procedural infection
- postpartum infection
- haematogenous (rare), tuberculosis, schistosomiasis
- spread from adjacent organs; for example, ruptured appendix (rare)

Physiological barriers to infection
- cervix
  - mechanical: diameter of endocervix, downward flow of mucus
  - biochemical: production of antibacterial lysozymes
  - immunological: local immunoglobulin A (IgA)

- endometrium
  - cyclical shedding
  - uterotubal junction: a mechanical barrier

Risk factors

- increased risk in adolescents and young women due to sexual behaviours and immaturity of the cervical epithelium with wide transformation zone
- early sexual debut, multiple partners, lack of condoms, past PID

Clinical presentation

- variable presentation which may be acute (≤ 30 days), subacute, or subclinical or chronic infection (> 30 days)
- often very subtle
- symptoms can include acute pelvic pain, febrile illness, vaginal discharge, postcoital or intermenstrual bleeding; less frequent symptoms include urethral syndrome (dysuria and pyuria), bartholinitis, right upper quadrant pain due to perihepatitis and proctitis
- hallmark sign is uterine or cervical motion or adnexal tenderness in the presence of cervical inflammation and vaginal discharge (sensitivity > 95% but lacks specificity); signs can include fever (although systemic features not prominent), abdominal tenderness, adnexal tenderness or mass
- Centers for Disease Control and Prevention (CDC) 2015 guidelines recommend that empiric treatment be undertaken in sexually active women with lower abdominal pain if they meet at least one of the following criteria: cervical motion, uterine or adnexal tenderness
- laparoscopy useful in unwell subjects where diagnosis is unclear, or there is no improvement with antibiotics, and for surgical intervention; findings include erythema and oedema of tubes, purulent discharge, pyosalpinx, tubo-ovarian abscess and pelvic adhesions, but high inter-observer variability and can miss early disease

Microbiology

- is a polymicrobial infection
- in 70% of cases no pathogen identified
- Table 11.1 lists the microbiological aetiology of PID

Table 11.1 Microbiological aetiology of PID	
AETIOLOGY	**INCIDENCE**
Chlamydia trachomatis	40%–60%
Neisseria gonorrhoea	15%–18%
Mycoplasma species	10%–15%
anaerobic facultative bacteria: *Escherichia coli*, group B streptococcus (GBS), *Bacteroides* species, *Peptostreptococcus* species, *Staphylococcus aureus*, *Gardnerella vaginalis*, *Haemophilus influenzae*	30%
Mycobacterium tuberculosis *Actinomyces* species	rare, can cause chronic PID

Principles of management of sexually transmitted infections
- accurate risk assessment and education and counselling regarding prevention
- pre-exposure vaccination for vaccine preventable STIs
- identification, treatment, counselling, and follow-up of infected persons
- evaluation, treatment and counselling of sex partners

Neisseria gonorrhoea

Epidemiology
- prevalence in Australian women very low (0.2%–0.3%); therefore, routine screening not recommended but testing recommended for those with symptoms
- prevalence higher in men who have sex with men (MSM) (7.0%), remote Aboriginal communities (7.0%), sex workers, drug users, those who have sex overseas or contact with gonorrhoea; screening recommended in these groups
- notifications in Australia in 2012: 58/100 000, (65% increase since 2007)

Infection
- gram-negative diplococcus which invades the columnar epithelium; infection usually occurs in the first half of the menstrual cycle
- incubation period: usually 2–10 days
- period of communicability: months in untreated individuals
- high rates of coinfection with *Chlamydia*

Clinical symptoms
- 80% of women are asymptomatic
- vaginal discharge, postcoital/intermenstrual bleeding, dyspareunia, pelvic pain, PID, anorectal pain
- conjunctivitis, skin lesions, septic arthritis, rarely meningitis or endocarditis

Diagnosis
- In Australia, outside of high-prevalence populations, testing should be done by culture. Endocervical culture is almost as sensitive as endocervical nucleic acid amplification test (NAAT), but more specific and provides antibiotic sensitivities. Culture endocervix (or posterior fornix if pregnant), urethra and rectum pharynx. Send the slide for gram stain, and then place the second swab into Amies +/– charcoal transport medium. It needs to be received by the laboratory within 24 hours.
- NAATS are highly sensitive. Polymerase chain reaction (PCR) test on endocervical specimens has 95% sensitivity, 100% specificity. However, NAATS is not validated for non-genital sites. False positives with NAATS are high (60%) where prevalence of gonorrhoea is < 1%.
- A positive NAAT for gonorrhoea in a low-risk or asymptomatic individual should be regarded as doubtful and confirmatory cultures are required.
- First-pass urine (10–20 mL at least 1 hour after passing urine) has sensitivity around 10% lower than genital swabs; or self-collected vaginal swab PCR if examination can't be undertaken. If PCR is positive and culture was not taken, then obtain culture at time of treatment.

Treatment
- Antimicrobial resistance is considered an urgent threat globally by the CDC.
- Two-thirds of gonorrhoeal infection occurs in the Asia-Pacific region where antimicrobial resistance is high.

- In 2013, 35% of isolates retested at reference laboratories in Australia were penicillin resistant, 34% were resistant to ciprofloxacin, 2.1% were resistant to azithromycin and 8.8% had decreased susceptibility to ceftriaxone. Resistance is lower in remote Aboriginal communities, and higher in urban centres due to introduction of resistant strains from overseas. Reduced susceptibility to ceftriaxone is widespread and variable in Australian states and territories, ranging up to 24% in isolated areas.
- Treatment guidelines for uncomplicated infection (*Australian STI Management Guidelines*, 2015):
  - ceftriaxone 500 mg intramuscular injection immediately, mixed with 2 mL 1% lignocaine plus azithromycin 0 1 g immediately (dual treatment to create pharmacologic barrier)
  - alternative treatments not recommended due to resistance apart from remote locations or severe allergic reactions
- If patient has an IUD leave in place, treat and monitor.
- Other measures:
  - a notifiable disease
  - no sexual contact for 1 week after antibiotics
  - test of cure 1 week after treatment
  - partners of last 3 months need to be notified, tested and treated
  - safe sex
  - test for other STIs

Chlamydia trachomatis

Epidemiology
- *Chlamydia* the most common notifiable sexually transmitted infection (STI) in Australia
- mean of 76 758 notifications/year between 2011–2014, prevalence at least tripled over 10 years
- majority (80%) of infections occur in 16–29 year olds (prevalence 4.6%).

Risk factors
- young women aged 16–19 years
- Indigenous women < 25 years
- past *Chlamydia* within the year
- symptoms or partner with an STI
- people disengaged with school
- commercial sex workers
- increased number of MSM sexual partners
- early age first sex
- rural/remote communities

Screening
- only 12% young women screened annually
- 50% reduction in prevalence can be achieved in 10 years by screening 30% of 20–25-year-old females annually)
- also recommend annual testing for all 15–29 year olds, or those with recent partner change or inconsistent condom use

Infection
- It is a gram-negative obligate intracellular organism.
- Its lifecycle has two stages: 1. an infectious and metabolically inactive elementary body which penetrates the cell wall by endocytosis, where it is transformed into 2. the reticulate body, which reproduces by binary fission to form new elementary bodies in the vacuole, and eventually ruptures to release the organism.
- The incubation period is poorly defined: 7–14 days or longer.
- The period of communicability is unknown: perhaps months to years.
- Females have a 40% risk of infection after unprotected sex with a *Chlamydia*-positive person. Men have a 20% risk.

Clinical symptoms
- around 70% asymptomatic
- urethritis, cervicitis: discharge, postcoital bleeding (PCB)
- PID: (risk is 9.5% at 12 months after one episode of untreated *Chlamydia* compared to 1.3% if treated); PID risk is higher for women who had two (OR, 4.0) or three or more (OR, 6.4) *Chlamydial* infections
- causes ⅔ of tubal infertility, ⅓ of ectopic pregnancy; higher risk of ectopic pregnancy in women who had two (OR 2.1) or three or more (OR, 4.5) *Chlamydial* infections
- arthritis, perihepatitis
- in pregnancy: low birth weight, miscarriage, prematurity, neonatal conjunctivitis, pneumonia; leading cause of blindness in developing countries

Diagnosis
- NAATs detect 20%–50% more *Chlamydial* infections than could be detected by culture
- endocervical or vaginal swab into PCR transport tube (or send as dry swab), or self-collected vaginal swab (all have comparable sensitivity: > 90% sensitivity, > 99% specificity), or
- first-void urine PCR: may have less sensitivity than vaginal swabs

Treatment
- first-line uncomplicated infection
  - azithromycin 1 g orally, single dose, or
  - doxycycline 100 mg orally twice daily for 7 days, or
  - erythromycin 500 mg orally four times a day for 7 days
- anorectal infection
  - doxycycline 100 mg orally twice daily for 7 days, or
  - azithromycin 1 g orally, single dose repeat in one week
- other supportive treatment
  - a notifiable disease
  - contact tracing of partners of 6 months (www.letthemknow.org.au)
  - safe sex
  - avoid sex for 7 days
  - STI screening
  - test of cure is not effective when advice has been followed (DNA of dead bacteria give false-positive results)
  - test of cure at 4 weeks acceptable in pregnancy and after anorectal disease
  - rescreen for reinfection at 3–4 months (reinfection rates are high)
  - if IUD in place leave in place, treat and monitor

Mycoplasma genitalium

- well-established cause of non-gonococcal urethritis in men
- largely asymptomatic in women
- meta-analysis demonstrates infection associated with around two-fold increased risk of cervicitis, PID, preterm birth, spontaneous abortion, infertility
- prevalence in low-risk populations around 2% so routine testing pregnancy not warranted

Diagnosis (*Australian STI Management Guidelines*, 2015)
- testing only available in specialised labs
  - testing should be limited to those with symptoms or known contact, rather than asymptomatic women
  - PCR on endocervical or HVS is recommended; first-pass urine less sensitive

Treatment
- azithromycin 1 g oral immediately
- doxycycline will only eradicate 30% of infections
- azithromycin resistance is increasing, in which case moxifloxacin is recommended to be used judiciously
- other: insufficient evidence for duration of contact tracing but recommended for 6 months
- test of cure in 4 weeks only if symptoms persist
- test for reinfection in 3 months and screen for other STIs

Other

- *Mycoplasma hominis* and *Ureaplasma urealyticum* are associated with bacterial vaginosis, possibly PID, but also may be non-pathogenic commensals
- Anaerobes: *Bacteroides* and *Peptostreptococcus* species
- treat with metronidazole 400 mg three times a day for 7 days

Investigations for PID

- serum human chorionic gonadotrophin (hCG) level
- full blood count, erythrocyte sedimentation rate, C-reactive protein (CRP), blood cultures
- urine for bacteriological studies
- vaginal wet prep
  - > 3 polymorphs on smear has sensitivity of 87%–91%
  - 0 polymorphs has a negative predictive value of 95%
  - presence of bacterial vaginosis (clue cells, whiff test amine odour on addition of KOH)
- bacteriological assessment of specimens from the vagina, endocervix, urethra, rectum, throat and pelvis (at laparoscopy), or first-pass urine as outlined above, screening for other sexually transmitted infections, including human immunodeficiency virus (HIV), hepatitis B and syphilis

- transvaginal ultrasound scan: adnexal mass, tubal oedema (thick wall, incomplete septum, cogwheel, beading): sensitivity 32%–85%, specificity 97%–100%
- power Doppler: increased fallopian tube flow highly sensitive
- Magnetic resonance imaging (MRI) highly sensitive but not routinely performed

Management of PID (*Australian STI Management Guidelines*, 2015)

- principles
  - requires high index of suspicion and low threshold for treatment
  - broad-spectrum antibiotics for 14 days: cure rates of over 90%
  - rapid response to antibiotic treatment is highly suggestive of PID
  - investigation and empiric treatment of sexual partners
  - notifiable diseases must be reported to Department of Health
  - counsel regarding safe sexual practices
  - advise avoidance of sexual intercourse for duration of treatment
  - test of cure is not cost-effective where the above advice has been followed
- outpatient treatment for mild to moderate PID
  - azithromycin 1 g orally, immediately
  - plus metronidazole 400 mg orally twice daily for 14 days
  - plus doxycycline 100 mg orally twice daily for 14 days
  - plus ceftriaxone 500 mg intramuscular injection with 2 mL 1% lignocaine or 500 mg intravenously (IV) immediately
- inpatient treatment for severe PID
  - cefotaxime 2 g IV 8 hourly, or ceftriaxone 2 g IV daily
  - plus metronidazole 500 mg IV twice daily plus azithromycin 500 mg IV daily until the patient is afebrile and improved; then continue doxycycline or roxithromycin for 2–4 weeks
- outpatient treatment of mild to moderate procedure-related PID
  - doxycycline 100 mg orally twice daily for 2–4 weeks, or
  - amoxycillin 500 mg orally three times a day, plus metronidazole 400 mg orally three times a day for 2–4 weeks
- inpatient treatment of severe septicaemic procedure-related PID
  - amoxycillin 2 g IV 4 hourly, plus gentamicin 1.5 mg/kg IV 8 hourly, plus metronidazole 500 mg IV 8 hourly until afebrile; then doxycycline 100 mg orally twice daily for 2 weeks
- other
  - if cannot tolerate doxycycline then provide azithromycin 1 g oral and repeat in 1 week
  - remove IUD if no response to treatment in 48–72 hours
  - contact tracing
  - notification if positive for a notifiable condition
  - avoid sex for 1 week or until improved

Consequences of PID

- short term
  - pyosalpinx

- tubo-ovarian abscess (TOA): accounts for 30% of hospitalisations with PID; treat initially with parenteral antibiotics; surgery if poor response; rupture of TOA is medical emergency
  - pelvic peritonitis
  - perihepatitis, colitis
  - acute infection with *Chlamydia* and gonorrhoea increases susceptibility to HIV infection
- long term
  - recurrent PID: in 74%; repeat infection significantly impacts on outcome
  - infertility
    — historical data suggests after one episode of PID is 10%–15%, after two episodes is 20%–35%, after three episodes is 40%–75%
    — more recent data suggests 18% by 3 years post-treatment
    — most with tubal factor infertility have no history of diagnosed PID, suggesting subclinical infection; however, history of pelvic pain is increased suggesting PID diagnosis is also missed
  - chronic pelvic pain (in 20%–30% of cases)
  - ectopic pregnancy: (historical data suggested 9%), recent data suggests 0.6%; Fitz-Hugh–Curtis syndrome (perihepatitis) (1%–30% of cases)

Toxic shock syndrome (TSS)

Epidemiology

- historically associated with use of superabsorbent tampons in presence of exotoxin producing *Staphylococcus aureus* colonisation
- non-menstrual TSS related to infected wounds, foreign bodies, viral infection
- menstrual TSS declining, annual incidence 1–2 in 100 000, with a 3% case fatality rate
- incidence of non-menstrual TSS remains relatively constant, with a 6% case fatality rate

Aetiology

- caused most commonly by *S. aureus*, which produces TSS toxin 1 (TSST-1); accounts for 90% of menstrual cases and 60% of non-menstrual cases of TSS or *S. aureus* producing enterotoxin B
- can also be caused by *Streptococcus pyogenes* (group A streptococcus), non-group A beta-haemolytic streptococcus, and *Streptococcus viridans* (more fulminant disease with higher mortality)

Presentation

- fever, hypotension
- erythroderma of palms, soles, hands, desquamation, multi-organ dysfunction including coagulopathy, renal failure, adult respiratory distress syndrome and abnormalities in electrolytes and liver biochemistry

Investigations

- full septic and biochemical screen
- isolation of TSST-1 pathognomonic for *S. aureus* TSS; however, testing infrequently performed and not freely available in Australia

Management
- resuscitate, ventilate if required
- intravenous antibiotics
- remove tampon if present
- open and debride infected wounds
- prevention: change tampons 4–8 hourly
- if previous TSS or a prior serious staph or strep infection, avoid tampons as recurrence is possible

Actinomyces israelii

- a gram-positive, non-acid, mycelium-bearing, anaerobic bacterium; is a normal commensal of mouth and gastrointestinal and genital tract
- causes infection after disruption of mucous membrane and spreading through tissue planes, causing PID and pelvic mass; can extend to parametrium, deep pelvic structures abdominal wall
- actinomyces-like organisms (ALOs) may be identified on cervical smears, but this is not diagnostic of pelvic disease
- 80% of pelvic actinomycosis found in women with intrauterine device IUD > 3 years but can be found in women without IUD
- if a woman is symptomatic, or has a pelvic mass, the IUD should be removed, and long-term treatment with antibiotics penicillin, tetracycline or erythromycin, +/– surgical intervention, is required

Genital herpes

Epidemiology
- prevalence 13–25% in developed countries
- caused by herpes simplex virus (HSV)
- HSV-2 tropism for genitalia
- HSV-1 tropism for skin and oro-genital region: more than 50% of genital HSV due to HSV-1 (increasing in prevalence in genital infection due to increasing orogenital sex and decreasing peri-oral infection in childhood)
- HSV infection increases the risk of HIV transmission

Infection and latency
- infects skin and mucous membranes through microabrasions
- travels along sensory nerves to sensory root ganglia where there is viral replication
- latency occurs for the life of the host
- trauma to skin results in reactivation of latent state with release of virus particles onto skin (recurrent infection)

Clinical symptoms
- primary infection
  - can be symptomatic in 10%–25% with the typical bilateral painful genital blisters and ulcers, labial oedema, dysuria, urinary retention, systemic symptoms
  - remainder are asymptomatic or have atypical short-lived symptoms

- secondary infection
  - mostly asymptomatic: minor itch or irritation but infectious particles spread through skin
  - can be symptomatic: localised blister/ulcer/skin splits on labia/anus/thighs/buttocks; only 4% are bilateral
  - many 'first episodes' are actual recurrences of a subclinical infection
  - after primary infection, recurrence and asymptomatic viral shedding is less frequent with HSV-1 (20%–50%) compared to HSV-2 (70%–90%)
- oral HSV infection (cold-sore): almost always HSV-1 in a healthy person, rarely HSV-2

Diagnosis

- swab base of ulcer or de-roofed vesicle for PCR for HSV-1 and HSV-2
- direct immunofluorescence, culture less sensitive
- type specific serology may assist with determining if a presentation is primary or secondary (important in the context of pregnancy)
- serology lacks positive predictive value in low-prevalence populations and is not recommended for asymptomatic screening; type-specific serology may be useful in counselling couples

Treatment (*Australian STI Management Guidelines*, 2015)

- primary infection
  - valaciclovir 500 mg twice daily for 5–14 days without delay will reduce severity and duration of episode
  - alternative acyclovir 400 mg three times daily, as effective
- infrequent recurrences
  - episodic therapy: valaciclovir 500 mg twice daily for 3 days at first sign of itching or redness
  - alternative famciclovir 1 g twice daily for 1 day
- frequent recurrences
  - suppressive therapy: valaciclovir 500 mg daily for 6 months reduces risk of transmission
  - alternative: famciclovir 250 mg twice daily for 6 months
  - review need for suppressive treatment 6 monthly as recurrences become less frequent
- other supportive treatment
  - provide written information and reduce stigmatisation
  - analgesia
  - saline baths
  - topical lignocaine
  - catheterisation if required
  - not required: contact tracing, notification to Department of Health, test of cure

Reducing the risk of transmission

- risk of HSV-2 transmission 5%–20% per year
- most occur within first 3 months of relationship
- risk of HSV-2 transmission is increased if:
  - there is no prior history of HSV-1: prior infection with HSV-1 give some cross protection (males with prior HSV-1 risk of acquiring it HSV-2 is 5% per year; females without prior HSV-1 risk is 20% per year)

- acquisition of HSV-2 occurred in the last 12–18 months
- there is a lesion present: infectivity arises in prodrome of lesion formation, viral titre peaks within first 24 hours of lesion development, and falls when lesions crust over
- for the first 6-12 months consider:
  - condoms: reduce risk by 50%
  - suppressive antiviral therapy: reduces risk by 50%
  - minimise skin trauma: use silicone-based lubricants

Pregnancy and genital HSV

(*See Ch 29.*)
- primary infection
  - risk of vertical transmission 50%, highest if primary infection within last 3 months
  - caesarean section if lesion present and membranes ruptured < 6 hours; or if primary infection within last 6 weeks.
- secondary infection
  - risk of transmission 1%–3% if lesions present, 0.04% if asymptomatic; consider caesarean if lesions present at time of delivery and membranes ruptured for less than 6 hours
  - suppressive treatment from 36 weeks reduces risk of recurrence
- partner
  - avoid orogenital sex if partner has cold sores
  - if partner has genital herpes, consider partner having suppressive therapy using condoms and silicone-based lubricant during pregnancy

References and further reading

Australian Government Department of Health, 2015. National Notifiable Diseases Surveillance System, 1 October to 31 December 2014. Commun. Dis. Intell. E158–E164.

Australian Sexual Health Alliance, 2015. Australian STI management guidelines for use in primary care. Available at: <www.sti.org.au> (updated January 2015; accessed 18 October 2015).

Brunham, R., Gottlieb, S.L., Paavonen, J., 2015. Pelvic inflammatory disease. NEJM 372, 2039–2048.

Centers for Disease Control and Prevention, 2014. Recommendations for the laboratory-based detection of *Chlamydia trachomatis* and *Neisseria gonorrhoeae*—2014. MMWR Recomm. Rep. 63 (RR–02), 1–19.

Centres for Disease Control and Prevention, 2015. Sexually transmitted diseases treatment guidelines, 2015. MMWR Recomm. Rep. 64 (3).

Chow, E.P., Fehler, G., Read, T.R., et al., 2015. Gonorrhoea notifications and nucleic acid amplification testing in a very low-prevalence Australian female population. Med. J. Aust. 202 (6), 321–323.

Cunningham, A.L., Taylor, R., Taylor, J., et al., 2006. Prevalence of infection with herpes simplex virus types 1 and 2 in Australia: a nationwide population based survey. Sex. Transm. Infect. 82 (2), 164–168.

Garland, S.M., Steben, M., 2014. Genital herpes. Best Pract. Res. Clin. Obstet. Gynaecol. 28 (7), 1098–1110.

Lahra, M.M., Lo, Y.R., Whiley, D.M., 2013. Gonococcal antimicrobial resistance in the Western Pacific Region. Sex. Transm. Infect. 89 (Suppl. 4), iv19–iv23.

Lis, R., Rowhani-Rahbar, A., Manhart, L.E., 2015. Mycoplasma genitalium infection and female reproductive tract disease: a meta-analysis. Clin. Infect. Dis. 61 (3), 418–426.

Menon, S., Timms, P., Allan, J.A., et al., 2015. Human and pathogen factors associated with *Chlamydia trachomatis*-related infertility in women. Clin. Microbiol. Rev. 28 (4), 969–985.

Molander, P., Sjoberg, J., Paavonen, J., et al., 2001. Transvaginal power Doppler findings in laparoscopically proven acute pelvic inflammatory disease. Ultrasound Obstet. Gynecol. 17 (3), 233–238.

Royal Australian College of General Practitioners, 2012. Guidelines for Preventive Activities in General Practice, 8th ed. RACGP, East Melbourne.

Sexual Health Australia, 2015. Pelvic inflammatory disease. Available at: <www .sexualhealthaustralia.com.au/pelvic_inflammatory_disease.html> (accessed 20 October 2015).

Workowski, K.A., Bolan, G.A., 2015. Sexually transmitted diseases treatment guidelines, 2015. MMWR Recomm. Rep. 64 (RR–03), 1–137.

Chapter 12

Menopause and premature ovarian failure

Michael Flynn

Definitions. Menopause is the permanent ceasing of menstruation resulting from the loss of ovarian follicular activity. Menopause is, by definition, only after 12 months of amenorrhoea with no other pathological cause; therefore, it is diagnosed only in retrospect. Leading into menopause is:
- early perimenopause, characterised by a change in cycle frequency
- late perimenopause, characterised by cycles up to 3–12 months apart
  The median age for menopause is 51.4 but it can occur between 45 and 55.
  Premature menopause is said to occur before age 40 and has a frequency of approximately 8%.

Aetiology and endocrinology

Menopause is due to the exhaustion of primordial follicles, with a subsequent failure of ovulation causing a fall in oestrogen and progesterone levels and a rise in follicle stimulating hormone (FSH).

Follicular development and menstrual cycles then become irregular. At menopause, insufficient ovarian follicular development results in insufficient oestrogen to cause endometrial growth. In the postmenopausal state, oestradiol decreases with a normal or slightly raised level of oestrone.
- Maximal rises in FSH and luteinising hormone (LH) occur in the first 2–3 years.
- After 20 years, FSH and LH may return to reproductive life levels.

Diagnosis

The diagnosis of menopause is made on the history of amenorrhoea in combination with vasomotor symptoms. There is no value in general checking of FSH, oestradiol or antimüllerian hormone (AMH) levels to confirm menopause. The differential diagnosis of some menopause symptoms include depression, anaemia or hypothyroidism.

Typical menopause symptoms include:
- hot flushes
  - a hot flush lasts between 1 and 4 minutes and is associated with a rise in temperature, peripheral vasodilatation and a slight rise in pulse rate
  - hot flushes are synchronous with, but are not caused by, LH pulses
  - up to 80% of women suffer from vasomotor effects at the menopause and 25% of these women complain of severe hot flushes; 9% continue to have hot flushes after the age of 70
- night sweats, disturbance in sleep quality, unusual tiredness
- crawling sensations under the skin (formication)
- anxiety, irritability, mood changes
- decreased concentration and changes in cognition
- decreased libido, dry vagina and uncomfortable intercourse
  - urogenital atrophy results in reduced glycogen and lactobacilli, causing a rise in vaginal pH, dryness and increased risk of infection
  - vaginal dryness and dyspareunia due to atrophy and responds to vaginal oestrogen
- urinary frequency
- muscle and joint pains

An initial menopause consultation should include assessment of:
- severity of menopause symptoms and their effect on quality of life
- recognition that women may also be at increased risk of heart disease, osteoporosis and thyroid disease
- contraindications of treatment: menopause hormone therapy (MHT)
- other routine screening: breast and cervix

Investigation

Hormonal assessment in peri- and postmenopause is rarely required and is of no use to monitor treatment when on menopause hormone therapy (MHT).

General health assessment and advice appropriate for middle-aged women are advised. Investigations include:
- pap smear
- mammogram
- blood profile including lipids, glucose tolerance test, thyroid function, renal and liver function, full blood examination
- bone density assessment
- pelvic ultrasound (if indicated)

Management

The management of the menopausal woman is aimed at a full treatment regimen to optimise quality of life. The concept of risk and benefit should be fully explained. The general issues that may require assessment and management include:
- moderate to severe vasomotor symptoms
- urogenital symptoms
- sexual dysfunction
- risk of bone density loss

MHT relates to the use of oestrogen in the management of menopause symptoms. Oestrogen is the best short-term treatment for women with vasomotor symptoms but each menopause symptom will have a response to oestrogen replacement. Oestrogen only is required if the uterus has been removed. Combined oestrogen and progesterone is indicated where the uterus is intact for the prevention of hyperplasia.

Selective oestrogen receptor modulators (SORMs) are synthetic molecules that bind to oestrogen molecules in either an agonist or antagonist mode, depending on the target organ. Tibolone is MHT that can be used in women with a uterus.

Vaginal oestrogen therapy is indicated for the use of local urogenital symptoms. Note that this is not therapeutic to prevent bone loss or vasomotor symptoms.

Once commenced, MHT should be reviewed yearly.

Contraindications to MHT include:

- oestrogen-dependant cancer
- high risk of venous thromboembolic event
- undiagnosed vaginal bleeding
- liver disease
- uncontrolled hypertension

Trials

Menopause management has been influenced by the continuing publication of a number of significant studies.

The women's health initiative (WHI)

This has been a long-term research program to address the most common causes of death, disability and quality of life in postmenopausal women. There have been many publications using these data. The main criticism of this study relates to the recruitment of older women to start MHT who may already have had established cardiovascular disease.

The study showed increased adverse events related to breast cancer, heart disease, stroke and venous thromboembolism in the arm of the study where patients took combined oestrogen and progestagen therapy. This was not replicated in the study arm of women who had a hysterectomy and required oestrogen only. Further reanalysis may suggest the adverse effects are not seen if MHT is commenced within 10 years of menopause.

Million women study

Coordinated in Oxford, UK, women were recruited between 1996 and 2001 to investigate women's health specifically in those over age 50. The focus was on hormone replacement therapy (HRT) and its effects on the breast and other aspects of health.

Other trials

Within a clinical field where advice is changing as more data emerge, the International Menopause Society provides consensus advice on the trials. Other studies which continue to influence menopause management include the *Nurses' health study* and the *Heart and estrogen/progestin replacement study (HERS) I and II*.

Current recommendations

- The main indication for MHT is to control menopausal symptoms.
- Initiate therapy when symptoms occur or as close to the menopause as possible.

- HRT reduces fracture risks and is therefore appropriate for women with osteoporosis.
- HRT is not appropriate for primary or secondary cardioprotection.
- Review each patient's management annually with risk–benefit assessment. Consider ceasing therapy at 60 years of age or after 5 years of treatment.

Premature ovarian dysfunction

Incidence. Incidence is 1%. It is associated with primary amenorrhoea in 10%–30% of cases.

Aetiology

GENETIC
- idiopathic (> 90%), familial (20%–30%)
- chromosomal
  - Turner's syndrome 45,XO; 45,XO/XX
  - pure gonadal dysgenesis 46,XX; 46,XY
  - trisomy 13 and 18, 47,XXX
  - deletions/inversions

METABOLIC
- 17-hydroxylase deficiency, galactosaemia, myotonic dystrophy
- autoimmune
  - thyroid disease 25%: Hashimoto's disease, Graves' disease, hypothyroidism, thyroiditis, silent thyrotoxicosis
  - Addison's disease
  - others: myasthenia gravis, hypoparathyroidism, autoimmune haemolytic anaemia/thrombocytopenia, pernicious anaemia

INFECTIOUS
- mumps (the commonest)
- tuberculosis
- malaria
- *Shigella*
- varicella

ENVIRONMENTAL
- smoking (there is a dose-related effect of smoking on age of menopause)
- increasing parity
- poor health and nutrition

IATROGENIC
- irradiation, chemotherapy (methotrexate, actinomycin)
- posthysterectomy (ovarian failure may be advanced by 6 years)

Pathophysiology
Ovarian biopsy shows a reduced number of preantral follicles. The lack of gonado-trophin receptors may be the underlying cause of premature ovarian failure, because

follicles require gonadotrophins and gonadotrophic receptors to develop beyond the preantral stage.

Diagnosis of premature ovarian failure

Diagnosis is based on a triad of amenorrhoea, raised gonadotrophins and signs/symptoms of oestrogen deficiency.

- age < 40 years
- primary or secondary amenorrhoea
- FSH levels of > 15 IU/L indicating perimenopausal levels
- hot flush and genital atrophy present in 50% of cases

Examination and investigations

EXAMINATION

- stigmata of Turner's syndrome
- secondary sexual characteristics
- body mass index, blood pressure, thyroid
- signs of hypo-oestrogenism
- signs of thyroid disease

INVESTIGATIONS

- to exclude pregnancy as a cause of amenorrhoea
- FSH of > 40 IU/L diagnostic
  - repeat if results borderline (e.g. three assays at 2–4-week intervals)
- karyotype (required for all patients with primary amenorrhoea and early-onset premature ovarian failure)
- adrenals/thyroid function

Consequences and their management

Treat the underlying disease, such as an autoimmune disorder.
  Consequences:
- short term: vasomotor symptoms, vaginal dryness, stress incontinence, psychological effects
- long-term: infertility, osteoporosis, cardiovascular effects
  MHT should be continued until the age of 50 years and then the woman should be reviewed.

References and further reading

Australasian Menopause Society: <www.menopause.org.au>.

De Villiers, T.J., et al., 2013. Global consensus statement on menopausal hormone therapy. Climacteric 16 (2).

International Menopause Society: <www.imsociety.org>.

Jane, F.M., Davis, S.R., 2014. A practioner's toolkit for managing the menopause. Climacteric 17 (5).

Jean Hailes for Women's Health: <www.jeanhailes.org.au>.

Million Women Study: <www.millionwomenstudy.org>.

Nurses' Health Study: <www.channing.harvard.edu/nhs>.

Women's Health Initiative (WHI): <www.nhlbi.nih.gov/whi/index.html>.

Chapter 13

Intersex variations

Yasmin Jayasinghe

Definition. Intersex people are born with variations in chromosomal, gonadal or anatomic sex that do not meet the stereotypical definitions of male or female. The terms 'hermaphrodite' or 'intersex condition' are not uniformly accepted by the intersex community. Intersex people have the same range of gender identities and sexual orientations as non-intersex people. The term now encompasses all variations in development (e.g. müllerian agenesis).

Incidence. Incidence is 1 in 5000 live births; therefore, it is rare. However, the situation requires rapid and sensitive assessment, knowledge of which is important.

Typical sexual differentiation

Undifferentiated gonads begin to develop during the fifth week after conception. During the sixth week, migration of primordial germ cells into the gonad is completed. Over 20 genes have been found to be involved in testicular and ovarian determination. Presence or absence of sex-determining region on the Y chromosome (SRY gene) leads to determination of gonadal sex (testis or ovary), followed by sex differentiation.

Male phenotypic development

Expression of the SRY gene causes differentiation of the gonad into a testis. (Several other genes are also involved in testicular development, mutations of which will result in 46XY sex reversal or ambiguous genitalia—for example, SRY, SOX9 and Wilms' tumour 1 (WT1).) Testis produces fetal testosterone and antimüllerian hormone (AMH), which act in exocrine fashion causing ipsilateral regression of müllerian ducts and development of wolffian structures. 5-alpha-reductase converts testosterone to dihydrotestosterone in order to virilise the cloaca.

Female phenotypic development

Two X chromosomes are required for normal ovarian development. The absence of SRY and the presence of DAX1 gene on the X chromosome inhibit testicular development. AMH is absent and müllerian development occurs into upper vagina, uterus and tubes.

The genital tubercle becomes the clitoris, urogenital folds become labia minora and labioscrotal swelling becomes labia majora.

Variations in sexual development

- Sex chromosome abnormalities can interfere with gonadal differentiation (e.g. mutations in WT1 SRY, SOX 9, DAX 1).
- Lack of testosterone is due to failure of testicular differentiation or biosynthetic (Leydig cell) defects.
- Reduction or absence of 5-alpha-reductase causes impaired cloacal response to testosterone, but there is normal response by the wolffian structures.
- An androgen receptor defect (androgen insensitivity) causes lack of cloacal response to androgens, regression of müllerian structures due to AMH, and no development of male internal genitalia (vas deferens, seminal vesicles, epididymis).
- Deficiencies in AMH (produced by Sertoli cells) cause growth of müllerian structures.
- A 46XX male occurs when the SRY gene is present on the X chromosome due to atypical crossover during meiosis.

Classification of intersex variations

Classification is according to chromosomes, gonadal histology and phenotype.

Sex chromosome variations
- 45XO Turner's syndrome
- 47XXY Klinefelter's syndrome

Undervirilisation of 46XY individuals
- faults of androgen production: 3-beta-hydroxysteroid dehydrogenase deficiency (3βHSD II), 17-beta-hydroxysteroid dehydrogenase deficiency (17βHSD III)
- end-organ receptor defect: androgen insensitivity syndrome (AIS)
- defects in testosterone metabolism: 5-alpha-reductase deficiency
- XY gonadal dysgenesis, SOX9 or WT1 mutations
- drugs: spironolactone

Virilisation of 46XX individuals
- congenital adrenal hyperplasia (CAH)
- exposure in utero to androgen-producing tumour (fetal or maternal)
- maternal drugs: danazol, methyltestosterone, androgenic progesterone

Ovotesticular variations
- Gonads are ovotestis.
- Diagnosis is by gonadal biopsy.
- Commonest chromosomes are 46XX; also associated with 46XX/XY, 45XO/46XY and 46XY.

Unclassified anatomical abnormalities
- Mayer-Rokitansky-Küster-Hauser syndrome (müllerian agenesis)
- cloacal exstrophy

Presentations of intersex

- ambiguous genitalia
- apparent female genitalia: clitoromegaly (> 9 mm length or > 6 mm width in full-term infant), posterior labial fusion, inguinal/labial mass
- apparent male genitalia: non-palpable testes, micropenis (< 2.5 cm stretched length in full-term infant), hypospadius
- genital karyotype discordance
- delayed puberty, primary amenorrhoea
- inguinal hernia in female
- virilisation
- pelvic tumour

Newborn investigation of ambiguous genitalia

Key points

- There needs to be an immediate referral to experts in a collaborative multidisciplinary team including paediatric endocrinology, gynaecology, surgery, psychology and clinical ethicist.
- Postpone gender affirmation in infants born with ambiguous genitalia prior to expert consultation. An answer is usually available within 2–3 days. Refer to the child as 'the baby' until then. The first interactions families have with healthcare providers are remembered, and have long-lasting consequences.
- Gender identity, gender role and sexual orientation are distinct entities. It is hoped that gender affirmation in childhood will be congruent with gender identity; however, gender dissatisfaction may manifest later in life. Gender dissatisfaction is not predictable by karyotype, androgen exposure, degree of genital virilisation or assigned sex.
- Ongoing psychological support, family-centred care and education, and full disclosure to the family and young patient that evolves over a developmental time line, are standards of care.

History

- past maternal pregnancy history, drug ingestion in pregnancy, maternal virilisation, relevant antenatal tests (e.g. imaging karyotype)
- familial history of consanguinity (increases risk of autosomal recessive disorders), other intersex conditions or neonatal death (e.g. salt-wasting CAH)

Examination

- vital signs and hydration (CAH), dysmorphic features (to suggest genetic causes), midline defects (to suggest hypothalamic pituitary hypogonadism), jaundice (thyroid/cortisol issue)
- genitalia: external genitalia, palpable gonads, phallic length, presence of hypospadias, assess for urogenital sinus, location urethral meatus, clitoral size, vaginal opening, pigmentation and rugosity of genital skin; masculinisation score using Prader staging may be used

Investigations

- monitor weight and fluid balance, and check electrolytes, glucose and plasma 17-renin activity (PRA)

- 17 hydroxyprogesterone, testosterone, dihydrotestosterone, DHEAS, gonado-trophins, 11 deoxycortisol
- serum AMH: if undetectable, absence of testicular tissue; if elevated, then defect in androgen synthesis or androgen receptor defect
- karyotype with microarray for SRY and other deletions, duplications
- abdominopelvic and renal ultrasound/magnetic resonance imaging (MRI)
- urogenital sinogram to evaluate urethra and vagina
- adrenocorticotrophic hormone (ACTH)/HCG stimulation tests as per endo-crinology

Gender affirmation

Controversy exists around early surgical management. Surgery is offered in the context of restoring anatomy or reducing future risks (such as risk of malignancy). Results from an Australian paediatric surgical centre suggest generally positive physical and psycho-social outcomes, with low risks for gender dysphoria. Influencing factors include diag-nosis, therapeutic options, fertility potential, cultural practices and pressures, and parental views. There are some who advocate waiting until the child can make their own decision. Surgery is guided by stringent ethical protocols, should only be under-taken at specialised centres and may require family court involvement.

Turner's syndrome (TS)

Incidence. Incidence is 1 in 2000 to 1 in 5000 live born.

Clinical presentation
- 45XO or mosaicism 45,X/46,XX or 45,X/46,XY
- clinically short stature and pubertal failure along with other stigmata
- diagnosis: clinical, karyotype (note that follicle-stimulating hormone [FSH] levels may be markedly elevated up to 2 years of age, then nadir to near normal levels at age 4–10 years before rising again)
- spontaneous puberty with menses may occur in 9% of XO (and up to 30%–50% of mosaics)
- 2% may conceive spontaneously; pregnancy may be achieved through oocyte dona-tion, but there is a high risk of pregnancy complications (30% miscarriage; 7% stillbirth; 34% of live births will have a malformation [e.g. Down syndrome, TS]) and maternal complications (preeclampsia, caesarean section, aortic dissection with maternal mortality of 2%)
- medical complications must be monitored: osteoporosis, hypertension, diabetes, obesity, thyroid disorders, Crohn's disease, sensorineural hearing loss, cardiovascular anomaly including aortic root dilatation and risk of dissection

Management
- gonadectomy if Y component (present in 6% on karyotype) to avoid malignancy
- growth hormone
- optimal to start oestrogen therapy at bone age of 12 years in those on growth hormone, and 11 if not (although coordination with paediatric endocrinologist is advised); start with very low doses, and aim to complete feminisation over 2–3 years (may add progesterone when withdrawal bleeding occurs)

Complete gonadal dysgenesis (Swyer syndrome)

- 46 XY
- no testicular development
- normal müllerian structures, female phenotype, streak gonads, presenting with delayed puberty or primary amenorrhoea
- mutations in SRY in 10%–20%

Congenital adrenal hyperplasia (CAH)

Incidence. Incidence is 1 in 14 500.

Clinical presentation
Clinical presentation varies, although it is often diagnosed after birth, and includes:
- ambiguous genitalia
- salt-losing crisis
- hypertension
- virilisation and amenorrhoea in late-onset CAH
- > 90% identify as females

Pathophysiology
- autosomal recessive disorder
- enzymatic defect in the synthesis of cortisol with loss of adrenal–pituitary feedback control
- result: an increase in ACTH, adrenal hyperplasia, increase in adrenal androgen production

21-hydroxylase deficiency
- accounts for ≥ 95% of cases of CAH
- due to mutations in CYP21 gene
- classic CAH (both alleles affected) presents in newborn period with ambiguous genitalia and three-quarters are salt losing
- diagnosis: based on raised 17-hydroxyprogesterone, +/– decreased Na, increased K, decreased aldosterone, increased PRA
- treatment: corticosteroids and, if salt losing, fluorohydrocortisone
- monitor with 17-hydroxyprogesterone and PRA
- increase glucocorticoids during stress, illness, surgery
- surgery at 6 weeks to 6 months of age at specialised centres: clitoroplasty, labioplasty, vaginoplasty
- in pregnancy, administration of maternal dexamethasone, starting in the first trimester; may prevent virilisation in up to one-third of female babies, although management is controversial
  - degree of suppression of the fetal pituitary–adrenal axis can be gauged by maternal oestriol and 17-hydroxyprogesterone levels
  - prenatal testing for mutations in CYP21 is available

11-beta-hydroxylase deficiency
- due to mutations in CYP11B1
- 11-deoxycortisol and 11-deoxycorticosterone levels high, resulting in salt-retention

- presentation: with ambiguous genitalia, cryptorchidism, hypertension and hypernatraemia

3-beta-hydroxysteroid dehydrogenase

- mutations in HSD3B2 gene
- very rare, severe adrenal insufficiency, may be salt losers, mild virilisation of female or undervirilisation of male (testosterone deficiency)

20,22-desmolase deficiency

- addisonian crisis

Androgen insensitivity syndrome (AIS)

Incidence. Incidence is 1 in 20 000 to 1 in 64 000 XY births.

Clinical presentation

- XY karyotype, mutation in androgen receptor gene

COMPLETE AIS

- phenotypic female, testes may be present in inguinal hernias at birth
- testes function normally, resulting in production of AMH; therefore, absent müllerian structures and blind-ending vagina
- normal androgen production; however, target tissues are unresponsive and male phenotype does not develop
- absent axillary and pubic hair
- female gender identity: manage with gonadectomy, vaginal dilators or vaginoplasty when mature enough; hormone replacement therapy

PARTIAL AIS

- spectrum of ambiguous genitalia, pubic and axillary hair present
- gender identity may be male or female

Müllerian agenesis

- XX karyotype, absent uterus, blind-ending vagina, axillary and pubic hair present
- often diagnosed in puberty due to primary amenorrhoea
- rudimentary müllerian structures may cause pelvic pain
- associated renal and skeletal anomalies may be present
- creation of neovagina
  - Frank method (vaginal dilatation)
    — in Australia, this is the first-line of management when the patient is ready
    — success is around 80% and vaginal length of around 6–7 cm can be reached
    — coitus may also achieve dilatation
  - other methods described
    — Sheares vaginoplasty: blunt dissection into rectovaginal space
    — McIndoe (split-skin graft)
    — bowel segments
    — Creatsas modification of Williams vaginoplasty

— Davydov: surgical inlay of peritoneum into vaginal space

— Vecchietti: laparoscopic upward traction of perineum with object (olive)

— plastic surgery flaps

A systematic review of 162 articles (including 1 available RCT), demonstrated that bowel vaginoplasty was the most commonly used method internationally, Vecchietti procedures had the highest injury rate (2%) and split-thickness skin graft had the highest infection rate (4.2%) and reoperation rate 7%.

Surgery in intersex

Role of surgery

- goals: restore anatomy for menstruation, sexual function; promote sexuality and reproductive function; prevent urologic complications
- feminising genitoplasty—may involve:
  - clitoroplasty with preservation of neurovascular bundle
  - labioplasty
  - neovaginal construction or simple Y–V flap vaginoplasty
  - gonadectomy in XY containing karyotypes due to risk of dysgerminoma, gonadoblastoma
    — high risk of malignancy (15%–50%): intraabdominal dysgenetic gonads, partial AIS with non-scrotal gonads
    — low risk 2%–3%: complete AIS, ovotesticular variations
  - may defer removal of gonads until after puberty in complete AIS (peripheral conversion of androgens to oestrogen allows spontaneous induction of puberty); however, risk increases over time

Timing of surgery

- At large Australian multidisciplinary centres of excellence, with defined protocols, most surgery in females born with ambiguous genitalia is performed up to and including 6 months of age, collaboratively between the surgeon and gynaecologist, with excellent long-term outcomes compared to other countries (6% require revision in adolescence, and around 25%–30% may need to use dilators, compared to around 50% revision rates worldwide). Positive psychosocial and psychosexual outcomes were also seen.
- Parents must be informed that there are those who advocate no sex assignment, allowing the child to choose for themselves when old enough; however, data are limited.
- When diagnosis of vaginal agenesis is made in later childhood or early puberty, vaginoplasty is best deferred, as most women can create a neovagina with the use of dilators alone (80% success rate). If surgery is required, success in the older population depends on successful use of a vaginal mould or dilators postoperatively (inappropriate to perform in young children).

References and further reading

Australia, O.A.-I., 2009. Style guide: on intersex and terminology. Organisation Intersex International Australia, Newtown. Available at: <www.oii.org.au> (accessed 17 November 15).

Crawford, J.M., Warne, G., Grover, S., et al., 2009. Results from a pediatric surgical centre justify early intervention in disorders of sex development. J. Pediatr. Surg. 44 (2), 413–416.

Hewitt, J.K., Jayasinghe, Y., Amor, D.J., et al., 2013. Fertility in Turner syndrome. Clin. Endocrinol. (Oxf) 79 (5), 606–614.

Lean, W.L., Deshpande, A., Hutson, J., et al., 2005. Cosmetic and anatomic outcomes after feminizing surgery for ambiguous genitalia. J. Pediatr. Surg. 40 (12), 1856–1860.

McCann-Crosby, B., Sutton, V.R., 2015. Disorders of sexual development. Clin. Perinatol. 42 (2), 395–412, ix–x.

McQuillan, S.K., Grover, S.R., 2014. Dilation and surgical management in vaginal agenesis: a systematic review. Int. Urogynecol. J. 25 (3), 299–311.

Warne, G., Grover, S., Hutson, J., et al., 2005. A long-term outcome study of intersex conditions. J. Pediatr. Endocrinol. Metab. 18 (6), 555–567.

Chapter 14

Paediatric and adolescent gynaecological disorders

Yasmin Jayasinghe

Gynaecological problems encountered in children and adolescents are unique to these age groups and involve sensitivity and skills differing from those utilised for adults.

Paediatric gynaecology

Normal genital anatomy in the prepubertal child

- Maternal oestrogenisation wanes by 6 months; however, endogenous hormone production due to activation of the hypothalamic–pituitary (HP) axis continues in infants for a few years. Female infants can have palpable breast tissue for around 2 years (in 50% the tissue regresses by 1 year). HP axis become quiescent thereafter until around 8 years.
- Hypooestrogenisation causes labia to be atrophic, and hymen to appear erythematous.
- Hymen may be crescentic, annular (circumferential), microperforate or cribriform.
- Other normal external genital findings:
  - hymenal ridges and tags: common at birth often resolve
  - hymenal bumps: localised bump anywhere on hymen
  - notches: U- or V-shaped indentations do not extend to vaginal wall; common at 3 and 9 o'clock
  - linea vestibularis: pale avascular midline streak on posterior vestibule
  - failure of midline fusion: at fossa navicularis (can extend towards anus, smooth edge).
- Cervix is often flush with the vaginal vault or protrudes slightly.
- Uterus may be so small that it may be difficult to identify on ultrasound in inexperienced hands.

Examination of a prepubertal child

- examine after parental consent and rapport established
- start with a general examination
- appropriate explanation to child and parent is important: it will not involve internal examinations, it should not hurt, there is no use of force, listen to the child if she wants you to stop
- with appropriate rapport and explanation, these examinations are usually tolerated very well: if very resistant, consider deferring examination; if symptoms of vaginal bleeding, consider going to examination under anaesthesia (EUA)
- frog-leg position (on mother's lap if more comfortable that way)
- genital inspection then traction on labia majora (slightly lateral but mainly towards you) will usually enable hymen to open; ask child to cough while inspecting lower vagina

Vulvovaginal abnormalities

VULVOVAGINITIS
Clinical features
- symptoms: pruritis, dysuria, soreness of the vulvar area, vaginal discharge, occasionally vaginal bleeding if severe infection
- signs: non-specific discharge, vaginal drip, mild vulvar erythema secondary to discharge

Causes
- usually non-specific inflammation with no identifiable pathogen (80% of cases)
- specific pathogens: group A beta-haemolytic streptococci and *Haemophilus influenzae*, from the upper respiratory tract, are the most common
- underlying factors: hypo-oestrogenism causing overgrowth of normal flora, close proximity of vagina to anus, alkaline vaginal pH
- moisture: synthetic fibre underwear, obesity
- irritants (bubble baths, irritant soaps)

Differential diagnosis of vaginal discharge and irritation
- pinworms: itchy bottom
- vulvar dermatoses
- foreign body
- sexual abuse
- ectopic ureter
- vulvar Crohn's: can present with fissures and erosions, swelling, painful red papules, plaques, ulcers

Management
- only take introital swab if moderate to severe offensive discharge, or bloody discharge
- perineal hygiene (vinegar baths: $\frac{1}{2}$ cup white vinegar in shallow bath as required)
- cotton underwear and change soon after sport
  - barrier cream (e.g. zinc and castor oil); hypoallergenic paraffin-based moisturiser if needs moisturising
- antibiotics if severe symptoms, including bloody discharge; if symptoms do not promptly settle, EUA

- treat empirically for *Enterobius vermicularis* (pinworms) if persistent significant pruritis
- reassurance, as symptoms settle with age

LABIAL ADHESIONS

- labia adherent in midline, midline raphe seen
- due to hypooestrogenisation and denudation of thin labial skin, avascular bridge develops
- present in 0.6%–5% of prepubertal girls
- usually present 6 months to 6 years, not seen in the newborn
- often asymptomatic, but may cause urinary dribbling due to narrow vaginal opening, vulvitis and rarely urinary tract infections
- differential diagnosis
  - imperforate hymen or disorder of sexual differentiation, where no midline raphe will be seen
  - lichen sclerosus may present with adhesions generally more anteriorly and in older girls
  - very rarely secondary adhesions may develop due to healing of straddle injury
- management
  - reassurance, vinegar baths and barrier cream for symptoms
  - manual separation not indicated in hypo-oestrogenised child: 40% recurrence rate, fibrotic scarring may occur
  - oestrogen creams may cause breast budding, vulvar pigmentation and spotting, and are also associated with recurrence after cessation of use
  - adhesions usually resolve with age and increasing oestrogen levels

GENITAL ULCERS

- may raise suspicion for sexual abuse, but most are *not* sexually transmitted
- often associated with non-specific viral illness
- causes
  - aphthous ulcers
  - viral: HSV via autoinoculation, Epstein-Barr virus (EBV), cytomegalovirus (CMV), varicella zoster virus (VZV)
  - group A strep, mycoplasma
  - autoimmune: Crohn's disease, Behçet's disease other vasculitis
  - dermatological, drugs
  - sexual: HSV, syphilis, chancroid, lymphogranuloma venereum
- history and examination: primary or recurrence, systemic symptoms, ulcers elsewhere, ancestry, family history, social history, sexual history
- investigation: viral, bacterial fungal swabs, (HSV, VZV PCR); serology (EBV, CMV, HSV) consider CRP, erythrocyte sedimentation rate (ESR), antinuclear antibody (ANA), HLA-B51, consider biopsy if ongoing, STI screen where appropriate
- treatment depends on cause: supportive care, sitz baths, analgesia, lignocaine topical ointment, catheter if required, antiviral, steroids, antibiotics as required; if Behçet's disease is suspected, rheumatology review

GENITAL WARTS

- Genital warts may raise suspicion for sexual abuse, particularly in children over 3 years; however, they may be transmitted in other ways (e.g. vertical and latent infection may possibly reactivate later in life).

- Warts are found in up to 0.2%–3% of children who have been sexually abused.
- The presence of warts alone without supporting clinical or social information is not diagnostic of abuse.
- Human papillomavirus (HPV) typing is not recommended. The viral subtype alone cannot determine the mode of transmission, as the virus does not display 100% site specificity in children.
- DNA fingerprinting to test for clonality is not useful. HPV 6 and HPV 11 are stable viruses, and do not vary markedly between hosts. Viral variants between the child and an alleged perpetrator are likely to be identical, as they represent circulating type for that area, and would not indicate the mode of transmission or the source.
- Get expert advice.

VULVODYNIA
- vulvar pain in the absence of physical findings
- childhood vulvar pain usually has a cause but may occasionally be neuropathic
- poorly understood in this age group, can be misdiagnosed
- pain may affect development of positive body image and self-esteem
- associated with psychological distress, anxiety
- in adolescents can be associated with tampon insertion, dyspareunia, OCP use > 2 years and intercourse prior to 16 years, recurrent candida infections, past traumatic experiences; overlap in symptoms with interstitial cystitis and painful bladder syndrome
  - management: cotton garments, avoid fragrances and irritation, apply oil to vulva prior to bathing and moisturise (e.g. with hypoallergenic paraffin-based moisturiser) after bathing, minimise liners, bladder and bowel retraining, physiotherapy in older teens, tricyclic antidepressants (e.g. amitriptyline, can consider weaning at 6 months)

VAGINAL BLEEDING
- generally pathological and warrants further investigation

Differential diagnosis of vaginal bleeding
- severe vaginitis
- foreign body
- trauma
- lichen sclerosus
- urethral prolapse
- sarcoma botryoides
- müllerian papilloma
- precocious puberty

Vaginitis
- commonest cause of vaginal bleeding in children
- if suspected, may treat with antibiotics alone initially; but if recurrent bleeding do EUA to exclude another cause

Foreign body
- commonly toilet paper
- EUA and removal of the object

Genital trauma

- Straddle injuries may cause haematomas and genital lacerations (usually involving labia or fourchette) and associated with bruising of labia or thigh. A consistent history is important.
- Labial fat pads generally protect the hymen and vagina. Hymenal, vaginal or perianal lacerations, without labial or thigh bruising, are unusual and suspicious for non-accidental penetrating injury, unless there is a clear witnessed history. Note that ano-genital injuries heal quickly often completely. Most children who have been sexually abused have normal clinical findings (< 5% have abnormal findings). Any concerns regarding sexual abuse should be immediately referred to a skilled professional in the field so that appropriate investigation, documentation and follow-up can be organised.
- Management of accidental genital trauma:
  - ensure voiding is possible, sitz baths
  - EUA if ongoing bleeding expanding haematoma, concerns about anatomical integrity.

Lichen sclerosus

- commonest age of presentation in premenarcheal girls is 5–7 years
- symptoms, signs: dysuria, pruritus vulvar soreness, dyschezia, bleeding (due to petechial haemorrhages, fissures, papules), sharp demarcation: figure of 8 hypopigmentation around vulva and anus, loss of architecture
- may have family history of autoimmune disease
- mistaken for sexual abuse
- Advantan fatty ointment (methylprednisolone aceponate); or 0.05% betamethasone dipropionate twice a day for 6–12 weeks until resolution, then low-dose maintenance for 3 months
- recurrences common, 75% improvement in symptoms after menarche

Urethral prolapse

- oedematous ring of mucosa prolapsed around urethral meatus, sometimes associated with ulceration, necrosis, bleeding, difficulty passing urine
- precipitants: hypo-oestrogenisation, chronic straining
- treat with oestrogen cream every night and sitz baths; regression seen over days to weeks
- if persists and symptomatic, may require surgical excision

Sarcoma botryoides (embryonal rhabdomyosarcoma)

- presents with lower abdominal mass and vaginal bleeding
- may sometimes see grape-like lesions at introitus
- most commonly presents under 5 years, with vaginal disease
- presentation in teenage years is usually cervical disease
- treated with neoadjuvant chemotherapy, surgery and radiotherapy
- over 90% survival in children

Müllerian papilloma

- rare benign soft tissue polypoid tumour of cervix or vagina
- median age of presentation 5 years

Precocious puberty

- normal pubertal development often occurs in sequence: growth acceleration, thelarche, adrenarche, menarche, although there is cultural variation

- time between onset of breast development to menarche is around 2 years; mean age of menarche in Australian girls is 13 years (range 12.2–14.2 years)
- precocious puberty: pubertal symptoms before 7 years
- central (activated hypothalamic–pituitary–ovarian [HPO] axis, gonadotropin dependent) or peripheral (non-activated HPO axis, gonadotropin independent)
- causes of central precocious puberty
  - constitutional precocious puberty (no organic abnormality; accounts for 90% of cases), caused by premature release of gonadotrophins from the anterior pituitary with no organic lesions, signs of puberty appear in correct order, bone age and height advanced for chronological age
  - intracranial lesions, meningitis, encephalitis, tumours, hydrocephalus, tuberous sclerosis
- causes of peripheral precocious puberty
  - feminising ovarian tumours (e.g. granulosa cell, malignant teratoma)
  - signs of puberty do not appear in the normal order: breast enlargement occurs with little body hair because adrenal function is not mature
  - McCune-Albright syndrome: spontaneous mutation of GNAS1 gene
    — syndrome is multisystem and requires two of the following: 1. polyostotic fibrous dysplasia (bone deformities and fractures); 2. café au lait spots; 3. autonomous endocrine hyperfunction (including peripheral precocious puberty, acromegaly, hyperthyroidism, Cushing's)
    — may develop autonomous ovarian function due to dominant ovarian cysts producing oestrogen
  - adrenal cortical tumours, congenital adrenal hyperplasia causing precocious virilism
  - ingestion of drugs containing oestrogen
- preliminary investigations for precocious puberty: growth chart, bone age, follicle-stimulating hormone (FSH), luteinising hormone (LH), oestradiol, pelvic ultrasound to look for ovarian activity, androgens if virilised; review by an endocrinologist may be indicated for complete endocrine profile including GnRH assessment and formal cranial and adrenal imaging
- treatment depends on underlying cause and may include GnRH analogues for central causes, aromatase inhibitors (to block conversion of testosterone to oestradiol), aldactone, ketoconazole, tamoxifen, surgery

Adolescent gynaecology

Adolescent health principles

- accessible, non-judgmental, confidential, adolescent-friendly care
- only some exceptions to the duty of confidentiality, including the risk of self-harm or harm to others, or abuse

Consent to treatment

- a young woman under 18 years can give consent to treatment if judged a 'mature minor', if she is assessed to be mature and competent and where she fully comprehends the nature of the specific condition for which treatment is sought, the purpose, methods, risks, potential benefits of treatment and alternatives to treatment, and the potential outcomes if the treatment is not implemented
- such a person can be deemed 'Gillick competent'

- assessment of maturity (checklist)
  - age
  - level of schooling
  - level of independence from parental care
  - general maturity of speech and bearing
  - information gained from prior knowledge of the patient
  - why they came to see you about the issue on their own
  - functioning in other aspects of their life
  - their ability to explain the clinical problem for which treatment is sought, by providing an appropriate clinical history, and
  - their ability to understand the gravity and complexity of the treatment proposed
- assessment of competence (checklist); the young person has sufficient understanding of
  - the nature of their clinical problem
  - the nature and purpose of the proposed treatment
  - the effects of the treatment including side effects
  - the consequences of non-treatment
  - other treatment options
  - possible repercussions of treatment (e.g. if someone found out)
  - how to carry through the proposed treatment
- important issues around consent and confidentiality
  - exceptions: confidentiality clause does not apply if it is to safeguard the young person or the public (e.g. in cases of self-harm or sexual abuse); seek advice if you are not sure
  - assessment of maturity and competence is specific to the scenario at hand, and does not necessarily apply across all situations of differing complexity and gravity, so assessments are made on a case-by-case basis

Adolescent heavy menstrual bleeding (HMB)

The commonest cause is anovulatory dysfunctional uterine bleeding.

BLEEDING DISORDERS

- about 10% of 'healthy' adolescents presenting to a tertiary clinic in Australia with HMB (up to 20% if known bleeding disorders included)
- family history is important risk factor
- HMB may be the only symptom of a bleeding disorder in a young person
- causes: Von Willebrand's disease 5%, platelet function disorders 6%, factor deficiencies are rare but can present with life-threatening bleeding
- bleeding screen: Von Willebrand's factor, platelet function analysis, coagulation profile and full blood count
- management: avoid non-steroidal anti-inflammatory drugs (NSAIDs), all of the usual hormonal measures, such as OCP, Mirena (menstrual suppression if necessary), Cyklokapron, intranasal desmopressin acetate if necessary; as young women get older and develop ovulatory cycles, impact of a mild bleeding disorder on menses will be less pronounced

ADOLESCENT METROSTAXIS (ACUTE HEAVY LOSS)

- The commonest cause is still dysfunctional uterine bleeding, but consider pregnancy complication, genital tract trauma, coagulopathy, arterio-venous malformation and malignancy (all rare).

- In the acute phase, vital signs may remain stable despite significant blood loss, and then drop very quickly. Aggressive medical management is required.
- Resuscitate with intravenous fluids, transfuse and get haematological opinion.
- Tranexamic acid.
- If hypo-oestrogenic (perimenarcheal, slim, poor breast development), and if stable enough, consider oestrogen first (e.g. Progynova for 24 hours prior to starting progesterone treatment).
- If clinically normo-oestrogenic, then try Provera 10 mg or Primolut 5 mg every 2 hours until bleeding stops (including overnight), and then wean slowly over a few weeks.
- Eventually maintenance hormonal treatment with menstrual suppression thereafter (extended cycle OCP, Mirena) may be beneficial.
- If already on the OCP consider a twice-daily dose for 2–3 days (under supervision) and then wean to daily.
- Investigations to consider: full blood count (FBC), iron, beta-HCG if appropriate, bleeding profile but not in the setting of acute loss or transfusion, FSH, LH, oestradiol may be useful to assess degree of hypo-oestrogenism, ultrasound scan for endometrial thickness (be careful to exclude clot).
- Surgical investigation/intervention is rarely required.

MENSTRUAL MANAGEMENT IN DEVELOPMENTAL DISABILITY

- Menses can be associated with great distress, and may interfere with important lifestyle and health measures (e.g. attending school, physical activity, swimming).
- These young women may already be at risk of low bone density due to issues with immobility and nutrition.
- Depending on the level of disability, education regarding normal development, the fact that menses signify good health, and preparation for menses can assist with reducing fear (e.g. practicing wearing pads, having a special toiletry bag to take to school, accessing educational material from family planning).
- Hysterectomy is not legal unless applications are made to the family court and all other measures to assist menstrual concerns have been tried and failed.
- Can reassure parents that other measures are usually very successful (e.g. menstrual suppression with the OCP if not contraindicated).
- The Mirena IUCD has been used with good success and is likely to be better for bone health than other progesterone-only options.

Adolescent dysmenorrhoea

- Prostaglandin-mediated primary dysmenorrhoea is the commonest cause, and can be managed with medical therapy.
- Endometriosis: difficult to establish prevalence as intervention rates vary significantly between institutions. Reported to be prevalent in 47%–67% of adolescents with refractory chronic symptoms but potential bias due to study population. Usually early stage and atypical lesions present. A study of 55 adolescents with *surgically managed* endometriosis reported positive family history in first-degree relatives in 25%, superficial implants in 56%, endometrioma in 33%, deep infiltrating endometriosis in 10%; recurrence rates were high for those with DIE or endometrioma. Five per cent had an infertility issue at initial laparoscopy.
- While it is clear that the vast majority of dysmenorrhoea in young women is prostaglandin-related and can be managed successfully medically, it is important to acknowledge that the women who go on to develop endometriosis often report delayed diagnosis and review by multiple providers.

- Current standard of care at the Department of Gynaecology in the Royal Children's Hospital, Melbourne, is to manage pain proactively with medical therapy (menstrual suppression if cyclic is not helpful) and to resort to diagnostic laparoscopy in refractory cases.
- Uterine anomaly: always consider in severe refractory primary dysmenorrhoea and pain in an adolescent.

Uterine anomaly

IMPERFORATE HYMEN

- amenorrhea, cyclic pain, urinary retention, bluish introital bulge with abdominal pressure, treat with cruciate incision
- consider microperforate hymen in someone with scant vaginal loss and similar symptoms

TRANSVERSE VAGINAL SEPTUM

- incidence: 1 in 70 000
- amenorrhea, bulge at introitus absent with abdominal pressure, yet haematocolpos seen on ultrasound
- correct diagnosis is crucial, as requires Z-plasty, and possibly use of vaginal dilators preoperatively and vaginal mould postoperatively (can only be done when the young woman is psychologically ready)
- menstrual suppression with the OCP prior to this to manage pain is successful

OBSTRUCTED LONGITUDINAL VAGINAL SEPTUM, UTERINE DIDELPHYS, RENAL AGENESIS

- incidence: 1 in 35 000
- menstruating from normal side, unilateral haematocolpos
- menstrual suppression for pain management until septum resected vaginally
- mould not required

RUDIMENTARY UTERINE HORN

- found in around 74% of unicornuate uteri
- can be communicating, non-communicating, separated (from unicornuate uterus), non-separated
- 92% are non-communicating
- generally present around 23–26 years of age
- only around half present with dysmenorrhoea
- functioning horns can have hypoplastic endometrium; therefore, haematometra does not always develop
- non-cavitary solid horns can cause pain through pressure atrophy or adenomyosis
- sensitivity for detection on ultrasound scan only about 26%
- 36% associated with renal anomaly
- non-communicating horns, even with little endometrium, may carry a pregnancy and rupture in the second or third trimester causing fetal loss and significant maternal morbidity
- recommended that rudimentary non-communicating horns be removed prior to childbearing when there is a good unicornuate uterus on the other side

VAGINAL AGENESIS

- incidence: 1 in 5000
- associated with renal spinal cardiac anomalies and hearing problems

- 80% success with use of dilators to create neovagina (when the young woman is ready)
- modified Sheares vaginoplasty may be used in other cases with use of mould and dilators postoperatively (timing driven by the young woman)
- important not to misdiagnosis late presentation of complete androgen insensitivity syndrome, by performing karyotype, and asking/checking for presence or absence of axillary or pubic hair, inguinal hernias

Adolescent polycystic ovarian syndrome (PCOS)

- Incidence is 3% in the adolescent population.
- Rotterdam criteria will overdiagnose PCOS in adolescence. Adolescents typically have relative androgenaemia, insulin resistance, cystic ovaries and anovulatory cycles. However, the pathway towards metabolic syndrome may be developing in some. Primary amenorrhoea may occasionally even be a presenting feature of severe PCOS. The key is to not miss the diagnosis in a young person at risk for severe metabolic disease, while not overdiagnosing normal physiological changes in adolescence.
- Therefore, special considerations regarding PCOS in adolescents are:
  - Persistence of menstrual irregularity for some years postmenarche (it takes around 4 years for 80% to become ovulatory), premature pubarche and adrenarche, insulin resistance as determined by acanthosis nigricans and a fasting insulin : glucose ratio < 7 (as opposed to 4.5 in an adult) may be predictive of development of PCOS. Clinical hyperandrogenism (hirsutism, alopecia) associated with irregular cycles (> 45 days) may also be predictive.
  - Of the adolescents who meet the diagnostic criteria, 16% may have impaired glucose tolerance and 1.8% may have diabetes.
  - A follicular phase morning 17-alpha-hydroxyprogesterone is useful to exclude non-classic congenital adrenal hyperplasia.
  - Lifestyle measures for all young women are important regardless of diagnosis.
  - Small studies with the use of metformin have shown a favourable effect on ovulation, resumption of menses and reduction of central adiposity, but treatment is generally reserved for those who have failed other lifestyle measures.

References and further reading

Audebert, A., Lecointre, L., Afors, K., et al., 2015. Adolescent endometriosis: report of a series of 55 cases with a focus on clinical presentation and long-term issues. J. Minim. Invasive Gynecol. 22 (5), 834–840.

Bacon, J.L., Romano, M.E., Quint, E.H., 2015. Clinical recommendation: labial adhesions. J. Pediatr. Adolesc. Gynecol. 28 (5), 405–409.

Berenson, A.B., Chacko, M.R., Wiemann, C.M., et al., 2000. A case-control study of anatomic changes resulting from sexual abuse. Am. J. Obstet. Gynecol. 182 (4), 820–831, discussion 31–4.

Berenson, A.B., Grady, J.J., 2002. A longitudinal study of hymenal development from 3 to 9 years of age. J. Pediatr. 140 (5), 600–607.

Clare, C.A., Yeh, J., 2011. Vulvodynia in adolescence: childhood vulvar pain syndromes. J. Pediatr. Adolesc. Gynecol. 24 (3), 110–115.

Coles, N., Bremer, K., Kives, S., et al., 2015. Utility of the oral glucose tolerance test to assess glucose abnormalities in adolescents with polycystic ovary syndrome. J. Pediatr. Adolesc. Gynecol.

Dun, E.C., Kho, K.A., Morozov, V.V., et al., 2015. Endometriosis in adolescents. JSLS 19 (2).

Gibbs, N.F., 1998. Anogenital papillomavirus infections in children. Curr. Opin. Pediatr. 10 (4), 393–397.

Gillick v West Norfolk and Wisbech Area Health Authority [1984], Q.B. 581.

Heppenstall-Heger, A., McConnell, G., Ticson, L., et al., 2003. Healing patterns in anogenital injuries: a longitudinal study of injuries associated with sexual abuse, accidental injuries, or genital surgery in the preadolescent child. Pediatrics 112 (4), 829–837.

Jayasinghe, Y., Cha, R., Horn-Ommen, J., et al., 2010. Establishment of normative data for the amount of breast tissue present in healthy children up to two years of age. J. Pediatr. Adolesc. Gynecol. 23 (5), 305–311.

Jayasinghe, Y., Garland, S.M., 2006. Genital warts in children: what do they mean? Arch. Dis. Child. 91 (8), 696–700.

Jayasinghe, Y., Moore, P., Donath, S., et al., 2005. Bleeding disorders in teenagers presenting with menorrhagia. Aust. N. Z. J. Obstet. Gynaecol. 45 (5), 439–443.

Jayasinghe, Y., Rane, A., Stalewski, H., et al., 2005. The presentation and early diagnosis of the rudimentary uterine horn. Obstet. Gynecol. 105 (6), 1456–1467.

Laufer, M.R., Goitein, L., Bush, M., et al., 1997. Prevalence of endometriosis in adolescent girls with chronic pelvic pain not responding to conventional therapy. J. Pediatr. Adolesc. Gynecol. 10 (4), 199–202.

McQuillan, S., Grover, S., Pyman, J., et al., 2015. Literature review of benign müllerian papilloma contrasted with vaginal rhabdomyosarcoma. J. Pediatr. Adolesc. Gynaecol. In press.

Medical Practitioner's Board of Victoria, 2014. Consent for treatment and confidentiality in young people. Melbourne.

Powell, J., 2006. Paediatric vulval disorders. J. Obstet. Gynaecol. 26 (7), 596–602.

Reed, B.D., Cantor, L.E., 2008. Vulvodynia in preadolescent girls. J. Low. Genit. Tract Dis. 12 (4), 257–261.

Royal Children's Hospital. Clinical practice guidelines: Vulval Ulcers. Melbourne. Available at: <www.rch.org.au/clinicalguide/guideline_index/vulval_ulcers/> (accessed 9 November 2015).

Savasi, I., Jayasinghe, K., Moore, P., et al., 2014. Complication rates associated with levonorgestrel intrauterine system use in adolescents with developmental disabilities. J. Pediatr. Adolesc. Gynecol. 27 (1), 25–28.

Sultan, C., Paris, F., 2006. Clinical expression of polycystic ovary syndrome in adolescent girls. Fertil. Steril. 86 (Suppl. 1), S6.

Villarroel, C., Lopez, P., Merino, P.M., et al., 2015. Hirsutism and oligomenorrhea are appropriate screening criteria for polycystic ovary syndrome in adolescents. Gynecol. Endocrinol. 31 (8), 625–629.

Chapter 15

Chronic pelvic pain

Judith Goh
Sue Croft

- Pelvic pain is the most common indication for laparoscopy. For chronic pelvic pain, the pain is present for at least 6 months severe enough to interfere with normal daily activities.
- Definition of pain (International Association for Study of Pain): a sensory and emotional experience that encompasses both tissue nociception and the interpretation of the pain experience.

Physiology and innervation

Pain
- Somatic innervation from the vulva, perineum and lower vagina is via the pudendal nerve (S2–S4).
- Visceral innervation from the uterus, tubes, ovaries and visceral peritoneum is via the autonomic nervous system (T10–L1).
- The assessment of pelvic pain requires a detailed pain history and system review.

Origin
- gynaecological
- gastrointestinal
- urological
- musculoskeletal
- neurological

Viscera
- Viscera are not sensitive to thermal and tactile sensation.
- Pain is poorly localised.
- Pain is referred from the overlying peritoneum via dermatomes of the same nerve root.

Stimuli that produce pain
- distension/contraction of an organ
- stretching of organ capsule
- irritation of the parietal peritoneum
- ischaemic tissues
- inflammation, neoplasia or fibrosis stimulating nerves

Examination

- general examination: look for signs of malignancy, lymphadenopathy, oedema
- abdominal palpation: feel for masses, ascites, organomegaly
- vaginal speculum examination
  - check for discharge
  - cervical pathology
  - vulva: inspect, Q-tip swab—tenderness over vestibular glands (*see Ch 23*)
  - bimanual examination: check uterine size and position, adnexal pathology, cervical motion pain, pouch of Douglas
  - uterosacral ligament nodularity, thickening or tenderness
  - vaginal: lateral over pelvic muscle pain, tight and painful to palpate
  - rectal examination for masses
  - lumbosacral and hip joints
- assess anatomical locations of tenderness and correlate these with areas of pain

Gynaecological causes of pelvic pain

- cyclical: dysmenorrhoea, ovulation pain, endometriosis, adenomyosis; some aetiologies of pelvic pain can be exacerbated during menses (irritable bowel syndrome and interstitial cystitis)
- chronic pelvic inflammatory disease
- polycystic ovarian syndrome
- residual ovary, ovarian remnant syndrome
- neoplasia
- pelvic venous congestion
- levator muscle spasm
- vulvodynia
- painful bladder
- pelvic adhesions

Non-gynaecological causes of pelvic pain

- gastrointestinal tract
  - diverticulitis, malignancy, obstruction
  - inflammatory bowel disease, irritable bowel syndrome, pelvic floor dyssynergia
- urinary tract
  - calculus, infection, retention, malignancy
  - interstitial cystitis (painful bladder)

- musculoskeletal
  - osteoarthritis
  - prolapsed disc
  - fibromyalgia
  - myofascial pain
  - peripartum musculoskeletal pain

Clinical presentation

Cyclical

Dysmenorrhoea is severe in 5% of women and is often associated with endometriosis, adenomyosis.

OVULATION

- Acute onset of lower abdominal pain is followed by a dull ache for several hours.
- The pain corresponds to the luteinising hormone (LH) peak (1 day before ovulation).
- The pain is due to prostaglandin F_2 causing contractility of ovarian perifollicular smooth muscle.

Pelvic inflammatory disease

- Only about 60% can be correctly diagnosed on history alone.
- The gold standard for diagnosis is by laparoscopy.
- Long-term sequelae include chronic infection, pelvic pain, dyspareunia, menstrual changes, infertility and ectopic pregnancy.

Endometriosis

- associated with dysmenorrhoea, dyspareunia and chronic pain

Neoplasia

- benign: degenerating fibroid, ovarian cyst complications
- malignant: weight loss, nausea, abdominal/pelvic pain, ascites, lymphadenopathy, irregular mass in pelvis

Pelvic venous congestion

- has been implicated as a cause of pelvic pain
- may be due to oestrogen causing dilatation of the thin-walled, unsupported pelvic veins

Residual ovary syndrome

- occurs in about 3%–4% of ovaries not removed during hysterectomy
- 75% of patients present with chronic pelvic pain and dyspareunia

Polycystic ovarian syndrome

- pelvic pain/discomfort may be a presenting complaint

Uterovaginal prolapse

- dull ache, dragging lump in vagina

Gastrointestinal
- change in bowel habit, rectal bleeding

Urinary
- infection, calculus causing dysuria, loin pain
- bladder pain syndrome: urgency, frequency, pain/tenderness around bladder/vagina, dyspareunia, pain often increases as bladder fills; may worsen with caffeine, alcohol, acidic foods

Musculoskeletal
- low back ache of musculoskeletal origin, radiating commonly to lower limbs and not abdomen or pelvis

Investigation for pelvic pain

Laparoscopy
- the most informative investigation for chronic pelvic pain

Radiology
- ultrasound scan of the pelvis
- X-ray of lumbosacral spine and hip joints
- other imaging (e.g. upper gastrointestinal series, barium enema, renal tract) if indicated
- cystoscopy

Others
- mid-stream urine
- *Chlamydia*
- pelvic congestion is difficult to diagnose

Treatment

Identify specific cause if evident and treat appropriately. Ongoing management of chronic pelvic pain involves a multidisciplinary approach and often includes: gynaecologist pelvic floor physiotherapist, pain management, sexual counsellor, support groups. Chronic pain is better managed with a bio-psychosocial model of treatment that works on interactions between the brain and body and acknowledges multiple causes from biological, psychosocial and sociological domains.

Treatment of chronic pelvic pain
- pharmacological: dependent on the cause of pain
  - non-steroidal anti-inflammatory drugs (NSAIDs)
  - oral contraceptive pill
  - gonadotrophin-releasing hormone (GnRH) agonist
  - amitriptyline: low dose
- physiotherapy
  - pain education
  - learning to down-train and relax pelvic floor muscles

- education on use of dilators: desensitisation, trigger point muscle release
- general exercise, movement: important management strategies
- bladder training
- correct postures for bladder/bowel emptying: pelvic floor dyssynergia
- psychological: pain clinics and management
- pain assessment forms may benefit in long-term management

Further reading

Butler, D., Mosely, L., 2013. Explain Pain. NOI Publications, Adelaide, Australia.

Gambone, J.C., Mittman, B.S., Munro, M.G., et al., 2002. Consensus statement for the management of chronic pelvic pain and endometriosis: proceedings of an expert-panel consensus process. Fertil. Steril. 78, 961–972.

Gelbaya, T.A., El-Halwagy, H.E., 2001. Chronic pelvic pain in women. Obstet. Gynecol. Surv. 56, 757–764.

Howard, F.M., 2003. Chronic pelvic pain. Obstet. Gynecol. 101, 594–611.

2011. IUGA Interstitial cystitis & painful bladder syndrome. International Urogynecological Association, Washington. Available at: <http://www.iuga.org/?patientinfo> (accessed 10 June 2016).

Chapter 16

Lower urinary tract symptoms

Judith Goh

Urinary incontinence is the complaint of involuntary urinary leakage. Lower urinary tract symptoms include complaints regarding urinary storage, voiding or postmicturition symptoms. When a woman presents with urinary symptoms, a detailed history on lower urinary tract symptoms is required.

History

- daytime frequency (normally up to 8 times a day): increased frequency is associated with increased fluid intake, detrusor overactivity, poor bladder compliance or increase in bladder sensation
- nocturia: complaint of interruption of sleep one or more times because of the need to pass urine
- urinary urgency: sudden desire to pass urine, which is difficult to defer
- urinary stress incontinence: involuntary leakage on effort or physical exertion
- urinary urgency incontinence: involuntary loss of urine associated with urgency
  - may present with frequent losses or large leakage
  - commonly associated with 'triggers' causing urgency and incontinence (e.g. turning on taps, coming home with 'key-in-the-door')
- continuous urinary incontinence: complaint of continuous involuntary loss of urine
- voiding problems
  - slow stream: urinary stream perceived as slower compared to previous voids or in comparison to others
  - straining to void: effort required to initiate, maintain or improve urinary flow
  - intermittency: complaint of urine flow that stops and starts
  - hesitancy: complaint of a delay in initiating micturition
- postmicturition
  - sensation of incomplete emptying
  - postvoid dribble: leaking after voiding (e.g. when standing from the toilet)
- other urinary history
  - dysuria (burning or discomfort during micturition), haematuria, previous urinary tract infections

- suprapubic pain
- coital incontinence: involuntary loss of urine with coitus; may occur during penetration or at orgasm
- other history
  - constipation
  - caffeine intake
  - symptoms of prolapse: needing to reduce the prolapse to void
  - previous gynaecological/urological procedures

Examination

A physical examination is performed to exclude transient causes and to evaluate other disease and functional ability.
- general, weight
- vulva (excoriation or urine dermatitis)
- gynaecological, vaginal prolapse, vaginal atrophy, urine in vagina
- local neurological
- urethra
  - urethral diverticulum, scarring around urethra and anterior vaginal wall
  - mobility of urethra
  - cough test and/or reduce prolapse and ask the woman to cough to assess for urinary stress incontinence

Investigation

This would depend on the history and examination.
- bladder diary
  - very useful tool
  - over a 2–3-day period, the woman is asked to record the times of micturition and her voided volumes, together with symptoms (e.g. urgency, incontinence)
  - fluid intake is also recorded
- urinalysis and culture, cytology
- postvoid residual volume
- blood sugar, renal function
- dye test: if a urinary tract fistula is suspected

Further evaluation

Further evaluation includes urodynamics assessment, cystoscopy and imaging. Criteria for further evaluation include uncertain diagnosis, failure of response to initial therapy, consideration of surgical intervention and suspicion of other pathology.

URODYNAMIC ASSESSMENT

The tests are designed to determine the functional status of the urinary bladder and urethra. The main components of urodynamics assessment are uroflowmetry, cystometry and urethral closure pressure/Valsalva leak point pressure.
- Uroflowmetry is a timed measure of voided urine volume.
  - a simple and non-invasive tool
  - cannot distinguish between obstruction and detrusor weakness as cause of voiding dysfunction without simultaneous measurement of detrusor function

- Cystometry is a test of detrusor function consisting of an observation and/or recording of the pressure/volume relationship during bladder filling.
- Maximal urethral closure pressure is the highest pressure, relative to bladder pressure, generated along the functional length of the urethra.
- Valsalva leak point pressure is the intravesical pressure at which urinary leakage occurs due to an increase in intra-abdominal pressure and in the absence of detrusor contraction.

Common causes of urinary incontinence

- urodynamic stress incontinence: diagnosis by symptom, sign and urodynamic investigation with the finding of involuntary leakage of urine associated with increased intra-abdominal pressure, in the absence of a detrusor contraction
- urgency incontinence
  - idiopathic detrusor overactivity (detrusor instability)
  - overactive bladder
  - neurogenic detrusor overactivity (detrusor hyperreflexia)
- mixed incontinence (combined stress and urgency incontinence)
- overflow incontinence: atonic detrusor, impaired bladder compliance
- extraurethral incontinence: genito-urinary fistula, urethral diverticulum, congenital abnormality
- functional disorders: cognitive impairment, physical disorder, psychological
- reversible causes (temporary causes)
  - conditions affecting lower urinary tract: infection, atrophy, constipation
  - drugs, diuretics, caffeine, alcohol
  - increased urine production: hyperglycaemia, excessive fluids
  - impaired mobility

Treatment of urinary incontinence

Aims are to:
- determine cause of incontinence
- detect and treat related urinary tract pathology
- evaluate the woman and available resources

The extent and interpretation of evaluation must be tailored to the individual. A multidisciplinary team approach optimises outcomes. Not all detected conditions can be cured and simple interventions may be effective even in the absence of a diagnosis. Many women with urinary incontinence develop undesirable bladder habits, which often exacerbate the problem and/or provoke other urinary symptoms (e.g. 'going just in case', voiding too often, reducing oral fluids). There is evidence to suggest that in women with mixed incontinence, detrusor overactivity should be treated prior to continence surgery, as this optimises overall outcomes.

In Australia, resources are available to women, including government-funded or subsidised schemes such as home assessments and continence products. The Continence Foundation of Australia provides a 24-hour helpline for men and women with urinary and faecal incontinence.

Overactive bladder

- overactive bladder (OAB) syndrome: urinary urgency usually associated with urinary frequency/nocturia, with or without urgency urinary incontinence, in the absence of urinary tract infection and other pathology
- detrusor overactivity
  - diagnosis by symptoms and urodynamic assessment: commonly OAB symptoms with detrusor muscle contractions during filling cystometry
  - causes include neurogenic, outflow obstruction, ageing and idiopathic (most common)
- overactive bladder survey in Europe and United States: about 17% of women with symptoms suggestive of overactive bladder; increasing prevalence with increasing age

OVERACTIVE BLADDER AND IDIOPATHIC DETRUSOR OVERACTIVITY

The mainstay of treatment is non-surgical.
- initial management (multidisciplinary approach)
  - exclude other causes (e.g. infection, other pathology, voiding dysfunction, neurological)
  - bladder diary
  - bladder training, pelvic floor rehabilitation
  - treat constipation, weight loss, reduce/avoid caffeine
- pharmacological
  - major portion of neurohumoral stimulus for physiological bladder contraction is acetylcholine-induced stimulation of postganglionic parasympathetic cholinergic receptor sites on bladder smooth muscle
  - anticholinergic drugs: contraindicated in closed-angle glaucoma (availability limited in Australia)
    — oxybutynin (oral or patch): care with anticholinergics in the elderly (oral oxybutynin may impair cognitive function); consider overall antimuscarinic burden (e.g. medications for Parkinson's disease and dementia); drug distribution changes due to reduced muscle mass and renal impairment
    — solifenacin, darifenacin, tolterodine
  - Beta-3-adrenoreceptor agonists
    — detrusor relaxation and increased stability during bladder storage via direct activation of beta-adrenoreceptors
    — mirabegron 25 or 50 mg daily
  - tricyclic antidepressants (have anticholinergic effects): amitriptyline
  - oestrogen: topical
- others
  - peripheral nerve stimulation
- surgical
  - intravesical botox injection
  - sacral nerve stimulator implant
  - augmentation cystoplasty, diversion

Urodynamic stress incontinence

CONSERVATIVE MANAGEMENT
- multidisciplinary approach
- treat overactive bladder symptoms

- pelvic floor rehabilitation
- vaginal/urethral devices for urinary incontinence

SURGERY

There are over 100 described surgical procedures for the management of urodynamic stress incontinence. Common complications of these procedures include voiding difficulty, injury to lower urinary tract, infection, de novo overactive bladder symptoms and failure to treat the stress incontinence. Better results have been documented for the slings and colposuspension, with approximately 85% success rate. Commonly performed procedures today are: slings (mid-urethral, pubo-vaginal); retropubic urethropexy (Burch colposuspension, Marshall-Marshetti-Krantz [MMK]); and urethral bulking agent.

Slings

- Traditional slings are placed at the urethro-vesical junction.
- In the mid-1990s the mid-urethral sling was described, which allowed minimally invasive surgery, reduced hospital stays and a quicker return to daily activities, without a reduction in success rates.
- Slings are made of fascia (autologous, human donor or xenographs) or synthetic mesh (e.g. polypropylene). When synthetic mesh is to be used, current evidence recommends a macroporous, monofilamentous mesh. This reduces the risk of mesh extrusion/erosion and infection.
- Mid-urethral slings may be placed in the retropubic space (first generation) or through the obturator foramen (second generation). The third-generation slings are 'exit-less'.

Retropubic urethropexy

- The Burch colposuspension 'hitches' the paravaginal tissue to the iliopectineal ligament, whereas the MMK sutures are placed into the periosteum of the posterior part of the pubic symphysis.
- Colposuspension may be performed laparoscopically or via a laparotomy.

Urethral bulking agent

- This involves periurethral or transurethral injection of a bulking agent, under endoscopic control, imaging or using an introducer.
- Materials used as a bulking agent include bovine collagen, silicone microparticles, Teflon and autologous material (e.g. fat).
- As a primary procedure, the success rates are lower (about 50%).
- Advantages include minimal anaesthesia/analgesia, ability to redo or 'top-up'.

References and further reading

Continence Foundation of Australia Helpline. 1800 330 066.

Haylet, B.T., et al., 2010. An International Urogynecological Association (IUGA)/International Continence Society (ICS) joint report on the terminology for female pelvic floor dysfunction. Int. Urogynecol. J. 21, 5–26.

Chapter 17

Pelvic organ prolapse

Hannah Krause

Definition. Pelvic organ prolapse (POP) is the protrusion of pelvic organs into the vaginal canal. Prolapse of pelvic organs occurs when their attachments, neural connections and supports fail.

Incidence. POP is common and affects about 1 in 3 women who have had one or more children.

Causes and risk factors

- age, parity, childbirth, chronic straining (e.g. chronic cough, constipation), connective tissue disorder, genetic/familial, congenital factors, obesity

History

- presenting complaint: asymptomatic or symptomatic of prolapse
- symptoms of prolapse include:
  - lump or bulge
  - sensation of discomfort or dragging
  - voiding difficulty
  - incomplete bowel emptying (splinting, manual evacuation)
  - dyspareunia
  - vaginal 'wind'/flatus
- other pelvic floor history
- urinary symptoms
- sexual function: dyspareunia
- bowel function
- menstrual history: menopausal
- past medical history: may be unsuitable for surgery
- past surgical history: previous prolapse or continence surgery

Examination

- general examination, including body mass index (BMI)
- abdominal: exclude mass lesion
- vaginal
  - genital hiatus: widened
  - cough with and without prolapse reduced: assess for urinary leakage
  - use Sims' speculum: left lateral or lithotomy, Valsalva
  - POP-Q assessment (see below)
  - vaginal examination for pelvic organ assessment
  - assessment of pelvic floor muscles for defects, strength, endurance

POP-Q (pelvic organ prolapse quantification) classification

The POP-Q system evaluates descent relative to a fixed reference point, the hymen. Six points are measured in centimetres above or below the hymen, and three further measurements evaluate the genital hiatus, perineal body and total vaginal length (see Fig. 17.1). The six points are as follows.

1. Point Aa is located in the mid-line of the anterior vaginal wall, 3 cm above the external urethral meatus.
2. Point Ba is a point that represents the most dependent (distal) position of any part of the upper anterior vaginal wall down to point Aa.
3. Point Ap is located in the midline of the posterior vaginal wall, 3 cm above the hymen.
4. Point Bp is a point that represents the most dependent (distal) position of any part of the upper posterior vaginal wall down to point Ap.
5. Point C is the distal edge of the cervix or the vaginal cuff following a hysterectomy.
6. Point D is the location of the posterior fornix in women with a cervix present.

The three further measurements are:
1. Genital hiatus (GH) is measured from the middle of the external urethral meatus to the posterior midline hymen.
2. Perineal body (PB) is measured from the posterior margin of the GH to the mid-anal opening.
3. Total vaginal length (TVL) is the length of the vagina when points C or D are reduced to their normal positions.

STAGES

- Stage 0: no prolapse is demonstrated.
- Stage 1: most distal portion of prolapse is > 1 cm above the level of the hymen.
- Stage 2: most distal portion of prolapse is ≤ 1 cm proximal to or distal to the plane of the hymen.
- Stage 3: most distal portion is > 1 cm below the plane of the hymen, but protrudes to no further than 2 cm less than the TVL.
- Stage 4: complete eversion of total length of lower genital tract.

Investigations

- Urodynamics studies are useful to assess for preexisting voiding dysfunction and occult urodynamic stress incontinence.

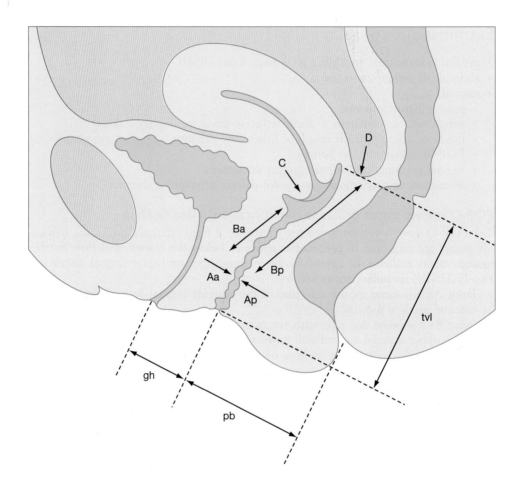

Figure 17.1 Reference points for the International Continence Society classification (1996) for vaginal prolapse. Source: Bill Reid, RCH Melbourne.

- Four-dimensional pelvic floor ultrasound scan is currently used as a research and adjunctive diagnostic tool to assess defects in the levator ani muscles. Evidence suggests that levator ani muscle defects and levator hiatal ballooning/enlargement are associated with prolapse development and a higher risk of recurrence of prolapse following surgery.

Conservative management

- pelvic floor exercises: may reduce symptoms of prolapse
- pessary
  - mechanical support for prolapse inserted into vagina
  - numerous types including ring, shelf, Gellhorn, cube
  - management of pessary: either self-manage or clinic care; both will require regular inspection of vagina for ulceration

- common issues with pessary:
  — sexual intercourse is possible depending on the type of pessary used; with self-management the pessary may be removed
  — vaginal discharge: usually physiological response, bacterial vaginosis or yeast infection
- complications of pessary
  — vaginal discharge
  — vaginal epithelial ulceration
  — occult stress urinary incontinence
  — vesico-vaginal fistula or recto-vaginal fistula
  — forgotten pessary

Surgical management

Identify which compartments require repair, and repair all defects. Options are vaginal or abdominal approach; conserve uterus or hysterectomy; and native tissue repair or augment with biomaterials. Biomaterials are biological or synthetic. Biological materials include autografts, allografts and xenografts. Synthetic materials may be absorbable or non-absorbable mesh (macroporous monofilamentous mesh).

Vaginal approach
- anterior compartment defects: anterior native tissue repair, anterior repair with bio-material augmentation, vaginal paravaginal repair
- posterior compartment defects: posterior native tissue repair, posterior repair with biomaterial augmentation
- vault or uterine descent: sacrospinous colpopexy or hysteropexy with sutures or mesh, high uterosacral plication, iliococcygeus fascial suspension, Manchester repair
  - obliterative procedure (colpocleisis) if not sexually active and not sexually active in future
- perineorrhaphy

Abdominal approach
- open, laparoscopic or robotic
- sacral colpopexy with biomaterials
- paravaginal repair

Risks and complications
- intraoperative complications: anaesthetic complications, bleeding and transfusion, damage to bladder, ureters or bowel
- immediate postoperative complications: infection, deep venous thrombosis, voiding difficulties, fistula formation
- long-term issues: recurrence of prolapse, dyspareunia, neuropathic pain
- biomaterials complications: vaginal exposure, erosion into bladder or bowel, contraction and scarring, vaginal and pelvic pain
- *Urogynecologic Surgical Mesh: Update on the Safety and Effectiveness of Transvaginal Placement for Pelvic Organ Prolapse* (US Food and Drug Administration statement, 2011)
  - in this update the FDA advised the public and medical community of complications related to transvaginal repair with mesh

- included in the update:
  — summary of adverse event reports; recommendations for patients; recommendations for healthcare providers
  — FDA activities
    – safety communication: the risks of serious complications associated with transvaginal POP repair with mesh are not rare; previously unidentified risk of vaginal shortening, tightening, and/or pain due to mesh contraction
    – regulatory changes: including reclassification of transvaginal surgical mesh products for POP from Class II to Class III; further clinical studies required to address risks and benefits of mesh used to treat POP and stress urinary incontinence; expanded post-market monitoring of device performance
  — subsequently, legal claims including individual and class actions worldwide regarding vaginal mesh complications; significant reduction in the use of vaginal mesh
  — Australian and New Zealand College of Obstetricians and Gynaecologists (RANZCOG) have provided a statement on polypropylene vaginal mesh implants for vaginal prolapse and a position statement on midurethral slings

Long-term considerations

Depending on the type of POP repair performed, there can be significant prolapse recurrence rates of more than 30%. While traditional native tissue repairs do have significant recurrence rates, they do avoid the risks associated with the use of biomaterials. Repair techniques using biomaterial augmentation aim to reduce recurrence rates and are continuing to be developed and modified in order to try to reduce such risks.

When counselling patients regarding prolapse treatment, conservative and surgical options should be fully discussed. An important aspect of counselling is the realistic expectations of outcomes, in particular of surgery.

Further reading

Bump, R.C., Mattieson, A., Bo, K., et al., 1996. The standardization of terminology of female pelvic organ prolapse and pelvic floor dysfunction. Am. J. Obstet. Gynecol. 175 (1), 10–17.

Royal Australian and New Zealand College of Obstetricians and Gynaecologists, 2014. Position statement on midurethral slings (C-Gyn 32). August. RANZCOG, East Melbourne.

Royal Australian and New Zealand College of Obstetricians and Gynaecologists, 2013. Polypropylene vaginal mesh implants for vaginal prolapse (C-Gyn 20). UGSA Executive. RANZCOG, East Melbourne.

US Food and Drugs Administration. Urogynecologic surgical mesh: update on the safety and effectiveness of transvaginal placement for pelvic organ prolapse. July 2011. Available at: <www.fda.gov/downloads/medicaldevices/safety/alertsandnotices/ucm262760.pdf> (accessed 10 June 2016).

Amy Tang

Chapter 18

Cervical neoplasia

Role of human papillomavirus

Over 100 different genotypes of human papillomavirus (HPV) have been identified. In some populations, it is present in over 70% of women and may be a vaginal commensal. More than 40 HPV types can be spread through direct sexual contact. Other cofactors, such as smoking, may be required to promote the development to cervical intraepithelial neoplasia (CIN).

Link with cervical cancer
- Sexually transmitted HPV types fall into two categories: low-risk and high-risk HPV.
- Low-risk types do not cause cancer but can lead to benign conditions (e.g. genital warts).
- Twelve types of high-risk HPV have been identified. They cause more than 99% of cervical cancer. The most common types are 16 and 18.
- Up to 10% of women will have HPV on cervical cytology at some stage. Most HPV infections clear up by themselves within 1–2 years without causing any problems.
- Persistent HPV infections can cause abnormal cell changes that may lead to cervical cancer and this process usually takes a long time, often about 10 years.
- There is no risk of cancer in patients with HPV without any CIN changes.
- There is no evidence that wearing condoms reduces the progression of HPV to CIN.

National cervical screening program updates

A new renewed screening program will begin on 1 May 2017 which, together with HPV vaccination, will reduce the number of cervical cancers by at least a further 15%. The key changes include the following.
- A primary HPV test every 5 years replaces the current 2 yearly Pap test program.
- All sexually active women aged 25 to 74 years now participate in the program instead of the previous 18 to 70 years age range.

- Women with positive HPV 16/18 now have a reflex liquid-based cytology and should be referred directly for colposcopy.
- Women with high-risk HPV other than 16/18 with negative or low-grade cytology have repeat HPV testing in 12 months. If a woman remains positive, she should be referred for colposcopy. Women with high-grade cytology should be referred for immediate colposcopic assessment.

The Cancer Council's clinical management guidelines for the prevention of Cervical Cancer is available online via the following link: http://wiki.cancer.org.au/australia/Guidelines:Cervical_cancer/Prevention

Screening for CIN

CERVICAL CYTOLOGY

- is 99.7% specific (i.e. has a false-positive rate of 0.3%)
- is 80% sensitive (with a false-negative rate of 20%)
- liquid-based cytology (ThinPrep) with automated image analysis technology can reduce the number of unsatisfactory smears and improve the sensitivity to detect cervical dysplasia

POSSIBLE REASONS FOR FALSE-NEGATIVES

- sampling error
- incorrect fixative (95% ethyl alcohol fixative is required)
- timing of smear (best at mid-cycle)
- amount of sample (too little/too much)
- screening error
- interpretive error

ENDOCERVICAL CELLS PRESENT

- means that the squamocolumnar junction is reached (i.e. the upper limit of the transformation zone)
- <1% of smears containing no endocervical cells (and no abnormal cells seen) is an abnormal result

HPV TESTING

- HPV testing is a feasible technique for primary screening for cervical cancer. As mentioned previously, the Medical Services Advisory Committee in Australia recommends that a HPV test every 5 years is more effective than, and just as safe as, screening with Pap smear every 2 years.
- It may be useful in the triage of equivocal cytology results or low-grade lesions.
- In Australia, it is currently used as a 'test of cure' for high-grade cervical dysplasias. Pap smear and HPV typing is carried out at 12 months after treatment and annually thereafter, until both tests are negative on two consecutive occasions. Patients can then have smears every 2 years.

Terminology for cervical cytology/pap smear reporting

THE AUSTRALIAN MODIFIED BETHESDA SYSTEM 2004

- possible low-grade squamous intraepithelial lesion
- low-grade squamous intraepithelial lesion (HPV and CIN1)

- possible high-grade squamous intraepithelial lesion
- high-grade squamous intraepithelial lesion (CIN2 and CIN3)
- squamous cell carcinoma

Cervical intraepithelial neoplasia (CIN)

Definition. Normally, as cells differentiate and mature they move towards the surface. Abnormalities result in mitotic figures, nuclear pleomorphism and changes in the nuclear-to-cytoplasmic ratio.
- CIN1: two-thirds or more of the upper epithelium showing good differentiation
- CIN2: maturation/differentiation in the upper half of the epithelium with mitotic figures in the basal half
- CIN3: less than one-third of the upper epithelium showing differentiation

Progression of CIN
- incidence varies in different studies
- CIN1 progressing to higher CIN lesions: about 16%–25% in 2–4 years
- CIN3 to invasive cancer: about 18%–35% in 1–23 years

Management

COLPOSCOPY
- Aims: identify abnormal area and exclude invasive disease.
- The transformation zone needs to be seen. This is the area between the original and existing squamocolumnar junction. The columnar epithelium undergoes metaplasia as the transformation zone extends. The squamocolumnar junction may recede up the endocervical canal (e.g. in postmenopausal women). The pathological process often occurs in the transformation zone.
- With 3%–5% acetic acid, abnormal epithelium turns acetowhite.
- Schiller's test: columnar or abnormal squamous epithelium has little or no glycogen and does not stain with iodine.
- Colposcopic changes seen with CIN lesions are punctation (vessels are perpendicular to surface), mosaic (capillaries parallel to surface), and atypical vessels irregular in size, shape and course.

CONSERVATIVE TREATMENT
Current Australian guidelines recommend that histologically proven low-grade squamous abnormalities can be safely managed by repeat Pap smears at 12 and 24 months. If persistent possible or low-grade squamous intraepithelial lesion (LSIL), annual smears should be continued until at least two are negative.

ABLATIVE TREATMENT
- A colposcopic-directed cervical punch biopsy is needed to confirm the diagnosis of CIN and to exclude invasive cancer before ablative treatment.
- Depth of ablation is up to 10 mm, as almost all lesions are <7 mm in depth.
- It takes 4–6 months to replace the transformation zone ablation.
- It should not be carried out if presence of glandular lesion or if entire transformation zone is not visualised.

EXCISION

- Large-loop excision of the transformation zone (LLETZ) or loop electrical excision procedure (LEEP) has a 96% cure rate.
- Its advantage over ablative treatment is the availability of a histological specimen.

CONE BIOPSY

Indications. At colposcopy, the lesion is not fully visualised, especially the upper limit; suspected adenocarcinoma in situ; colposcopic examination shows no evidence of dysplasia despite repeated cytology with high-grade dysplasia; or early invasive disease is suspected.

HYSTERECTOMY

- It may be indicated if other gynaecological problems are present.
- Yearly vault smears are required, as there is a risk of vaginal intraepithelial neoplasia.

PREGNANCY

- Perform colposcopy by an experienced colposcopist to exclude invasive cancer.
- If CIN, leave treatment until postpartum.
- If invasion is suspected colposcopically, biopsy should be performed.
- Cone biopsy of the cervix is associated with a 5% fetal loss.

FOLLOW-UP

- After treatment for low-grade squamous intraepithelial lesion (HSIL), perform colposcopy and Pap smear at 4–6 months.
- Repeat Pap smear and perform HPV typing at 12 months after treatment and annually thereafter until negative tests on two consecutive occasions.

Cervical intraepithelial glandular neoplasia

Adenocarcinoma in situ (AIS) coexists with CIN in 70% of patients. Up to 15% of CIN is associated with glandular abnormalities. AIS is present in 40%–45% of cervical adenocarcinoma.

Atypical glandular cells of undetermined significance (AGUS) refers to morphological changes in glandular cells beyond those suggestive of a benign reactive process, but insufficient for the diagnosis of AIS. Other terminology under the Australian Modified Bethesda System 2004 includes possible high-grade glandular lesion, endocervical adenocarcinoma in situ and adenocarcinoma.

Management of adenocarcinoma in situ

COLPOSCOPY AND BIOPSY

- Abnormal epithelium is often within the cervical glands with few or no surface changes.
- Most lesions are near the squamocolumnar junction.

TREATMENT

- Cone biopsy: requires a cone of up to 2.5 cm in length. Risk of skip lesion is about 30%.
- Hysterectomy should be considered if fertility is not desired due to continued risk of residual and recurrent disease.

Cervical cancer

Of cervical malignancies, 85% are squamous cell carcinoma and 15% are adenocarcinoma. The development of cervical cancer is in either the squamous epithelium or endocervix. Most squamous cancers originate in the transformation zone.

Spread of malignancy
- Direct extension: ureteric obstruction can occur if malignancy extends to the pelvic side wall.
- There may be lymphatic spread to the pelvic nodes.
- Haematogenous spread is less common.

Risk factors
- age: mean age at time of diagnosis is 52 years, with two peak frequencies at ages 35–39 years and 60–64 years
- early age of sexual activity
- multiple sexual partners
- smoking
- partner with previous partner with cervical cancer

Diagnosis and examination

PRESENTING COMPLAINT
- most common: abnormal vaginal bleeding such as menorrhagia, postcoital, irregular and postmenopausal bleeding
- vaginal discharge

EXAMINATION
- general, lymphadenopathy
- vaginal/pelvic findings depending on the stage of the disease
- speculum: check vaginal extension of tumour; cervix may be large, ulcerated, irregular, bleeding
- vaginal/pelvic examination: cervix expanded, firm, assess for parametrial spread
- rectal examination

Investigations and staging of cervical cancer
- full blood count, electrolytes, liver biochemistry, renal function
- radiology: chest X-ray, abdominopelvic computed tomography (CT) scan, magnetic resonance image (MRI) of pelvis
- positron emission tomography (PET) scan can delineate extent of disease more accurately
- staging examination under anaesthesia: vaginal/pelvic and rectal examination; cervical biopsy; cystoscopy; curettage and sigmoidoscopy if indicated

FIGO STAGING FOR CERVICAL CANCER
This is a clinical staging system. See Table 18.1 for correlation of stage and 5-year survival.
- Stage I: the carcinoma is strictly confined to the cervix; extension to corpus is disregarded.
  - IA: invasive cancer identified only microscopically
  - IA1: measured invasion of stroma not >3 mm in depth and 7 mm in diameter

Table 18.1 Correlation of stage and 5-year survival			
STAGE	**+ PELVIC NODES**	**+ PARA-AORTIC NODES**	**5-YEAR SURVIVAL**
I			85%
IA1	<1%	0	
IA2	5%	<1%	
IB	15%	2%	
IIA	25%	10%	70%
IIB	30%	20%	60%
III	45%	30%	35%
IV	55%	40%	<15%

Source: Berek, J.S & Hacker N.F. Practical Gynecologic Oncology 2004, Lippincott Williams & Wilkins.

- IA2: measured invasion of stroma >3 mm in depth and not >5 mm in depth and 7 mm in diameter
  - IB: clinical lesions confined to the cervix or preclinical lesions larger than stage IA
  - IB1: clinical lesions not >4 cm in size
  - IB2: clinical lesions >4 cm in size
- Stage II: the carcinoma extends beyond the cervix, but has not extended onto the pelvic walls. The carcinoma involves the vagina, but not the lower third.
  - IIA: no obvious parametrial involvement
  - IIB: obvious parametrial spread
- Stage III: the carcinoma has extended onto the pelvic side wall. On rectal examination there is no cancer-free space between the tumour and the pelvic wall. The tumour involves the lower third of the vagina. All cases with hydronephrosis or non-functioning kidney.
  - IIIA: no extension to the pelvic wall but involvement of the lower third of the vagina
  - IIIB: extension onto the pelvic wall and/or hydronephrosis or non-functioning kidney
- Stage IV: the carcinoma has extended beyond the true pelvis or has clinically involved the mucosa of the bladder or rectum.
  - IVA: spread to adjacent organs
  - IVB: spread to distant organs

Management of cervical cancer

SURGICAL TREATMENT
- radical surgery: removal of the uterus, cervix, parametrium, upper third of the vagina and pelvic nodes. This can be performed by laparotomy, laparoscopy or robot.

Complications
- haemorrhage
- prolonged theatre time, which increases risk of infection and thromboembolism (1%–2%)
- atonic bladder, which occurs in up to 3% of cases due to pelvic denervation
- ureteric fistula, which occurs in 1%–2%; vesicovaginal fistula in <1%
- urinary tract infection in 10%

- febrile morbidity, which affects 10%–20%, caused by pulmonary atelectasis, urinary tract infection, wound infection, haematoma, pelvic cellulitis
- pelvic lymphocyst, which affects 1%–2% (incidence may decrease with intraoperative drainage)
- nerve injury (obturator nerve injury causing weakness in adduction of thigh; femoral nerve compression)
- small bowel obstruction, which affects 1%

RADIATION THERAPY

- The limiting factor in getting the maximum dose to the tumour is normal tissue tolerance. Cellular DNA is damaged by a direct action of radiation or indirectly via water free radicals.
- Tumour cells undergo mitotic death and rate of tumour shrinkage is proportional to cell cycle time.
- The typical radical dose is 60 gray; a palliative dose is 30 gray. The total dose is delivered in multiple fractions to allow repair of normal tissues between fractions (e.g. 50 gray may be given in 30 fractions over 6 weeks for pelvic radiotherapy). The chance of eradication of the tumour depends on the dose and extent of disease.

Morbidity of pelvic radiotherapy

- About 5% severe morbidity is considered acceptable.
- Acute effects are proctitis, ileitis, diarrhoea, tenesmus, skin reaction (especially skin-folds) and bladder irritability.
- Late effects are chronic proctitis, ileitis with perforation or stricture, fistula or necrosis, lymphoedema, vaginal atrophy and contraction, radiation menopause, femoral head necrosis, induction of malignancy.
- Radiation morbidity may be reduced by field planning, barium contrast and gentle fractionation to allow normal tissue the chance to repair.

Treatment of early-stage cervical cancer

STAGE IA

- Microinvasion <1 mm may be treated with cone biopsy or simple hysterectomy.
- Less than 3 mm invasion may be treated with simple hysterectomy.
- Stage IA lesions >3 mm invasion require radical hysterectomy and lymphadenectomy, with adjuvant radiotherapy and concurrent chemotherapy if nodes are positive.

STAGE IB

- Identical survival rates obtained if managed primarily by radical hysterectomy/lymphadenectomy or radiotherapy when surgical margins and lymph nodes are clear.
- Radical hysterectomy and pelvic lymphadenectomy is often used to treat stage IB1 disease and chemoradiation reserved for stage IB2.
- Use radiotherapy and concurrent chemotherapy if the woman is unfit for surgery or as adjuvant therapy if the nodes are positive.
- Radical trachelectomy can be an option for a woman who wants to preserve fertility if the tumour is <2 cm.

STAGE IIA

- Surgery can be offered to patients with early-stage IIA cervical cancer. Otherwise, primary radiation therapy is the standard treatment for more advanced disease.

ADVANTAGES OF SURGERY

- In young women, the ovaries may be left if they appear normal, as the risk of ovarian metastasis is <1% in squamous cell carcinoma of the cervix, stage I.

Management of advanced-stage cervical cancer

- Radiation treatment with concurrent chemotherapy is used for stages IIB or greater. Radiation doses are normally quoted from point A (i.e. 2 cm lateral to the centre of the uterus and 2 cm above the lateral fornix).
- Hysterectomy and pelvic exenteration may sometimes be performed for central residual disease after completion of chemoradiation.

Follow-up management of cervical cancer

- Review the patient 4–6 weeks after surgery, then every 3 months for 2 years, then every 6 months to year 5, then yearly to year 10. Assessment requires general examination (breasts, nodes), vault smear, vaginal and rectal examination, and other investigations as appropriate, such as chest X-ray, colposcopy/biopsy.
- Recurrence usually occurs in the first 12 months, and most patients with recurrent disease die within 2 years.

POST-TREATMENT SURVEILLANCE

- vaginal cytology: poor sensitivity (15%) but up to 100% specificity
- physical examination: about 60% sensitivity and up to 95% specificity
- suspicious symptoms: 70% sensitivity and up to 95% specificity

Adenocarcinoma of the cervix

- This accounts for 15%–25% of cervical cancer. FIGO prognosis for this condition is poorer than for squamous lesions, due to greater tumour volume.
- Clinical behaviour of the disease is similar to that of squamous cell carcinoma.
- In young women with early-stage disease, the ovaries may be conserved, as < 2% metastasises to the ovaries.

Special circumstances

CERVICAL CANCER IN PREGNANCY

- It occurs in about 1 in 1500 pregnancies.
- Vaginal delivery is not advised, as this may disseminate disease through large cervical venous sinuses and dilated lymphatics, cause disease to be transmitted down the vagina or produce haemorrhage.

SMALL CELL CANCER

- metastasises early and requires local surgery in conjunction with combination chemotherapy

Further reading

Basil, J.B., Horowitz, I.R., 2001. Cervical carcinoma. Obstet. Gynecol. Clin. North Am. 28, 727–740.

Cancer Council Australia. National Cervical Screening Program: Guidelines for the Management of Screen Detected Abnormalities, Screening in Specific Populations and Investigation of Abnormal Vaginal Bleeding. 2016. Available at: <http://wiki.cancer.org.au/australia/Guidelines:Cervical_cancer/Prevention>.

Flowers, L.C., McCall, M.A., 2001. Diagnosis and management of cervical intraepithelial neoplasia. Obstet. Gynecol. Clin. North Am. 28, 667–684.

Grisby, P.W., Herzog, T.J., 2001. Current management of patients with invasive cervical carcinoma. Clin. Obstet. Gynecol. 44, 531–537.

Levine, L., Lucci, J.A., Dinh, T.V., 2003. Atypical glandular cells: New Bethesda terminology and management guidelines. Obstet. Gynecol. Surv. 58, 399–406.

National Health and Medical Research Council (NHMRC), 2005. Screening to prevent cervical cancer: Guidelines for the management of asymptomatic women with screen detected abnormalities. NHMRC, Canberra.

Chapter 19

Uterine neoplasia

Amy Tang

Benign tumours of the uterus

Uterine polyps

Polyps in the uterine corpus (the commonest site) may be part of a hyperplastic endometrium and present with changes in the menstrual cycle. Presenting symptoms include vaginal discharge and intermenstrual bleeding.

Uterine fibroids (leiomyomas)

These are present in 20%–30% of women and the aetiology is uncertain. Risk factors include nulliparity, family history, African race and hormonal influences, especially oestrogen.

Pathology

- macroscopic: firm, round, whorled masses
- sites: intramural, subserous, submucous, also in cervix and broad ligament
- microscopic: smooth muscle proliferation, fibrous tissue

Degenerative changes

These occur because of poor vascularity, and include:
- hyaline degeneration
- cystic degeneration
- calcification
- necrosis
- red degeneration/necrobiosis
- sarcomatous degeneration, rarely (< 0.5%)

Clinical features

- often asymptomatic or variable in presentation; usually shrink after menopause
- presentation: menorrhagia, intermenstrual bleeding, infertility, abdominal swelling, pressure effects on the bladder or on large pelvic veins, which can result in oedema of legs or deep venous thrombosis
- in pregnancy, may grow in size, undergo red degeneration and may obstruct labour

Management

- conservative with small or asymptomatic fibroids
- medical treatment
  - progesterone
  - gonadotrophin-releasing hormone (GnRH) analogues: cause rapid shrinkage of fibroids in the first 3 months, but they regrow to pretreatment size within 3 months of stopping therapy; reduction in volume is proportional to degree of oestrogen suppression; side effects include menopausal symptoms, pelvic pain from acute necrosis of fibroids, reduced bone density (6% trabecular bone loss in lumbar vertebrae after 6 months, but reversed 6 months after stopping therapy)
- surgery: hysterectomy; hysteroscopic resection, myomectomy with or without pre-treatment GnRH analogues

Fibroids in pregnancy

Fibroids become soft because of oedema and grow in size during pregnancy. If pedunculated, the fibroid may undergo torsion. There is an increased risk of red degeneration. This causes pain and a slight rise in temperature. Management of red degeneration of fibroids in pregnancy is conservative (rest, analgesia). Pain will abate in about 10 days.

EFFECT OF FIBROIDS ON PREGNANCY

- uterus is larger than dates; the growth of fibroid occurs mostly in the first trimester
- risk of abortion/miscarriage
- when present at lower parts of the uterus and cervix, fibroids can obstruct the presenting part and cause abnormal lie of the fetus
- risk of postpartum haemorrhage
- caesarean section may be difficult if the fibroid is in the lower uterine segment
- rupture of uterus after myomectomy is rare

Endometrial hyperplasia

Definition. Hyperplasia is an increase in the number of cells in an organ/tissue; it may be pathological or physiologically normal.

Endometrial hyperplasia consists of a variety of changes in endometrial glandular and stromal elements. It is characterised by proliferation of endometrial glands resulting in greater gland-to-stroma ratio than in normal endometrium. These glands vary in size and shape and may show cytological atypia.

World Health Organization classification of endometrial hyperplasia

- glandular/stromal architectural pattern
  - simple: cystically dilated glands with occasional outpouching
  - complex: back-to-back crowding of glands with minimal intervening stroma
- presence or absence of nuclear atypia

Risk factors

Endometrial hyperplasia is oestrogen-dependent but its precise role is unknown. Conditions such as polycystic ovarian syndrome (PCOS), unopposed oestrogen therapy, ovarian tumours (oestrogenic or virilising) and obesity are associated with an increased risk of hyperplasia. Other risk factors are infertility, nulliparity and medical conditions (liver disease, hyperthyroid).

Malignant potential

- cytological atypia is the most useful predictor of the likelihood of cancer progression
- simple hyperplasia without atypia: about 1% will progress to cancer; 80% regress after curettage and other treatment
- complex hyperplasia without atypia: 3% progress to cancer
- simple hyperplasia with atypia: 8% progress to cancer
- complex atypical hyperplasia: 29% progress to carcinoma; up to 25% of women have well-differentiated cancers when hysterectomies are done within 1 month of curettage

Diagnosis and screening

- common presentations: menorrhagia and abnormal bleeding per vagina
- investigations: ultrasound scan to assess thickness of the endometrium; hysteroscopy and endometrial curettage; endometrial sampling; cytological sample from the cervix and/or vagina (sensitivity is low: 35% for atypical hyperplasia, and 20% for adenomatous hyperplasia)

Management

- oral progesterone: by providing a more complete sloughing of the endometrium, reducing the number of oestrogen receptors on endometrial cells and by affecting the metabolism of oestrogen; when using cyclical therapy, the duration of therapy is important (i.e. at least 12 days per month)
- levonorgestrel-releasing intrauterine system (Mirena)
- stop unopposed oestrogen
- surgical treatment: dilatation and curettage; hysterectomy

Guides to treatment

- treatment dependent on the type/grading of hyperplasia, the age of the woman and her desire for future fertility
- simple hyperplasia: dilatation and curettage, hormone therapy, monitoring with yearly endometrial sampling
- complex hyperplasia: if fertility required, treatment with progesterone and induction of ovulation; if fertility not required, or in the older woman, treatment with progesterone or hysterectomy with or without oophorectomy; if conservative management used, an endometrial sample recommended in 3–6 months
- atypical hyperplasia: if fertility required, treatment with progesterone and induction of ovulation; if fertility not required, or in the older woman, treatment with hysterectomy and oophorectomy; if conservative management used, an endometrial sample recommended in 3 months

Cancer of the uterine corpus

This is the leading cause of genital cancer in developed countries, with a 1% lifetime risk.

Epidemiology and risk factors

- 80% postmenopausal (peak incidence at 61 years); < 5% aged under 40 years
- obesity: increased conversion of androstenedione to oestrone in fat (this lowers sex hormone-binding globulin and raises free oestrogen—a three-fold increased risk if

the woman is up to 25 kg overweight and ten-fold if the woman is > 25 kg overweight)
- medical conditions: hypertension, previous pelvic irradiation, immunodeficiency, diabetes (raises risk by two to eight times)
- hereditary non-polyposis colorectal cancer (HNPCC): 40%–45% risk
- abnormal hormonal status: unopposed oestrogen therapy, raised endogenous oestrogen (e.g. obesity, polycystic ovarian syndrome, oestrogen-producing tumours, use of tamoxifen)
- parity: up to 35% of women with endometrial cancer nulliparous, representing a two-fold risk compared with multiparous women; late menopause also a risk factor

Pathology of uterine cancer
- Adenocarcinoma accounts for 60%–80% of endometrial cancers.
- Adenosquamous malignancies occur in 15%.
- Papillary serous carcinomas are aggressive, with early peritoneal spread.
- Clear cell carcinoma is rare and the prognosis is poor.

Mode of spread of uterine cancer
- direct invasion of the myometrium and cervix
- at the time of diagnosis, at least 10% with extension of disease beyond the uterus
- lymphatic spread: para-aortic and pelvic nodes
- haematogenous spread in later stages: lungs, liver, bone

Clinical presentation
- postmenopausal bleeding in 90% of cases
- intermenstrual bleeding, menorrhagia

Diagnosis and investigations
- endometrial sampling
- examination under anaesthesia, hysteroscopy, curettage
- full blood count, electrolytes, blood sugar levels, liver biochemistry
- chest X-ray
- computed tomography (CT) of abdomen and pelvis to assess for metastatic disease
- CA125 can be useful to predict extrauterine disease once diagnosis of uterine cancer is confirmed

FIGO staging for uterine cancer (2009)
- stage I: tumour confined to the body of the uterus
  - IA: tumour with no invasion or ≤ half of the myometrium
  - IB: invasion of more than half of the myometrium
- stage II: tumour invasion into cervical stroma
- stage III: tumour with local spread and/or positive nodes
  - IIIA: tumour invades serosa and/or adnexa
  - IIIB: vaginal and/or parametrial metastasis
  - IIIC1: metastasis to pelvic node
  - IIIC2: metastasis to para-aortic node
- stage IV: tumour spread to pelvic viscera and beyond
  - IVA: invasion of bladder and/or bowel mucosa
  - IVB: distant metastasis, intra-abdominal and/or inguinal nodes

In addition, the stage will include the grade of the tumour (grade 1: well-differentiated; grade 2: moderately differentiated; grade 3: poorly differentiated).

SURGICAL STAGING ASSESSMENT

Myometrial invasion
- Survival rates with superficial myometrial invasion and no invasion are similar.
- There is reduced survival with deep myometrial invasion.

Adnexal spread
- This is present in 7%–8%, and often microscopic.

Lymph nodes
- Metastases increase with worsening differentiation of the tumour and increasing depth of myometrial invasion.

Survival rates
- The overall 5-year survival of women with uterine cancer is 65%. Survival depends on tumour stage, grade and cell type (the worst being clear cell).
- Table 19.1 lists survival rates for uterine cancer according to the FIGO stage.

Management of uterine cancer

SCREENING AND PREVENTION
- Positive cervical smear is found in < 50%.
- Aspiration endometrial sampling has up to 96% accuracy.
- Protect endometrium with hormone therapy in conditions of unopposed oestrogens.

STAGE I
- About 75% of patients have stage I disease. Survival is better with surgery than radiotherapy alone.
- Standard treatment is hysterectomy and bilateral salpingo-oophorectomy, which can be performed either by laparotomy or laparoscopy.
- Intraoperative frozen section is used to assess tumour grade and myometrial invasion to determine whether lymphadenectomy is required.
- Positive nodes are found in 10% and positive peritoneal cytology in 15%.
- Lymphadenectomy may be used as a prognosticator and treatment modifier (radiotherapy if nodes are positive).
- Incidence of vault recurrence rises with worsening tumour grade and increasing myometrial invasion. Postoperative brachytherapy may reduce vault recurrence from 10% to 3%, but has no effect on overall survival.

Table 19.1 Survival rates for uterine cancer according to FIGO stage	
STAGE	**5-YEAR SURVIVAL**
I	75%–90%
II	65%–75%
III	30%–40%
IV	10%

Source: Berek, J.S & Hacker N.F. Practical Gynecologic Oncology 2004, Lippincott Williams & Wilkins.

STAGE II

- Modified radical hysterectomy, bilateral salpingo-oophorectomy and pelvic and para-aortic lymphadenectomy is associated with better survival when compared with simple hysterectomy.
- Pelvic lymph nodes are positive in up to 20% of cases.
- Postoperative adjuvant radiation is individualised and is given if positive lymph nodes.

STAGES III AND IV

- Treatment must be individualised and may include total abdominal hysterectomy, bilateral salpingo-oophorectomy, debulking of macroscopic tumour, preoperative/postoperative chemotherapy and pelvic irradiation, and hormonal therapy.

RECURRENT DISEASE

- About 80% of recurrences occur within 2 years of primary therapy.
- It can be loco-regional or distant recurrence.
- Treatment is directed to the site of recurrence.
- Two common sites of vaginal recurrence are apex of vault and lower anterior third of the vagina in the retrourethral position.
- Management includes surgery, irradiation, hormone therapy, chemotherapy or combination.

HORMONE THERAPY AND CHEMOTHERAPY

- high-dose progesterone: gives a better response with well-differentiated carcinoma, as there is a reduction in receptor concentration with worsening histological grade; may be used in the treatment of pulmonary metastasis
- levonorgestrel-releasing intrauterine system (Mirena): suitable for a patient who is unfit for surgery
- anti-oestrogen
- chemotherapy: carboplatin, paclitaxel, doxorubicin, fluorouracil, cyclophosphamide

Uterine sarcomas

Uterine sarcomas are rare and account for about 3% of all uterine cancers. Sarcomas are mesodermal tumours with an overall 5-year survival rate of 30%.

Classification

LEIOMYOSARCOMA

- It accounts for 50% of uterine sarcomas.
- The mean age at diagnosis is 50 years.
- The risk of malignant change in fibroid is < 0.5%.
- Survival is better if it arises in a fibroid.
- It is usually intramural and 60% are solitary.
- Presentation: includes vaginal bleeding/discharge, pain, abdominal mass.
- Diagnosis: 10 or more mitotic figures per 10 high-power fields is associated with a 25% 5-year survival rate.
- There is a 95% 5-year survival rate in those with fewer than 10 mitotic figures per 10 high-power fields.

- Spread of the disease is mainly haematogenous; thus surgical staging is not as important.
- Overall 5-year survival rate is 20%.

ENDOMETRIAL STROMAL SARCOMA

- It accounts for 15%–25% of uterine sarcomas.
- The mean age of diagnosis is 45 years; only a third of patients are postmenopausal.
- It is divided into low-grade and high-grade categories.
- Low-grade type is called endometrial stromal sarcoma. They are relatively indolent and late recurrences may occur. Prolonged survival and even cure is possible even after recurrence. They are responsive to hormonal therapy with progesterone after surgery.
- High-grade type is now termed endometrial sarcoma. They are aggressive tumours. Prognosis is poor.

MALIGNANT MIXED MÜLLERIAN TUMOUR

- The mean age at diagnosis is 65 years.
- It is a mixture of sarcoma and carcinoma (thus also termed carcinosarcoma).
- Risk factors include increasing age, hypertension, diabetes, obesity and previous pelvic irradiation.
- Prognosis: metastasise early; overall 5-year survival rate is 25%.

Management of uterine sarcomas

SURGERY

- Staging: includes laparotomy, total abdominal hysterectomy, bilateral salpingo-oophorectomy.
- Radical hysterectomy has no significant effect on survival.
- Disseminated disease: value of debulking is uncertain.

RADIOTHERAPY

- Leiomyosarcoma is resistant to radiotherapy.
- In malignant mixed müllerian tumours, radiotherapy reduces pelvic recurrence but may not improve survival rates.

CHEMOTHERAPY

- The value of chemotherapy has yet to be proven.

Cancer of the fallopian tubes

Primary cancer of the fallopian tube is rare. It accounts for < 0.5% of all gynaecological cancers, and only about 1000 cases have been reported. The mean age at diagnosis is 55 years. The only identified risk factor is an inherited mutation in BRCA1 or BRCA2 gene.

Pathology

- Malignancy is mostly due to secondary disease.
- Most primary carcinomas are adenocarcinoma; very rarely there are sarcomas or choriocarcinomas.

Clinical presentation

- There is a classic triad of pelvic pain, pelvic mass and watery vaginal discharge in 15% of patients.
- It is often asymptomatic, but may present with a mass with ascites.
- The most common symptoms are abnormal vaginal bleeding (30%) and vaginal discharge (20%).

Treatment

- similar to that for epithelial ovarian cancer
- surgery: total abdominal hysterectomy, bilateral salpingo-oophorectomy, omentectomy, lymphadenectomy, appendicectomy, peritoneal washings and biopsy
- adjuvant platinum combination chemotherapy
- radiotherapy: may be used in palliative therapy

Five-year survival rate

- overall survival is 56%
- stage I, 70%; stage II, 50%; stage III, 30%; stage IV, 10%

Further reading

Hernandez, E., 2001. Endometrial adenocarcinoma. Obstet. Gynecol. Clin. North Am. 28, 743–757.

Marsden, D.E., Hacker, N.F., 2001. Optimal management of endometrial hyperplasia. Best Pract. Res. Clin. Obstet. Gynaecol. 15, 393–405.

Mutch, D.G., 2009. The new FIGO staging system for cancers of the vulva, cervix, endometrium and sarcoma. Gynecol. Oncol. 115, 325–328.

Chapter 20

Ovarian neoplasms

Amy Tang

Features of malignant versus benign ovarian neoplasms

- Age: in childhood and in older women, there is an increased risk of malignancy.
- Pain: pain can occur in both. Acute pain usually indicates torsion or haemorrhage.
- Rapid growth: suspect malignancy.
- Bilaterality: 75% of malignant disease and 15% of benign lesions are bilateral.
- Consistency: solid, nodular and/or irregular features are suggestive of malignancy.
- Fixation of the mass: suspect malignancy.
- Ascites: ascites is associated with malignancy.
- Leg/vulvar oedema, venous obstruction/thrombosis: this is strongly suggestive of malignancy.
- Evidence of distant metastasis: indicates malignancy.

Risk of malignancy index (RMI)

RMI is useful to help determine those women with a pelvic ovarian mass who would benefit from direct referral to a tertiary gynaecological oncology unit.

RMI = menopausal status (1 or 3) × ultrasound features (0, 1 or 3) × CA125
- menopausal status: premenopausal = 1; postmenopausal = 3
- ultrasound features (multiloculated, solid areas, bilateral pathology, ascites, metastases): no features = 0; one feature = 1; more than one feature = 3

If RMI ≥ 200, there is a high risk of malignancy and the woman should be referred to a gynaecological oncologist.

Screening for ovarian cancer

Screening for ovarian cancer has not been proven to reduce ovarian cancer deaths in the general population. It may have a role in high-risk patients (e.g. a strong family history).
- Bimanual pelvic examination: low-cost, requires no special equipment but not specific or sensitive in the detection of ovarian cancer.

- Ultrasound scan: malignant features include semisolid or cystic areas, thick septa, surface papillary growths, neovascularisation, bilateral masses and/or ascites.
- Cytology: routine cervical cytological tests give abnormal results in 10%–30% of advanced ovarian cancer cases. Peritoneal cytology is not specific or sensitive, and is time-consuming and painful to perform.
- Prophylactic salpingo-oophorectomy: this should be considered in women with a strong family history of ovarian cancer or women who are BRCA carriers; 7% of women with ovarian cancer have had a previous laparotomy; 0.2% of women who have had their ovaries conserved during operations for benign gynaecological disorders develop ovarian cancer.

Tumour markers for ovarian cancer
- Markers are used in diagnosis, prognosis and to detect subclinical disease.
- The four types of potential markers for ovarian cancer are oncodevelopmental markers, carcinoplacental, metabolic and tumour-specific/tumour-associated antigens. None has sufficiently high specificity for screening.
- CA125 tumour-associated antigen is a high molecular weight glycoprotein expressed in coelomic epithelium during embryogenic development; 80% of patients with ovarian carcinoma have levels > 35 IU/mL. It is elevated in about 1% of healthy women and also in non-malignant conditions such as endometriosis, inflammation, benign tumours and pregnancy. CA125 levels fall with age. It is a good marker for epithelial carcinoma, except mucinous tumours, but has poor specificity (not useful for screening).
- CA19.9 is usually elevated in mucinous tumours and pancreatic cancers.
- CEA is useful to exclude metastatic bowel primary if patient has bowel symptoms.
- Human epididymis protein 4 (HE4) is often used together with CA125 to detect ovarian cancer using the risk of malignancy algorithm (ROMA).
- The markers may be used in combination to improve specificity and sensitivity.
- False-negative results can occur in early-stage disease.

Ovarian cancer

Epidemiology
There are geographical variations in the incidences of ovarian cancer. The peak incidence by age group occurs in the seventh to eighth decade. Ovarian cancer accounts for up to 35% of all gynaecological cancers.

Risk factors
- nulliparity, infertility
- family history: a woman with a mother or sister with ovarian cancer has a twenty-fold increased risk; increased risk is associated with inherited mutations in the BRCA1 and BRCA2 genes
- previous other cancers: breast, endometrial
- oral contraceptive pill affords protection
- other risk factors: blood group A, Peutz-Jeghers syndrome

Pathology of ovarian cancer
- epithelial tumours: make up 90% of ovarian malignancies
- types of epithelial ovarian cancer: serous, mucinous, endometrioid, Brenner, clear cell

- sex cord stromal tumours: granulosa cell, Sertoli-Leydig cell (androblastoma, arrhenoblastoma), fibroma, sex cord tumours with annular tubules
- germ cell tumours: dysgerminoma, non-dysgerminoma (endodermal sinus tumour, embryonal carcinoma, choriocarcinoma, mature and immature teratomas)
- secondary tumours: Krukenberg (gastrointestinal, especially stomach), breast

Presentation
- Ovarian cancer is often asymptomatic in early disease.
- The woman may present with:
  - abdominal pain, pelvic pressure, frequency of urine
  - abdominal swelling, dyspepsia, back pain
  - constipation, deep venous thrombosis

Examination
- general examination
- assess for lymphadenopathy
- examination of breasts, thyroid, abdomen/liver, ascites
- pelvic and rectal examination

Investigations for ovarian masses
- tumour markers: CA125, CA19.9, CEA, HE4
- consider human chorionic gonadotrophin (hCG), alpha-fetoprotein, inhibin, lactate dehydrogenase (LDH) if suspect non-epithelial ovarian tumours
- full blood count, electrolytes, liver biochemistry
- radiology: abdominopelvic ultrasound and/or computed tomography (CT) scan, chest X-ray, colonoscopy

FIGO staging for ovarian cancer
Staging is based on clinical examination, laparotomy, histology and cytology findings.
- stage I: growth limited to ovaries
  - IA: growth limited to one ovary, capsule intact, no ascites, negative peritoneal cytology
  - IB: growth limited to both ovaries, no ascites, no tumour on the external surfaces, capsule intact
  - IC: tumour either stage IA or IB, but with tumour on surface of one or both ovaries; or capsule ruptured; or with ascites present containing malignant cells or with positive peritoneal washings
- stage II: growth involving one or both ovaries with pelvic extension
  - IIA: extension and/or metastases to the uterus and/or tubes
  - IIB: extension to other pelvic tissues
  - IIC: tumour either stage IIA or IIB, but with tumour on surface of one or both ovaries; or with capsule(s) ruptured; or with ascites present containing malignant cells or with positive peritoneal washings
- stage III: tumour involving one or both ovaries with peritoneal implants outside the pelvis and/or positive retroperitoneal or inguinal nodes; superficial liver metastasis equals stage III; tumour is limited to the true pelvis but with histologically proven malignant extension to the small bowel or omentum
  - IIIA: tumour grossly limited to the true pelvis with negative nodes, but with histologically confirmed microscopic seeding of abdominal peritoneal surfaces

- IIIB: tumour involving one or both ovaries with histologically confirmed implants of abdominal peritoneal surfaces; none > 2 cm in diameter
- IIIC: abdominal implants > 2 cm in diameter and/or positive retroperitoneal or inguinal nodes
- stage IV: growth involving one or both ovaries with distant metastases; if pleural effusion present, there must be positive cytology to allot a case to stage IV; parenchymal liver metastasis equals stage IV

Epithelial ovarian tumours

These account for 90% of ovarian cancer.

FIVE-YEAR SURVIVAL RATES

- stage I: 80%
- stage II: 50%
- stage III: 25%
- stage IV: 10%

SEROUS TUMOURS

- are the commonest epithelial tumours, malignant or benign
- 50% are bilateral and usually unilocular

MUCINOUS TUMOURS

- large, unilateral multilocular cysts
- 5%–10% are malignant
- *Pseudomyxoma peritonei*: a rare complication of perforation and spillage of cyst contents

ENDOMETRIOID TUMOURS

- 20% associated with endometrial carcinoma
- may be associated with endometriosis
- account for 15% of ovarian cancers
- usually well-differentiated, with good prognosis

CLEAR-CELL TUMOURS

- arise in the cervix, vagina, endometrium, broad ligament and ovaries
- may be associated with endometriosis
- large, solid/cystic, unilateral tumours with poor prognosis

BRENNER TUMOURS

- usually benign, small and unilateral

PROGNOSTIC FACTORS FOR EPITHELIAL OVARIAN CANCER

- stage at time of diagnosis is important
- cell types:
  - poor prognosis: clear-cell and serous tumours
  - moderate prognosis: mucinous
  - good prognosis: endometrioid
- tumour grade is an important prognostic factor: grade 1, well-differentiated; grade 2, moderately differentiated; grade 3, poorly differentiated
- ability to achieve optimal surgical debulking with no residual disease is a major prognostic factor

MANAGEMENT
Preoperative preparation
- optimise health if other medical problems are present
- admit for bowel preparation and anaesthetic review
- employ prophylactic antibiotics and anticoagulation therapy

Surgical treatment
- vertical abdominal incision
- assessment for free fluid and collection of peritoneal washings
- systematic exploration and biopsy of all intraperitoneal surfaces
- diaphragmatic sampling
- total abdominal hysterectomy and bilateral salpingo-oophorectomy; debulking tumour (primary cytoreduction), preferably to < 1 cm to achieve optimal debulking
- omentectomy and appendicectomy
- pelvic and para-aortic node sampling
- the insertion of intraperitoneal port if optimal debulking and if intraperitoneal chemotherapy is considered

Chemotherapy
- used for adjuvant treatment and palliation
- most commonly used agents are combination carboplatin and paclitaxel
- can be given intravenously or intraperitoneally
- used at an earlier stage in cases with poorer prognostic factors, such as poorly differentiated tumours, cyst rupture or ascites
- can be used as neoadjuvant treatment in stage IV disease or in those patients who are not fit for initial upfront surgery (e.g. recent pulmonary embolism)

Aims of surgery
- improve tumour response to further therapy
- delay/prevent inevitable complications, such as gastrointestinal obstruction
- alter immunological state and immunosuppression
- relieve symptoms and to achieve psychological benefit from the removal of a large mass

Sex cord stromal tumours
Stromal cells retain the potential for differentiation into any of the cells/tissues from mesenchymal gonad (i.e. granulosa, theca, Leydig and Sertoli cells).
- Some tumours produce sex steroid hormones
  - feminising: granulosa and theca cell tumours
  - masculinising: Sertoli-Leydig (androblastoma)

GRANULOSA CELL TUMOURS
- These account for 2% of ovarian tumours and occur at any age.
- These solid tumours are usually unilateral (bilateral in 2%–5%).
- They vary in size, with an average of 10 cm in diameter.
- Rupture or haemorrhage into the tumour may occur.
- They can produce oestrogen and inhibin.
- Histopathology: Call–Exner bodies are granulosa cells arranged around small spaces containing nuclear fragments.

- They are associated with endometrial hyperplasia and even endometrial cancer in 5%–6% of cases.
- They are mostly diagnosed at stage I disease, are usually a slow-growing tumour, and late recurrences are not uncommon.

Management
- surgery: if childbearing complete, total abdominal hysterectomy and bilateral salpingo-oophorectomy; if early-stage and the patient still requires fertility, uterine curettage and removal of the affected ovary and fallopian tube
- chemotherapy: for disease beyond the ovary or for late recurrences

ANDROBLASTOMA
- These are solid tumours with low malignant potential, composed of Sertoli and/or Leydig cells (pure Sertoli cell tumours are rare; Leydig cell tumours are hilar or lipoid cell tumour).
- They present with masculinisation, abdominal pain and menstrual dysfunction.

FIBROMA
- This large, firm and lobulated mass consists of fibroblast-like cells.
- It is usually benign; bilateral in 10% of cases.
- It is associated with Meigs' syndrome (ascites and right hydrothorax), which resolves with removal of the tumour.
- If marked atypia and mitosis, it is termed fibrosarcoma; this tumour is very aggressive.

Germ cell tumours

Germ cell tumours are the second largest group of ovarian neoplasms. They occur predominantly in childhood and adolescence. The commonest germ cell tumour in all ages is the mature cystic teratoma/benign dermoid. This is derived from multipotent germ cells (i.e. from primitive germ cells before sexual differentiation occurs).
- Treatment intent is curative with conservation of ovarian function and fertility.
- Tumour markers: alpha-fetoprotein is produced by yolk sac cells; hCG is produced by syncytiotrophoblast.

DYSGERMINOMA
- This is the commonest malignant germ cell tumour.
- Peak age incidence is 10–30 years, especially in patients with developmentally abnormal gonads.
- It is hormonally inert.
- It is associated with elevated lactate dehydrogenase.
- Rapid growth can occur; most tumours are over 10 cm in diameter at time of diagnosis.
- It is solid, rubbery and bilateral in 15% of cases; most (75%) present in stage I.

Management
- The tumour is very radiosensitive and chemosensitive.
- Stage IA: unilateral salpingo-oophorectomy, peritoneal cytology, exploration of abdomen and removal of retroperitoneal lymph nodes, biopsy of contralateral ovary if suspicious. No adjuvant chemotherapy is required.

- All other stages: conservative surgery can be offered, but will need chemotherapy. BEP (bleomycin, etoposide and cisplatin) is recommended.
- Overall 5-year survival rate is over 90%, but prognosis is worse if the tumour is at an advanced stage and other germ cell elements are present.
- Careful follow-up is required, as 15%–20% of tumours recur.
- Consider karyotyping the patient.

CHORIOCARCINOMA

- This is the rarest of the germ cell group. It can be mixed with other germ cell elements.
- It secretes hCG.
- It may present with precocious puberty.
- Choriocarcinoma in the ovary can occur as metastasis from gestational trophoblast disease in the uterus, malignant change in an ovarian ectopic pregnancy or as a primary ovarian germ cell tumour.
- It is highly malignant, with early local and lymphatic spread compared with gestational trophoblast.
- Management comprises combination chemotherapy.

EMBRYONAL CARCINOMA

- This is the least well-differentiated of the germ cell tumours.
- It can differentiate along somatic line to produce teratoma, or extraembryonal to endodermal sinus or choriocarcinoma.
- It can produce tumour markers such as hCG, alpha-fetoprotein.
- It is highly malignant with early metastasis.
- Management: remove ovary for tissue diagnosis. These tumours are not radio-resistant, but treatment is usually with combination chemotherapy.

INTERSEX

- Dysgenetic gonad has high malignant potential.
- The commonest tumours are dysgerminoma and gonadoblastoma.
- The greatest risk occurs when associated with the Y chromosome.

ENDODERMAL SINUS TUMOUR

- This is a yolk sac tumour with alpha-fetoprotein as the tumour marker.
- The median age at presentation is 18 years.
- It is the most aggressive of germ cell group tumours, with rapid growth.
- Presentation: acute abdomen, a large mass with haemorrhage and necrosis; 50% of patients complain of symptoms for < 24 hours, and rarely symptoms are present for > 2 weeks.
- Management: radical surgery produces no better results than local tumour removal. Irradiation is not helpful. Combination chemotherapy may be curative. The ideal management is conservative surgery and combination chemotherapy. Alpha-fetoprotein is the marker to gauge the woman's response to treatment and is also used as a marker for recurrence.

TERATOMA

All but 1% are cystic, mature teratomas or benign dermoid cysts. Cells are derived from all three germ cell layers of the embryo: the ectoderm, mesoderm and endoderm. Teratomas are often asymptomatic, unilateral and large at time of diagnosis.

Malignancy

- occurs in solid immature teratomas
- occurs in the first two decades of life
- very rarely found in the postmenopausal woman
- immature teratomas with neurogenic elements have better prognosis
- stage IA grade 1 immature teratoma can be managed by surgery alone without BEP

Mature cystic teratoma/dermoid cyst

- accounts for 20%–40% of ovarian tumours in pregnancy
- presentation: asymptomatic; torsion in pregnancy or puerperium; rupture, especially with torsion; infection is uncommon; malignant change is found in up to 3% of cases, most commonly squamous cell carcinoma, to be managed by surgery (prognosis depends on the presence of extraovarian disease)

Struma ovarii

- a monodermal teratoma which is usually benign
- usually involves non-functioning thyroid tissue
- treatment: surgery

Carcinoid tumour of the ovary

- a rare monodermal teratoma, usually occurring in older women
- one-third present with the carcinoid syndrome of flushes due to histamine release, diarrhoea, tachycardia, hypertension
- slow-growing and rarely metastasises
- investigation: raised urinary 5-hydroxyindole acetic acid
- treatment: surgical excision

Borderline (low malignant potential) tumours

Low malignant potential tumours account for 15% of all epithelial ovarian cancers. Up to 20% occur with metastases. Metastases may represent disease of multifocal origin, rather than spread from a single site. The average age at time of diagnosis is the late 40s. About 30% of women are nulliparous.

FIGO and World Health Organization criteria for diagnosis of low malignant potential tumour are the presence of epithelial stratification, cellular atypia, mitotic activity with multilayering and nuclear pleomorphism, but with absence of ovarian stromal invasion.

PATHOLOGY

- 80%–95% are serous or mucinous
- 50%–80% are stage I at diagnosis
- 8%–35% are stage III at diagnosis

MANAGEMENT

- Initial management is similar to that for any patient with a pelvic mass.
- Perform a thorough physical examination.
- Test for tumour markers, renal and liver biochemistry.
- Ultrasound scan and/or CT scan of the pelvis.
- Laparotomy/laparoscopy: staging and debulking as indicated.
- Management of early-stage disease: when fertility is desired and disease is localised, conservative surgery is indicated. This includes unilateral salpingo-oophorectomy and

biopsy of the contralateral ovary if suspicious and omental biopsy. In older patients, or if fertility is not required, treatment is with total abdominal hysterectomy/bilateral salpingo-oophorectomy.
- Recurrence in stage I disease: if managed by cystectomy alone, this is associated with a 25% recurrence rate; with oophorectomy of the affected ovary alone, a 10% recurrence rate. If total pelvic clearance, the recurrence rate is < 5%.
- Management of advanced disease: treatment is similar to that for invasive ovarian cancer (total abdominal hysterectomy, bilateral salpingo-oophorectomy, debulking of tumour deposits, omentectomy, lymphadenectomy and appendicectomy).
- Chemotherapy is not indicated for stage I. In advanced stages, chemotherapy does not appear to be as effective as in invasive ovarian cancer because the tumour is slow-growing with poor clinical response to chemotherapy or radiotherapy.

PROGNOSTIC FEATURES
- *Pseudomyxoma peritonei* with mucinous tumours is associated with a poor prognosis.
- Ploidy (DNA analysis by flow cytometry): most tumours are diploid and follow an indolent course. Two-thirds of ovarian cancer are aneuploid, compared with 5%–12% in low malignant potential tumours.

Further reading

Berek, S., Hacker, N. (eds), 2014. Practical Gynecologic Oncology, 6th ed. Lippincott Williams & Wilkins, Philadelphia.

Shafi, M., Luesley, D., Jordan, J. (eds), 2001. Handbook of Gynaecological Oncology. Churchill Livingstone, London.

Chapter 21

Premalignant and malignant vulvar diseases

Amy Tang

Vulvar intraepithelial neoplasia (VIN)

VIN was once classified according to the degree of abnormality into VIN 1, VIN 2 and VIN 3 (or mild, moderate and severe dysplasia). Since there is no evidence to suggest VIN 1 is precancerous, it is now called low-grade VIN, while VIN 2 and VIN 3 are referred to as high-grade VIN.

Classification

The International Society for the Study of Vulvovaginal Diseases 2015 classifies all types of vulvar squamous intraepithelial lesions (SIL) as follows.

- Low-grade SIL of the vulva or vulvar LSIL; for example, flat condyloma or human papillomavirus (HPV) effect.
- High-grade SIL of the vulva or vulvar HSIL (used to be called VIN usual type). This is often related to HPV16, 18 and 31, is often multifocal and occurs in younger, premenopausal women.
- VIN differentiated type. This is non-HPV related, usually unifocal and is seen in older women with chronic vulvar dermatosis, such as lichen sclerosus or squamous cell hyperplasia.

General

- The incidence of VIN is increasing worldwide, especially in younger women.
- Risk factors are smoking, immunosuppression and HPV infection.
- There are up to 50% with associated cervical or vaginal intraepithelial neoplasia.
- Clinical presentation includes pruritus, perineal pain and vulvar lesion, with 50% asymptomatic.
- Diagnosis is by tissue biopsy after colposcopic examination. The entire lower genital tract and perianal area should be examined.

Treatment

- Treatment should be individualised depending on histology, location and extent of disease.
- The goal of treatment is to prevent development of cancer and to relieve symptoms.
- Surgical treatment is preferable, and this includes wide local excision, skinning vulvectomy and laser ablation.
- Medical treatment is reserved for situations where surgery is not feasible. This includes topical imiquimod cream (Aldara) or 5-fluorouracil (5-FU).
- The response rate for medical therapy has been reported to be 75%.
- The recurrence rate for VIN is about 30%. Therefore, long-term follow-up is necessary.

Paget's diseases of vulva

Paget's disease is an intraepithelial neoplasia. About 10% of patients have invasive Paget's disease, and 4%–8% have an underlying adenocarcinoma.

- It mostly affects postmenopausal Caucasian women in their 60s and 70s.
- Symptoms include pruritus and vulvar pain.
- The lesion is well demarcated and has an eczematoid appearance with slightly raised edges.
- Diagnosis is by tissue biopsy.
- Patients should be investigated for synchronous cancer, as 25% may have a non-contiguous cancer involving the breast, rectum, bladder, urethra, cervix or ovary.
- Treatment is by wide local excision, including underlying dermis. Positive margins can be common, as Paget's disease usually extends well beyond the gross lesion.
- Recurrent local recurrences are common and they are treated with surgical excision.

Vulvar cancer

Vulvar cancer accounts for 3%–5% of all gynaecological cancers.

Aetiology

- There is no clear aetiological agent. Smoking is a risk factor.
- It mainly occurs in postmenopausal women with a long history of vulvar irritation/pruritus.
- It is often associated with vulvar skin dermatosis which may also be a consequence of irritation and scratching.
- Oncogenic HPV infection may be associated.
- There is common association with other squamous intraepithelial lesions of the lower genital tract.

Histopathology of vulvar cancer

SQUAMOUS CELL CARCINOMA

- the commonest type of vulvar cancer (up to 90% of cases)

MELANOMA
- the second commonest: up to 5% of cases
- as with melanoma found elsewhere, prognosis is dependent on depth of disease

BARTHOLIN'S GLAND
- up to 1%–3% of vulvar cancers
- associated with higher groin node metastases and poorer prognosis than squamous cell cancer due to late diagnosis

OTHERS
- basal cell carcinoma: low propensity for lymph spread
- sarcoma: rare
- invasive Paget's disease: low lymphatic spread
- secondary spread from vagina, ovary, breast, kidney, thyroid and gastrointestinal tract

Presentation and spread of vulvar cancer

It usually presents in the seventh decade of life. Often there is significant delay (mean of 10 months) in the diagnosis, as the woman does not seek attention early. Another contributing factor is the failure of adequate assessment.

PRESENTATION
- pruritus and irritation occurring in up to two-thirds of patients; often present for months to years before diagnosis
- mass or ulcer
- bleeding or discharge
- pain
- the most common site affected is the labia; it may also present on the clitoris and perineum

SPREAD OF VULVAR CANCER
- The major route of spread is local invasion and via the lymphatic system.
- Lymphatic spread usually occurs in an orderly fashion (i.e. to the inguinofemoral nodes, then to the pelvic nodes, and then to the para-aortic nodes).
- About 25% of patients have local spread to the vagina, urethra, anus and rectum.
- Haematogenous spread to distant sites (e.g. lungs, liver and bone) can also occur.

FIGO staging for vulvar cancer (2009)

- stage IA: tumour confined to the vulva or perineum, ≤ 2 cm in size with stromal invasion not > 1 mm; no nodal metastases
- stage IB: tumour confined to the vulva or perineum, > 2 cm in size with stromal invasion > 1 mm; no nodal metastases
- stage II: tumour of any size with adjacent spread to lower $\frac{1}{3}$ urethra and/or lower $\frac{1}{3}$ vagina or anus; no nodal metastases
- stage IIIA: tumour of any size with positive inguino-femoral lymph nodes
  - 1 lymph node metastasis greater than or equal to 5 mm
  - 1–2 lymph node metastases less than 5 mm
- stage IIIB:
  - 2 or more lymph node metastases greater than or equal to 5 mm
  - 3 or more lymph node metastases less than 5 mm
- stage IIIC: positive node(s) with extracapsular spread

- stage IVA:
  - tumour invading any of the following: upper ⅔ urethra, upper ⅔ vagina, bladder mucosa, rectal mucosa, or fixed to pelvic bone
  - fixed or ulcerated inguino-femoral lymph nodes
- stage IVB: distant metastasis, including pelvic lymph nodes

Up to 70% of patients present in stage I and II disease (i.e. with no nodal spread). The overall 5-year survival rate is 60%. Women with stage I disease have a 90% 5-year survival rate.

Management of vulvar cancer

SUPERFICIALLY INVASIVE STAGE IA

- Radical wide local excision is used when < 2 cm in diameter, < 1 mm invasion, no lymphvascular space involvement, no abnormal nodes clinically.
- The risk of inguinal node involvement is almost zero.

OTHER EARLY-STAGE DISEASE

- For stage IB disease, risk of inguinal node metastases is > 8%. If lesion is unifocal, > 1 cm from midline, and not located in the anterior portion of labia minora, a radical wide local excision plus ipsilateral groin node dissection is performed. If positive nodes, then contralateral node dissection or irradiation is indicated.
- For other stage IB disease, bilateral groin node dissection is performed.
- When two or more microscopically positive inguinal nodes are found, bilateral groin and pelvic radiotherapy is indicated.

REASONS FOR LESS RADICAL SURGERY

- Wound healing is superior with separate incisions, compared with the butterfly incision radical vulvectomy, and results are not inferior.
- Superficial groin node dissection may be sufficient, as metastatic progression along the inguinal node chain occurs in an orderly fashion.
- Surgical node dissection is more a prognostic indicator and treatment modifier than a definitive therapy.
- There is less morbidity with superficial dissections.
- Groin dissection is very important, except in early superficial disease, as there is a high mortality in those who develop recurrence in the undissected groin.

SENTINEL LYMPH NODE BIOPSY

- Promising data from large prospective observational studies have suggested that this approach is safe to assess early stage cancer less than 4 cm. It incurs less morbidity compared with inguinofemoral dissection, without compromising detection of lymph node metastases.
- Use of a combination of blue dye and radiolabelled colloid yields more accurate results.

ADVANCED VULVAR CANCER: STAGES II, III AND IV

- Radiotherapy and surgery can be combined.
- It may require pelvic exenteration and radical vulvectomy if the anus, rectum, rectovaginal septum or proximal urethra is involved.
- Irradiation is associated with severe vulvar necrosis and poor survival rates in those treated with irradiation alone as primary therapy.

COMPLICATIONS OF VULVAR SURGERY

- lower extremity lymphoedema 30%
- wound breakdown and infection 30%
- thromboembolism
- haemorrhage
- urinary tract infection
- femoral nerve trauma
- hernia
- osteitis pubis
- lymphocyst
- psychosexual problems

Further reading

Berek, J.S., Hacker, N.F. (eds), 2014. Practical Gynecologic Oncology, 6th ed. Lippincott Williams & Wilkins, Philadelphia.

Bornstein, J., Bogliatto, F., Haefner, H.K., et al., 2016. The 2015 International Society for the Study of Vulvovaginal Disease (ISSVD) Terminology of Vulvar Squamous Intraepithelial Lesions. Obstet. Gynecol. 127 (2), 264–268.

Hopkins, M.P., Nemunaitis-Keller, J., 2001. Carcinoma of the vulva. Obstet. Gynecol. Clin. North Am. 28, 791–804.

Mutch, D.G., 2009. The New FIGO Staging System for Cancers of the Vulva, Cervix, Endometrium and Sarcoma. Gynecol. Oncol. 115, 325–328.

Sideri, M., Jones, R.W., Wilkinson, E.J., et al., 2005. Squamous vulvar intraepithelial neoplasia: 2004 modified terminology, ISSVD Vulvar Oncology Subcommittee. J. Reprod. Med. 50 (11), 807–810.

Chapter 22

Vaginal disease

Amy Tang

Benign conditions

Vaginal epithelium changes in different phases of life.
- In the newborn, it is thick with much glycogen due to the maternal oestrogen effect; then, with the withdrawal of oestrogen, the vaginal epithelium atrophies and the basal layer is covered by a thin, cornified epithelium.
- At menarche, the epithelium regenerates.
- At climacteric, the epithelium reverts to its prepubertal state.

Vaginal discharge

Physiological vaginal discharge is a product of vaginal mucosal transudate, cervical mucus and secretions from Bartholin's and Skene's glands. Excess physiological discharge occurs during pregnancy, sexual arousal, at mid-cycle/ovulation, with use of a high-oestrogen oral contraceptive or an intrauterine contraceptive device, and with large cervical ectropion.

Abnormal vaginal discharge may originate from diseases of the vagina, cervix, uterus or fallopian tubes. Causes of abnormal vaginal discharge include infections, foreign body, atrophic vaginitis and neoplasia of the upper and lower genital tract.

History
- colour, consistency, odour and duration of discharge
- blood-stained discharge
- pruritus, pain
- associations with menstrual cycle, coitus
- medical history (e.g. diabetes)
- medications, contraception
- cervical cytology

Examination
- general examination
- genital/pelvic: vulvar examination

- speculum: examining vagina and cervix, checking discharge (colour, odour), cervical ectropion, malignancy, cervical cytology, microbiological swabs
- pelvic examination for cervical excitation and palpable masses

Vaginal infections

During the reproductive life, the vaginal pH is < 4.5, and this offers some protection against infections.

TRICHOMONAS

- It is a flagellate, about 20 microns in size.
- It presents with vaginal discharge and pruritus.
- Examination reveals a yellow/green frothy discharge, punctate injection of vagina with pH > 5.0.
- Treat with metronidazole 400 mg orally three times a day for 7 days or a 2 g dose immediately, and treat the partner.

CANDIDA

- It presents with vaginal discharge and vulvar pruritus, and curd-like patches which are adherent to the epithelium.
- Predisposing factors include pregnancy, premenstrual period of cycle, glucose intolerance, and the use of the oral contraceptive pill, antibiotics and corticosteroids.
- It may be distinguished as uncomplicated (isolated episodes, albicans species and normal host), and complicated (severe, recurrent, non-albicans *Candida* species, abnormal host).
- Treatment: miconazole, econazole or clotrimazole inserted into the vagina for the short term, or single-dose oral fluconazole. Complicated *Candida* requires longer duration therapy.

GARDNERELLA VAGINALIS

- It is also called bacterial vaginosis.
- It is a highly prevalent polymicrobial syndrome.
- The vaginal epithelium is coated with the small bacteria; on microscopy, clue cells are present.
- It is present in up to 40% of women.
- It presents with grey, frothy, offensive discharge and pruritus.
- Treat with metronidazole 400 mg orally three times a day for 7 days or 2 g dose immediately, or vaginal clindamycin cream.

Postmenopausal woman

- Atrophy secondary to oestrogen deficiency predisposes to bleeding and secondary infection.
- Perform microbiological swabs and cervical cytology.
- Treat with oestrogen if atrophic.

Other vaginal conditions

CYSTS

- Endometriosis: involves pain, dyspareunia, postcoital bleeding.
- Gartner's duct runs lateral and anterolateral, at any level from the cervix to urethra. If it is small, no treatment is required; marsupialise if large.

FISTULA
- It occurs between the vagina and gastrointestinal or genitourinary system.
- It may be congenital or acquired.

Vaginal intraepithelial neoplasia (VAIN)

VAIN coexists with cervical intraepithelial neoplasia in 1%–3% of cases. The mean age at diagnosis is 52 years. The cause is unknown, but it may be associated with the human papillomavirus (HPV).

Classification
- VAIN 1: low-grade squamous intraepithelial lesion
- VAIN 2 and VAIN 3: high-grade squamous intraepithelial lesion

  There is no adequate study to prove the progression of VAIN to cancer. If the lesion is small, treatment options include an excisional biopsy, topical chemotherapy with imiquimod (Aldara) or 5-fluorouracil (5-FU), laser or cryotherapy.

Vaginal carcinoma

It may be primary or secondary. It usually occurs by direct spread or metastasis from the cervix, uterus, vulva, bladder, rectum or sigmoid colon. It accounts for 1% of female genital tract cancer. Squamous cell cancer presents in the sixth to seventh decade of life.

Histopathology
- Primary disease is usually squamous cell (80%–90%) or adenocarcinoma.
- Clear-cell adenocarcinoma is related to maternal diethylstilboestrol ingestion.
- Rarer tumours include melanoma, sarcoma botryoides, verrucous squamous cell carcinoma and endodermal sinus tumour.

Presentation, site and spread
- It involves postmenopausal bleeding, vaginal discharge, pain and urinary symptoms.
- Diagnosis can be missed if the lesion is small. A Pap smear may detect malignant cells in 20% of cases.
- About 50% occur in the upper vagina, 30% in the lower vagina and 20% in the mid-vagina.
- Posterior-wall tumour is the most common, followed by anterior-wall and lateral-wall; therefore, the most common site is in the posterior upper third, and then anterior lower third of the vagina.
- Spread is by direct extension and via the lymphatic system.

Investigations
- examination under anaesthesia and biopsy
- cystoscopy, sigmoidoscopy
- chest X-ray, ultrasound scan, computed tomography (CT) scan, intravenous pyelogram

FIGO staging for primary cancer of the vagina

This is a clinical (not surgical) staging (same as for cervical cancer).
- stage I: limited to the vaginal wall
- stage II: involvement of subvaginal tissue, but not extending to the pelvic wall
  - IIA: subvaginal infiltration, but not to the parametrium
  - IIB: parametrial involvement, but not to the pelvic wall
- stage III: tumour extending to the pelvic wall
- stage IV: involves mucosa bladder/rectum; extends beyond the true pelvis
  - IVA: spread to adjacent organs and/or direct extension beyond the true pelvis
  - IVB: spread to distant organs

Five-year survival rates

- stage I: 70%–80%
- stage II: 30%–45%
- stage III: 25%
- stage IV: 0%–30%

Management of vaginal cancer

- Therapy is individualised depending on the stage and site of vaginal disease.
- Generally, radiotherapy and/or surgical excision are performed.
- Stage I upper vaginal < 2 cm lesions can be treated with either surgery (radical hysterectomy, upper vaginectomy, bilateral pelvic lymphadenectomy) or intracavitary radiotherapy.
- Less radical surgery may be appropriate as the primary treatment in some forms of vaginal cancer (e.g. basal cell carcinoma).
- Chemoradiation therapy is currently being assessed.

Further reading

Berek, S., Hacker, N. (eds), 2014. Practical Gynecologic Oncology, 6th ed. Lippincott Williams & Wilkins, Philadelphia.

Joura, E.A., 2002. Epidemiology, diagnosis and treatment of vulvar intraepithelial neoplasia. Curr. Opin. Obstet. Gynecol. 14, 39–43.

Shafi, M., Luesley, D., Jordan, J. (eds), 2001. Handbook of Gynaecological Oncology. Churchill Livingstone, London.

Stewart, E.G., 2002. Developments in vulvovaginal care. Curr. Opin. Obstet. Gynecol. 14, 483–488.

Chapter 23

Benign vulvar disease

Neroli Ngenda

Infections

Fungal

CANDIDA ALBICANS

- predisposed groups: newborns, females between puberty and menopause, postmenopausal women on hormone replacement therapy (HRT), women with diabetes mellitus
- risk factors: oral contraceptive pill, diabetes mellitus, iron deficiency, antibiotic use, immunosuppression
- symptoms: vulvar pruritus, cheesy discharge, dyspareunia
- premenstrual and postcoital exacerbation can occur
- diagnosis: on vaginal swab; clinical findings are also important as swabs can be negative especially in chronic candidiasis; swabs unreliable if antifungals used in the preceding week
- standard treatment: vaginal antifungals +/– single oral dose fluconazole (Diflucan)
- vaginal antifungals: clotrimazole (Canesten) vaginal cream daily for 6 days; nystatin (Nilstat) vaginal cream 100 000 U or twice daily for 7–14 days; miconazole (Resolve) vaginal cream daily for 7 days; 1- or 3-day treatments are usually not fully effective except in mild cases; vaginal boric acid may be used
- antifungals applied intravaginally only, not to the vulva (can cause irritation externally)
- longer term vaginal or oral therapy may be required for recurrent candidiasis (e.g. fluconazole, itraconazole); ketoconazole is no longer used
- chronic candidiasis (symptoms > 6 months)
  - daily oral fungals for 3–6 months with regular liver function test monitoring
  - gradually decrease the dose to the lowest level that controls symptoms
  - any flare-ups are treated with an increased dose until symptoms have settled
  - once remission of 6 months is achieved, cease treatment
  - caution patients regarding risk of relapse

- vaginal or oral antifungals are used when taking antibiotics if candidiasis is recurrent or chronic

NON-ALBICANS YEAST INFECTION
- *Candida glabrata, C. krusei, C. parapsilosis, C. guillermondii*
- relatively resistant to imidazoles (clotrimazole, miconazole)
- boric acid is used for treatment: 9600 mg in a gelatine capsule daily for 10–14 days vaginally (needs to be organised through a compounding chemist)

TINEA CRURIS
- This is a fungal infection which is an uncommon cause of vulvar disease.
- It produces a well-demarcated erythematous lesion extending from the labia to the inner aspect of the thigh.
- Diagnosis is via microscopy of scrapings.
- Topical treatment with imidazoles (clotrimazole, miconazole) may help; however, oral antifungal treatment is required for cure (e.g. griseofulvin 500 mg/day or terbinafine 250 mg/day). Antifungals are used until there is complete clearance of the rash (usually 4–6 weeks) and a repeat scraping is negative.

PITYRIASIS VERSICOLOR (TINEA VERSICOLOR)
- mild fungal infection caused by *Malassezia furfur*
- may be asymptomatic or cause vulvar pruritus
- diagnosis is via microscopy of scrapings
- treatment: topical or oral antifungals

Viral
- herpes simplex virus 1 and 2
- human papillomavirus (HPV)
- molluscum contagiosum

Bacterial
- pyogenic vulvar infection (impetigo, folliculitis, abscess, carbuncle, cellulitis), Bartholin's gland infection, chancroid, donovanosis, syphilis, lymphogranuloma venereum

Parasitic
- pediculosis pubis (pubic lice), scabies, worms, trichomoniasis, schistosomiasis, filariasis, hydatid disease

Non-infectious dermatoses

Vulvar dermatitis
- most common cause of chronic vulvar symptoms
- divided into:
  - endogenous dermatitis (atopic dermatitis, seborrhoeic dermatitis): inflammatory dermatoses of the skin intrinsic to the patient; often associated with a history of asthma, hay fever, dermatitis affecting other areas of skin, family history of atopy
  - exogenous dermatitis (contact/allergic dermatitis): inflammatory skin condition caused by exogenous agents such as allergens and irritants; may be triggered by

local irritants (e.g. perfumes, soaps, fabric softeners, detergents, feminine sprays, urine, pads and panty liners, toilet paper, topical creams, latex in condoms) or may also be triggered by local or systemic medication

- all forms of dermatitis have a common histological appearance known as 'spongiosis' (oedema of the epidermal layer of the skin)
- causes vulvar pruritis; symptoms often worse at night
- examination may reveal vulvar erythema and/or swelling; fissuring in the interlabial sulci may occur
- the vagina is not involved
- lichenification can occur from scratching
- important to exclude the presence of candidiasis and treat if present
- identify the trigger if possible
- if a topical cause cannot be found, may require allergy testing to find a systemic cause
- environmental modification is required: important to avoid the trigger and other irritants such as perfumes, soaps, powder, fabric softener, nylon underwear, tight clothing, excessive pad/panty liner use, toilet paper with fragrance
- use aqueous cream, sorbolene or non-soap wash to clean the vulva
- zinc may be useful to protect the skin in cases of urinary incontinence
- topical steroids can assist in resolution and control symptoms
  - usually a weak topical corticosteroid (e.g. 1% hydrocortisone [Dermaid, Sigmacort or Cortic]) is effective
  - ointment is preferable to cream
  - if lichenification is present, Advantan fatty ointment (0.1% methylprednisolone aceponate) is effective for initial treatment

Lichen sclerosus

- can occur at any age, but is most common in postmenopausal women in whom it is a chronic condition
- also can occur in childhood (usually regresses at puberty)
- autoimmune condition
- causes vulvar pruritus and eventually decreased clitoral sensation
- in advanced stages can result in dyspareunia due to introital stenosis
- sites of occurrence include the vulva, perineum and perianal area (spares the labia majora and vagina)
- examination includes the vulva and review of the perineum and perianal area
- the skin develops well-defined white sclerotic plaques; ecchymoses can develop
- the condition alters the vulvar architecture resulting in atrophy (resorption of labia minora, phimosis of clitoral hood, introital stenosis, fissuring of the fourchette and/ or vestibule during intercourse)
- malignant potential: 1%–4% risk of vulvar squamous cell carcinoma (if adequately managed, risk is reduced)
- biopsy is used to confirm the diagnosis
- histology reveals homogenised collagen in the upper dermis; basal layer vacuolar degeneration and lymphocytic inflammatory infiltrate; acanthosis of the epidermis
- in established lesions, histology reveals hyperkeratosis, dermal hyalinisation and fibrosis

MANAGEMENT

- Topical steroid therapy can be used for symptoms and to slow the progression of anatomical distortion.

- Treatment starts with potent topical steroids (e.g. betamethasone dipropionate [Diprosone], mometasone furoate [Elocon]) and may move to mid-strength topical steroids for maintenance (e.g. betamethasone valerate 0.02% [Betnovate], triamcinolone acetonide [Aristocort]). Ointment is preferable to cream.
- Use of topical pimecrolimus (Elidel) may be necessary in cases resistant to topical steroids.
- Vulvar care is important: gentle drying of the vulva after washing; cease use of perfumes, deodorants, douches, soaps, fabric softeners, nylon underwear, tight clothing, excessive pad/panty liner use.
- The condition will recur after surgical excision; therefore, vulvectomy has no place.
- Surgery, however, may be necessary to exclude malignancy or to treat introital stenosis.
- Regular follow-up is required due to malignant potential, at least yearly or more frequently if clinically indicated; biopsy any suspicious lesions.

Lichen planus
- Aetiology is uncertain.
- Most cases affect the mucosa of the mouth and gums; 25% of cases involve the vulva.
- Symptoms include pain, soreness, dyspareunia, heavy non-offensive discharge and bleeding from lesions; pruritus is not a prominent feature.
- It causes epithelial erosions, usually on the medial aspect of the labia minora, extending to a variable degree into the vagina.
- In severe cases, adhesions can cause partial obliteration of the vagina.
- Diagnosis is made on biopsy and/or clinical findings.
- Treatment is with intravaginal steroids or pimecrolimus.
- Oral steroids may be required.
- Steroid sparing agents may be required (e.g. oral retinoids, oral methotrexate).
- Lignocaine gel applied prior to intercourse may be helpful.
- Vaginal dilators may be required to help decrease vaginal scarring.

Lichen simplex chronicus (LSC)
- refers to lichenified skin where no other pathology is diagnosed
- also referred to as lichenified dermatitis
- causes vulvar pruritus especially at night
- skin thickening occurs in response to scratching
- the skin may appear white if moist; fissuring and excoriation may be present
- the condition may have commenced due to a pruritic process (e.g. dermatitis/allergic reactions; fungal infection; psoriasis)
- need to exclude other causes of vulvar pruritus to make the diagnosis
- biopsy can be helpful to confirm the diagnosis and to exclude lichen sclerosus
- check for iron deficiency, which may be present in LSC
- treatment: topical steroids; behaviour modification (breaking the itch–scratch cycle); eliminate exposure to any irritants
- usually a good resolution if the itch–scratch cycle can be broken

Psoriasis
- autoimmune disease
- causes intermittent vulvar pruritus
- lesions are erythematous and well demarcated
- no scale is present on vulvar lesions

- the vagina is not involved
- can extend to the natal cleft and perianal area
- look for extragenital lesions to help establish the diagnosis (knees, elbows, scalp) and check for family history
- treatment: topical steroids

Vulvodynia

- genital dysaesthesia described as pain, burning, stinging and irritation in the absence of visible findings or identified disease of the vulva or vagina
- neuropathic pain: increased concentration of nerve endings in the vestibule have been demonstrated
- can be provoked, unprovoked, mixed/generalised or localised
- may be triggered by: infection (recurrent candidiasis, herpes simplex virus, human papillomavirus), vulvar laser or diathermy, trauma, vaginal surgery
- often no apparent trigger
- superficial dyspareunia is a common presenting symptom
- on examination with a Q-tip swab, one can find tenderness over the vestibular glands and vestibule (which may be erythematous)
- exclusion of candidiasis is imperative; if candidiasis is present, treat with long-term oral antifungals
- a biopsy is only indicated if there is suspicion of other vulvar pathology (e.g. lichen sclerosus, vulvar intraepithelial neoplasia)
- management involves a multidisciplinary approach: gynaecologist, pelvic floor physiotherapist (to address secondary muscle spasm), psychologist (biofeedback), psychosexual counselling, pain management, support groups
- medication for treatment
  - low-dose amitriptyline (Endep) or nortriptyline (Allegron); pregabalin (Lyrica); gabapentin
  - use medication for 3–6 months (sometimes longer treatment is required)
  - if using amitriptyline or nortriptyline, explain to patient that it is not being used as an antidepressant
  - medication is started at a low dose and gradually increased to a therapeutic dose (to minimise any side effects)
- lignocaine gel may be helpful for intercourse (not a long-term strategy)
- surgery: rarely indicated, but vestibulectomy may be required for refractory cases

Further reading

Fischer, G., Bradford, J., 2010. The Vulva: A Clinician's Practical Handbook. Family Planning NSW, Sydney.

Dennerstein, G., Scurry, J., Brenan, J., et al., 2005. The Vulva and Vagina Manual. Gynederm Publishing, Melbourne.

Farage, M., Galask, R., 2006. Vulvar vestibulitis syndrome: a review. National Vulvodynia Association News, US. Winter.

Goldstein, A., 2006. Dermatological diseases of the vulval. National Vulvodynia Association News, US. Summer.

Chapter 24

Gestational trophoblastic disease

Amy Tang

Gestational trophoblastic diseases are disorders in which the normal regulatory mechanisms controlling the behaviour of trophoblastic tissue are lost.

Incidence. Incidence is 1 in 1400 pregnancies.

Hydatidiform mole

Risk factors

- varying between populations
- dietary factors
- maternal age > 35 years (complete mole)
- previous molar pregnancy

Complete hydatiform mole

CHROMOSOMES

- origin is entirely paternal
- is usually a 23X duplication, with a haploid sperm fertilising an empty egg and duplicating itself
- 46XY moles are rare

PATHOLOGY

- no identifiable fetal tissue
- chorionic villi with generalised hydatidiform swelling and diffuse trophoblastic hyperplasia

Partial hydatidiform mole

CHROMOSOMES

- It involves a triploid karyotype, paternal 46XX/XY and maternal 23X (i.e. a normal egg with dispermy).

- If maternal 46XX and paternal 23X or 23Y, the result is a triploid fetus.
- Thus, placental growth is dependent on paternal genetic material.

PATHOLOGY
- chorionic villi of varying size with focal hydatidiform swelling, cavitation and trophoblastic hyperplasia
- marked villous scalloping, prominent stromal trophoblastic inclusions
- identifiable fetal tissues

PRESENTATION
- most diagnosed on ultrasound scan
- vaginal bleeding, hyperemesis
- uterus large for dates, theca lutein cysts
- preeclampsia, hyperthyroidism

INVESTIGATIONS
- full blood count, blood group and cross-match, quantitative human chorionic gonadotrophin (hCG)
- ultrasound scan of the pelvis, chest X-ray

MANAGEMENT
- suction curettage with oxytocics
- hysterectomy is an option if the woman has completed childbearing
- register in the trophoblastic registry

FOLLOW-UP
- involves weekly quantitative serum or 24-hour urinary hCG until normal (usually takes 8–12 weeks); then monthly hCG levels for 12 months (6 months if partial mole)
- contraception is required, and the oral contraceptive pill may be used
- advise to avoid pregnancy for at least 9 months after hCG levels return to normal

Persistent gestational trophoblastic disease

This is a complication for about 20% of women with complete moles and in up to 4% of partial moles. This condition is also known as gestational trophoblastic neoplasia.

Diagnosis and presentation
- plateau or rising hCG levels over 3 weeks after suction curettage
- delayed postevacuation bleeding
- raised hCG longer than 6 months
- evidence of metastatic disease
- presence of histologic choriocarcinoma

Investigations
- Assess risk factors and arrange further work-up: computed tomography (CT) scan of abdomen and pelvis, chest X-ray, quantitative hCG, full blood count, electrolytes, liver biochemistry.
- CT brain scan will also be required if presence of neurological symptoms or if lung/liver metastases are present.

Modified World Health Organization (WHO) scoring system for FIGO 2000 staging

This is used to determine if a patient belongs to a high-risk or low-risk group so the appropriate treatment can be offered. The prognostic factors used to calculate this score include: age, type of antecedent pregnancy, interval from index pregnancy, pretreatment hCG level, largest tumour size including uterus, site and number of metastases, and presence of previous failed chemotherapy. A score < 7 indicates low-risk group and a score of ≥ 7 indicates high-risk group.

Management

- For low-risk patients, single-agent chemotherapy is the first-line treatment. Cure rate for these patients is almost 100%.
- Methotrexate and folinic acid: 2-weekly courses continuing for two courses after hCG returns to normal.
- About 10% of patients suffer from side effects (especially serositis and mucosal ulceration) and require a change of chemotherapy to actinomycin D every 2 weeks.
- Treatment failure rate is 10%, and this requires second-line therapy: actinomycin D if hCG levels are below 100 IU/L; etoposide, methotrexate, actinomycin D, cyclophosphamide and oncovin (EMACO) if hCG levels are over 100 IU/L. Potential side effects include thrombocytopenia, hepatotoxicity and hair loss.
- Follow-up patient with a weekly quantitative hCG until normal, and then monthly for 6–12 months.

High-risk gestational trophoblastic disease

Definition. This is a disease that is not cured by low-risk chemotherapy, or with a histological diagnosis of choriocarcinoma, or with other high-risk features such as metastatic disease in the brain or liver, over 12 months between the antecedent pregnancy and starting therapy and term antecedent pregnancy. WHO scoring ≥ 7.

Investigations

- quantitative hCG, full blood count, electrolytes, liver biochemistry
- CT scans of chest, abdomen, pelvis and brain
- lumbar puncture to measure blood-to-cerebrospinal fluid hCG ratio (normally the ratio is 65:1, but with metastases this is reversed)
- selective angiography of abdomen and pelvic organs if indicated
- histological confirmation not required

Management

- Follow the EMACO regimen.
- If the central nervous system is involved, use EMACO with 1000 mg methotrexate and intrathecal methotrexate 12.5 mg weekly.
- With a single large brain metastasis, seek neurosurgical review for possible removal before chemotherapy.
- Second-line therapy uses high-dose cisplatinum VP-16.

Follow-up

- weekly hCG tests
- four courses of chemotherapy continued after hCG returns to normal

- after chemotherapy, monthly hCG levels required for 2 years, and then 3-monthly levels for 3 years
- advise against pregnancy until hCG levels have been normal for 12 months
- cure in 80% of non-metastatic disease, 50% with metastatic disease
- if central nervous system metastases appear during or after high-risk chemotherapy, survival rate is 0%–20%

Theca lutein cysts

- These are present in 20%–25% of molar pregnancies.
- They are thin-walled benign cysts with an average size of 7 cm.
- They usually reduce in size with decreasing hCG levels.
- Complications include rupture, torsion and bleeding.
- If present after curettage, they are associated with a risk of persisting trophoblastic disease.
- Management of uncomplicated cysts is conservative.

Choriocarcinoma

- This is a malignant tumour of villous trophoblast with anaplastic syncytiotrophoblast and cytotrophoblast.
- It has a tendency to early vascular invasion and widespread dissemination.

Placental site trophoblastic tumour

- the least common form of gestational trophoblastic disease
- shows predominance of cytotrophoblast with little syncytium
- intermediate trophoblasts are present
- hCG levels are often low; human placental lactogen is produced by the tumour
- does not readily respond to standard chemotherapy
- diagnosis: by curettage
- treatment: surgically when disease confined to uterus

Further reading

Hancock, B.W., Tidy, J.A., 2002. Current management of molar pregnancy. J. Reprod. Med. 47, 347–354.

Royal College of Obstetricians and Gynaecologists, 2009. Guidelines and Audit Committee. The management of gestational trophoblastic disease. Green-top Guideline No. 38, 2nd draft, May. RCOG, London.

Shapter, A.P., McLellan, R., 2001. Gestational trophoblastic disease. Obstet. Gynecol. Clin. North Am. 28, 805–817.

Obstetrics

Chapter 25

Antenatal care

Michael Flynn

Prepregnancy care

Ideally, all couples should seek prepregnancy care. Most couples are not reviewed until after the critical fetal developmental period.

Aims of counselling before conception
- Advise the woman and her partner on general healthcare (e.g. on nutrition/diet/ folate, smoking, alcohol and drugs). These and factors such as obesity are thought to have a significant long-term epigenetic impact on the fetus.
- Carry out general screening, including rubella and varicella serology, and immunise when required; cervical cytology; blood pressure.
- Assess and advise on the effects of existing disease and its management on the pregnancy, and the effects of pregnancy on the disease. Treat preexisting diseases to minimise the problems that may arise in pregnancy.
- Assess and advise on the problems that may recur from previous pregnancies and deliveries.
- Provide genetic counselling with full genetic history, especially in high-risk racial groups.
- Review past obstetric history.
- Preconception care often requires a team of obstetricians, physicians, geneticists, dietitians and specialised educators such as diabetic educators.

Antenatal care

Antenatal clinics act as a screening tool to identify and then manage problems that arise during the pregnancy. As this is also often the first time healthy women are assessed, they may provide information for long-term healthcare.

Aims of antenatal care
- screen and manage/prevent maternal problems
- screen and manage/prevent fetal problems
- provide antenatal education regarding general health, nutrition and childbirth

Booking assessment

- history: age, gravidity, parity
- menstrual history
- problems so far in pregnancy, such as bleeding and nausea
- past obstetric and gynaecological history
- past medical/surgical history
- family and social history
- medication, drugs, alcohol and smoking
- allergies

Examination

- weight, height
- blood pressure, urinalysis
- general: teeth/gums, thyroid, breast, chest, heart, varicose veins
- abdomen: scars, fundal height, masses, pain
- pelvic: cervical cytology if indicated; vaginal examination

Investigations

FIRST VISIT

- full blood examination
- ABO blood type, Rh factor and antibodies (the antibody screen should be performed at the beginning of every pregnancy)
- rubella immunity (antibody titres may decline, so check at the start of each pregnancy)
- syphilis serology using specific *Treponema* assay (e.g. *T. pallidum* haemagglutination assay [TPHA])
- hepatitis B serology
- urine for culture and sensitivity
- hepatitis C and human immunodeficiency virus (HIV) serology, offered after appropriate counselling
- varicella serology
- cervical cytology if no normal smear within the previous 18 months

Other tests considered but not mandatory include:
- testing for vitamin D deficiency in dark-skinned or veiled women
- screening for haemoglobinopathies, especially if mean corpuscular volume (MCV) or mean corpuscular haemoglobin concentration (MCHC) are abnormal
- *cytomegalovirus* (CMV)/toxoplasma serology: recommended only in at-risk women and ideally as prepregnancy test
- thyroid-stimulating hormone (TSH)

DISCUSSION OF ANTENATAL SCREENING

Screening for potential adverse outcomes in pregnancy via:
- screening for pre-eclampsia risk factors
- assessed for risk factors of preterm birth
- antenatal screening for Down syndrome and other fetal aneuploidy should be discussed (*see Ch 27*).

At the conclusion of the first visit in pregnancy, all women should be clear as to estimated due date, have an understanding as to investigations available and understand a plan and model of care for the pregnancy.

OBSTETRIC ULTRASOUND SCAN AT 18–20 WEEKS GESTATION

All women should be offered fetal morphology assessment prior to 20 weeks gestation.

AT THE END OF THE SECOND TRIMESTER:

- full blood examination
- platelet assessment
- blood group and antibody status
- fasting 75 gm oral glucose tolerance test, except those considered high risk whereby this would be performed in the first trimester

GROUP B STREPTOCOCCUS DISEASE (GBS)

This is the leading cause of neonatal sepsis, which if left untreated would affect 1 in 200 newborns. Intrapartum chemoprophylaxis significantly decreases infection rates. The decision for prophylaxis comes from either screening via low vagina/anorectal swab at 35–37 weeks gestation or treating via clinical risk factor analysis.

Continuing antenatal visits

- routine antenatal visits every 4 weeks to 28 weeks gestation, then every 2 weeks to 36 weeks gestation, then every week until delivery
- at each visit, assessment of:
  - history of events since previous visit, fetal movements, blood pressure, review of risk factors
  - fundal height, clinical amniotic fluid assessment, fetal heart sounds, and (in the third trimester) fetal lie and presentation
  - discussion of anti-D prophylaxis at 28 and 34 weeks gestation, and at any time of blood loss in a Rh-negative woman

Indications for ultrasound scan in antenatal care

- First trimester: vaginal bleeding, abdominal pain, hyperemesis gravidarum, before procedures (e.g. amniocentesis, chorionic villus sampling or cervical suture). Down syndrome screening and definitive diagnosis of multiple pregnancies is offered early in the second trimester.
- Second trimester: at 18–20 weeks to confirm dates, assess fetal morphology and exclude multiple pregnancies; to assess complications of pregnancy, including antepartum haemorrhage, threatened premature labour and preterm prelabour rupture of membranes.
- Third trimester: fundal height small or large for gestation, previous intrauterine growth restriction, multiple pregnancies, antepartum haemorrhage, malpresentation, maternal medical conditions such as diabetes, renal disease, pre-eclampsia. Late pregnancy tests of fetal wellbeing for assessment of the fetoplacental function may be appropriate.

Chapter 26

Antenatal diagnosis of fetal and chromosomal abnormalities

Jackie Chua

Two to three per cent of children are born with a significant physical/mental handicap, and a further 3% have mild intellectual physical disability.

Major malformations are present in 10%–15% of miscarriages, 50% of stillbirths and 3% of newborns. One-third of malformations are associated with genetic abnormalities. Multifactorial causes of malformation include neural tube defects, congenital heart defects or cleft lip/palate. The recurrence rate is about 2%–4%. Table 26.1 shows a breakdown of the causes of fetal malformations.

Genetic counselling

All women who choose to have an antenatal screening test should have access to adequate counselling. Specialist genetic counselling clinics should be available for discussion of the following:
- abnormal screening tests
- abnormal ultrasound and karyotype findings
- patients with a family history of genetic disorders
- previously affected child
- advanced maternal age
- medical condition of the mother with possible fetal transmission (e.g. *human immunodeficiency virus* [HIV])
- three or more miscarriages (recurrent miscarriage)
- consanguinity
- chemical or radiation exposure in pregnancy (teratogen exposure)
- physically or mentally handicapped parent

Aims of genetic counselling
- make accurate diagnosis
- provide adequate pedigree information

Table 26.1 Causes of malformations	
CAUSE	**INCIDENCE**
single gene defect	9%
chromosomal defect	6%
multifactorial	20%
environmental	5%
unknown	60%

Source: Callen PW. Ultrasonography in Obstetrics and Gynecology. 2007. Philadelphia: Saunders.

- explain risks to family
- identify methods of avoiding or decreasing risks
- arrange follow-up
- explain options available: ignore risks, have no more children, adoption, sperm or ovum donation, prenatal diagnosis and selective termination

Indications for prenatal diagnosis

Every woman is at risk of having a fetus with a chromosome abnormality. Genetic testing allows the patient to be counselled about the possible fetal outcomes and the recurrence risk. The woman should be advised of prenatal screening and diagnosis to facilitate an informed choice. Preconception would be finding alternative genetic material, such as a donor. Prenatally, it would mean the decision to continue with the pregnancy, consider palliation or terminating the pregnancy.

The at-risk patient risk factors are:
- family history
- past obstetric history: affected pregnancy (live born or miscarriage)
- fetal anomaly
- maternal age

Preimplantation genetic diagnosis (PGD)
- biopsy of embryo at day 3, blastomere stage or at blastocyst stage at day 5
- preimplantation genetic diagnosis (PGD) at day 3 has higher risk of damaging the embryo and higher risk of mosaicism; this risk is lower with day 5 testing
- fluorescent in situ hybridisation (FISH) is used for fast turnaround time
  - accurate
  - limited number of chromosomes examined
- risk of confined placental mosaicism; therefore, invasive testing should still be offered

Tests available for antenatal diagnosis

Screening
- maternal age
- first trimester: combined nuchal translucency and non-invasive prenatal testing (NIPT)
- second trimester: triple/quadruple test, morphology test

Screening tests reaching clinical acceptability qualify with a sensitivity of greater than 75% and specificity of greater than 95%. The combination of tests reaching this standard is presented in Table 26.2. Many tests including maternal age alone have previously been used as a screening tool; however, those that fail to reach performance standard criteria are listed in Table 26.3.

Diagnostic

- first trimester: chorionic villus sampling
- second trimester: amniocentesis
- other: fetal blood sampling, microarray, comparative genomic hybridisation (CGH)

Distribution of chromosomal abnormalities

- first-trimester miscarriage: 50%–60%
- second-trimester miscarriage: 35%
- stillbirths: 5%
- live births: 0.5%

Table 26.2 Screening tests for trisomy 21 that meet the performance criteria (i.e. have > 75% sensitivity / > 95% specificity)

TEST	GESTATION FOR SCREENING	SENSITIVITY	SPECIFICITY	POSITIVE PREDICTIVE VALUE[#]
Combined first trimester screening: MA + NT + βhCG + PAPP-A	11^{+0}–13^{+6} weeks	85%	95%	~7–10%[5]
Quadruple test: MA + AFP + βhCG + UE3 + Inhibin	15–20 weeks	75%	95%	~2–3%
cell-free DNA screening*	> 10^{+} weeks	99%	99%*	~45%[6]

* In a small proportion (< 5%) of cases cfDNA testing is unable to provide a result
MA = maternal age; NT = nuchal translucency; βhCG = free B human chorionic gonadotrophin; PAPP-A = pregnancy associated plasma protein A; AFP = Alpha-fetoprotein; UE3 = oestriol.
# These positive predictive values are derived from test performance in the general pregnant population, but will vary according to the underlying prevalence of the condition.
Source: RANZCOG. Prenatal screening and diagnosis of chromosomal and genetic abnormalities in the fetus in pregnancy (C-Obs 59). March 2015. Updated guidelines will be published in 2017

Table 26.3 Screening tests for trisomy 21 that do not meet the performance criteria (i.e. have < 75% sensitivity / < 95% specificity)

TEST	GESTATION FOR SCREENING	SENSITIVITY	SPECIFICITY
Maternal age alone	Any stage	30–50%*	70%*
Double test: MA + AFP + βhCG	15–20 weeks	60%	95%
Triple test: MA + AFP + βhCG + UE3	15–20 weeks	70%	95%
Nuchal translucency alone (no biochemistry): MA + NT	11^{+1}–13^{+6} weeks	70%	95%

* Varies according to maternal age distribution in the population.
Source: RANZCOG. Prenatal screening and diagnosis of chromosomal and genetic abnormalities in the fetus in pregnancy (C-Obs 59). March 2015. Updated guidelines will be published in 2017

After two or more miscarriages, there is a 5% chance of chromosomal abnormalities in the parents. This rises to 10% with four or more miscarriages.
- Rate of fetal death for euploid fetuses is 1–2%.
- Risk of fetal death between 12 weeks and term is 30% for trisomy 21 and 80% for trisomy 18 and 13. The risk of delivering an affected baby decreases as pregnancy continues due to the fact aneuploidy fetuses selectively die.

Screening

Maternal age

Table 26.4 shows the corresponding risk of trisomy 201 with increasing maternal age.
- maternal age: > 35 years high risk for aneuploidy
  - incidence of trisomy 18 is 1 in 3000
  - incidence of trisomy 13 is 1 in 5000

COMBINED NUCHAL TRANSLUCENCY AND BIOCHEMICAL SCREENING
- A combined first-trimester screening test is performed between 11 weeks and 1 day gestation and 13 weeks and 6 days gestation. This correlates to a crown–rump length (CRL) measurement of 45 mm to 84 mm. This test has a detection rate (DR) of 90%, with a false-positive rate (FPR) of 5%.
- Operators are accredited by the nuchal translucency (NT) program through the Royal Australian and New Zealand College of Obstetricians and Gynaecologists (RANZCOG) and audits are performed yearly.
  - ultrasound assessment: CRL and NT are measured
  - biochemical screening
    — free beta-human chorionic gonadotrophin (free beta-hCG) and pregnancy-associated plasma protein A (PAPP-A) levels are converted to multiples of the median (MoM)
  - maternal age: background risk
  - additional bioinformation: weight, ethnicity, smoking, mode of conception, maternal diabetes
  - pathophysiology of increased NT measurement
    — cardiac failure in association with cardiac defects
    — venous congestion in head and neck due to constriction, mediastinal compression or narrow chest (e.g. diaphragmatic hernia or skeletal dysplasia)

Table 26.4 Risk of trisomy 21	
MATERNAL AGE	**RISK**
20	1 in 2000
25	1 in 1200
30	1 in 700
35	1 in 400
37	1 in 250
40	1 in 100
43	1 in 50

> — altered composition of extracellular matrix
> — abnormal development of lymphatic system
> — fetal anaemia or hypoproteinaemia
> — congenital infection
> * adverse pregnancy outcome in normal karyotype fetus with an NT measurement in the 99th percentile (3.5 mm) is 30%
* Additional markers used to increase sensitivity: 95% detection rate with a 3% false-positive rate.
  * presence or absence of nasal bone: currently used in the algorithm
  * presence or absence of tricuspid regurgitation
  * presence or absence of ductus venosus A-wave
  * fetal maxillary facial angle
* Biochemical markers may also be used to screen for pre-eclampsia, intrauterine growth restriction and fetal demise.
* Additional biochemical markers are being researched for early pre-eclampsia screening; PlGF (placental growth factor) combined with PAPP-A, mean arterial pressure, uterine artery Doppler and maternal risk factors.
* Additional ultrasound markers for screening.
  * intracranial translucency for spina bifida

Non-invasive prenatal testing (NIPT)

* Non-invasive prenatal testing (NIPT) identifies cell-free DNA in maternal blood. They originate from the trophoblast. The DNA fragments are unstable and have a half-life of about 16 minutes. They can be detected reliably from 9 weeks gestation; they are undetectable 2 hours after delivery and are therefore pregnancy specific. Due to next generation sequencing-techniques, the cell-free DNA is extracted from maternal plasma and copied millions of times. There are a few different techniques; one way is to calculate proportional representation of potential aneuploidy compared to a reference chromosome. An increase in proportional representation would indicate the presence of trisomy. Another technique uses single nucleotide polymorphism (SNP) as a statistical determination. Maternal genotype information and recombination frequencies construct billions of theoretical fetal genotypes and the software calculates the relative likelihood against the actual data from the sample.
* Screens for trisomy 21,18 and 13; X and Y chromosome; microdeletion panel (22q11.2 deletion, Angelman's syndrome, Prader Willi syndrome, Cri Du Chat 5p deletion, 1p36 deletion).
* Screening detection rate for trisomy 21 is 99% but less for the other trisomies.

Second-trimester screening

* Triple test is commonly known as the maternal serum screening (MSS):
  * maternal blood test done from 16–22 weeks gestation.
* Quadruple test:
  * alpha-fetoprotein, unconjugated oestriol, free beta-hCG and inhibin A.
* Screening is performed using alpha-fetoprotein (AFP), unconjugated oestriol, free beta-hCG and inhibin A combined with maternal age; sensitivity is 70%.
* AFP is the principal plasma protein of the fetus in early gestation. It is initially produced in the yolk sac, and then the fetal liver and gut.
  * Fetal AFP: plasma levels peak at 12–13 weeks gestation and fall throughout pregnancy.

- Maternal serum AFP rises in the second trimester, reaches maximum levels at approximately 30 weeks and then falls.
- Amniotic fluid AFP parallels levels in the fetal plasma, but in a ratio of 1:200.
- Raised AFP > 2.0 MoMs may be due to neural tube defects, gastrointestinal defects (omphalocele, gastroschisis, oesophageal and duodenal atresia), cystic hygroma, threatened abortion or antepartum haemorrhage, fetal death in utero, multiple pregnancy and advanced gestation.

Ultrasound screening

- There is 50% sensitivity for babies with Down syndrome.
- Nearly all trisomy 13/18 have ultrasound findings.
- Previous soft markers of echogenic focus in the heart, choroid plexus cysts and hypoplasia of the middle phalanx of the fifth finger are not generally used anymore.

Not all anomalies require definitive testing but for those with a high association with chromosome abnormalities, invasive testing should be offered.

Morphology ultrasound assessment

Under defined protocol, assessments are performed typically between 18 and 20 weeks gestation. Common anomalies screened include the following.

TRISOMY 21

- Detection features include short femur/humerus, cardiovascular lesions such as atrioventricular septal defect, duodenal atresia, hypoplastic nasal bone and growth restriction with polyhydramnios.

TRISOMY 18

- Diagnostic features include congenital heart disease, diaphragmatic hernia, omphalocele and growth restriction.
- Choroid plexus cysts are present in 1%–2.5% of normal fetuses (previously associated with trisomy 18, so look at previous screening and other ultrasound features for trisomy 18).

TRISOMY 13

- Diagnostic features include congenital heart disease, omphalocele, renal abnormalities, holoprosencephaly and intrauterine growth restriction.

Definitive diagnostic tests

- Routine karyotyping:
  - has been around since the 1960s
  - detects large chromosomal abnormalities.
- FISH analysis (fluorescent in situ hybridisation):
  - for trisomy and specific marker genes, may give rapid diagnosis
  - confirmation is from long-term karyotype.
- Microarray testing (CMA):
  - can detect at a higher chromosome resolution
  - eliminates the use of cell culture, decreases overall turnaround time and is less labour intensive
  - does not provide any information of structure like translocations, inversions or mutations causing single gene disorders.

- Comparative genomic hybridisation (CGH):
  - analyses copy number variant (CNV) to a reference sample
  - can detect unbalanced translocations
  - more expensive but will detect more chromosome abnormalities in the structurally abnormal fetus.

Amniocentesis

- It is usually performed after 16 weeks gestation when the amnion has fused with the chorion.
- Information gained includes chromosomes and DNA analysis, AFP and enzymology.
- Fetal loss between 1/500 and 1/1000.
- False-positive results occur in 0.3%, inadequate cell collection in up to 2% of samples and maternal contamination in 1 of 1000 samples.
- Anti-D prophylaxis is required if the woman is Rh-negative.

Chorionic villus sampling

- Chorionic villus sampling (CVS) is usually performed at 11–14 weeks gestation. As the sample is directly from the chorion, there is a 1% risk of mosaicism (i.e. the presence of a genetic cell line that is not fetal, but purely placental in origin and therefore a false-positive result). If this occurs, amniocentesis is required for fetal karyotyping.
- It is a test that gives the woman the advantage of early termination of pregnancy which could be possible operatively rather than induction in comparison with amniocentesis.
- The tissue may be collected transabdominally or transcervically. The risk of fetal loss from the procedure is may be between 1/500 to 1/1000.
- It has a false-positive rate of 2%, inadequate specimen collection in up to 8%, and maternal contamination in 1%–2%. Up to 4% of cases require follow-up by amniocentesis.
- The oromandibular limb hypogenesis syndrome has been reported with procedures performed at 56–66 days gestation and is probably due to vascular insult in early pregnancy.

Cordocentesis/fetal blood sampling

- collection of fetal blood sample from cord; performed in second and third trimester
- use: fetal karyotype, viral serology, full blood count, blood group, blood gases, metabolic abnormalities and DNA analysis, as well as treatment such as transfusion
- fetal loss of 1%–2%

Chromosomal abnormalities

Trisomies

After one affected fetus, the recurrence risk is 1% plus the risk for maternal age.

The only factor related to trisomy 21 is maternal age (see Table 26.4). The incidence of all chromosomal abnormalities is about twice that of trisomy 21. Women affected by trisomy 21 are often infertile. However, if the woman becomes pregnant, the risk of trisomy 21 to her offspring is 33%, which is less than the expected 50% because of an increased trisomic loss in early pregnancy.

Trisomy 18 and 13 are associated with severe anomalies and disability. The majority of fetuses affected will demise during the pregnancy, with a very small percentage born alive surviving for more than a month.

Translocations
- If the mother has a translocation, there is a 10% recurrence risk.
- If the father has a translocation, there is a 2% recurrence risk.

RECIPROCAL TRANSLOCATION
If this is demonstrated through an unbalanced translocation in the offspring, the risk of unbalanced translocation in another offspring is 10%–20% for female carriers and 5%–10% for male carriers. If amniocentesis shows a balanced translocation and the parents have normal chromosomes, the child will look normal, but there is a 1 in 8 risk of intellectual handicap, as some genes may be lost during the translocation.

ROBERTSONIAN TRANSLOCATION
This involves acrocentric chromosomes (13, 14, 15, 21 and 22). The carrier has 45 chromosomes. Be aware of the risk of uniparental disomy with the imprinted chromosomes (i.e. 14 and 15). Of people with Down syndrome, 4% have a parent with a Robertsonian translocation. When the translocation occurs on the same chromosome, the risk of another affected child is 100%.

Sex chromosome abnormalities

Turner's syndrome
- incidence: 1 in 2500 females
- karyotype: 45, XO
- affects development in females
- tend to have short stature
- infertile or premature ovarian failure
- webbed neck
- common heart association: coarctation of the aorta
- normal intellect
- no increased recurrence rate as not related to maternal age
- mosaic Turner's syndrome woman may have issues with reduced fertility

KLINEFELTER'S SYNDROME
- incidence: 1 in 500–1000 males
- karyotype: 47, XXY
- affects male sexual function
- associated with intellectual disability, distinctive facial features, skeletal abnormalities, poor coordination and severe problems with speech
- no increased recurrence risk

Other genetic syndromes

Fragile X syndrome
- incidence of 1 in 1000 male births; responsible for 25% of male intellectual handicap

- second only to trisomy 21 as a chromosomal cause of mental impairment; 35% of heterozygote females are mentally impaired
- prenatal testing available, though parental karyotype comparison important
- diagnosis by presence of nucleotide triplet repeat and expansion of > 220 repeats in males

Cystic fibrosis

This is an autosomal recessive disorder, with an incidence in Caucasians of 1 in 2500 and a carrier frequency of 1 in 25.

Genetics. The mutant gene is the cystic fibrosis transmembrane conductance regulator, situated on the long arm of chromosome 7 (CFTR gene). In 75% of cases, cystic fibrosis is due to the deletion of a single codon (delta F508 is the most common).

Screening. If one parent has a close relative with cystic fibrosis, then the carrier risk is reduced to a 1 in 99 chance by a negative result in tests for F508 and other common gene deletions. Prenatal diagnosis may be necessary if ultrasound abnormalities are discovered, such as hyperechogenic bowel. Prenatal diagnosis is possible. Test for one mutation or for multiple; 31 different mutations would cover 90% possibilities. The whole CFTR gene can be sequenced.

Muscular dystrophies

Duchenne muscular dystrophy has an incidence of 0.3 in 1000 male births. It is an X-linked recessive disorder with the mutant gene at Xp21. Presentation is one of progressive muscle wasting, with death in the second or third decade of life. Diagnosis is based on the absence of dystrophins on immunoblotting muscle biopsy.

Myotonic dystrophy is an autosomal dominant inheritance with associated abnormalities of mental retardation, cataracts, diabetes, cardiomyopathy and infertility. Pregnancy in an affected woman can increase the severity of disease, causing prolonged labour, uterine atony, postpartum haemorrhage and polyhydramnios.

Phenylketonuria

- Phenylketonuria has an incidence of 1 in 12 000 births. It is an autosomal recessive disorder.
- The pathology is that of an inborn error of metabolism with a deficiency of the enzyme phenylalanine hydroxylase. This enzyme converts phenylalanine to tyrosine. In phenylalanine hydroxylase deficiency, there is a rise in serum phenylalanine levels in children, leading to impaired myelination of the brain and subsequent mental retardation.
- The concentration gradient across the placenta produces fetal levels that are twice maternal levels.

Marfan's syndrome

Marfan's syndrome is an autosomal dominant connective tissue disorder.

Neurofibromatosis

Neurofibromatosis is an autosomal dominant disorder.

Thalassaemia

Alpha-thalassaemia is due to gene deletion. Beta-thalassaemia has more than 40 gene mutations. Both have lethal forms.

Incidence in ethnic and racial groups

Genetic disorders are more common in certain ethnic and racial groups. For example:
- Ashkenazi Jews: Tay-Sachs disease
- African Americans: sickle cell anaemia
- South-East Asians, Greeks, Italians: thalassaemia.

The morphology scan performed at 18–20 weeks gestation is a developmental screening test. It provides information about anatomy, number of gestation, placental site and cervical information. Where appropriate, further counselling or invasive testing should be offered.

Neural tube defects

- spectrum includes anencephaly and spina bifida
- detection rate: close to 100%
- incidence: 1 in 650 births
- prevention: 4 mg folic acid per day can reduce the risk of recurrence of neural tube defect from 3.5% to 1%; supplementation with folate should begin 3 months before conception and continue to the end of the first trimester; also helpful for cleft lip and palate
- increased risk of recurrence with a previous history of spina bifida and anencephalics
- diagnosis: uses ultrasound scan—open defect of the spine seen with or without intracranial ultrasound signs; maternal serum AFP (false-negative occurs in 12% of anencephalics and 21% of open spina bifida); amniotic fluid AFP has been used in the past; ultrasound markers of associated chromosome anomalies; closed spina bifida are difficult to detect antenatally

Gastrointestinal anomalies

- include tracheo-oesophageal fistula (polyhydramnios and absent stomach on ultrasound scan)
- omphalocele is a ventral wall with variable degree of herniation of abdominal contents with covering membrane present; can be associated with trisomies
- gastroschisis is a full thickness ventral wall defect, with no membrane present, which can be diagnosed after 12 weeks (after physiological herniation of the bowel has resolved); not usually associated with chromosome abnormalities
- duodenal atresia, on ultrasound scan, has a characteristic double-bubble sign; up to 50% of these fetuses will have other abnormalities and 30% are associated with trisomy 21

Renal tract anomalies

- Those detected on ultrasound scan include renal agenesis resulting in oligohydramnios, congenital polycystic kidneys and renal tract obstruction.
- A common renal finding is renal pelvis dilatation. Postnatal paediatric review is usually recommended.
- Renal function is reflected by liquor volume and is associated with pulmonary hypoplasia.

Cardiac abnormalities

- incidence of 4 in 1000 live births
- complex cardiac defects: paediatric cardiology review recommended as some anomalies have improved outcome with antenatal diagnosis

Dwarfism

- In the heterozygote for achondroplasia, bony abnormalities may not be obvious on ultrasound scan until 24 weeks gestation. It can be non-lethal.
- Bony characteristics for lethal skeletal dysplasias should be looked for, especially if early onset.
- Genetic counselling is recommended. Test for FGFR3 gene mutations recommended.

Cleft lip/palate

- higher incidence in males
- recurrence rate: 4% with one sibling
- simple cleft lip not usually associated with chromosome abnormality but median or bilateral cleft lip and palate can be, especially with trisomy 13

References and further reading

Genetic Home Reference. Klinefelter syndrome. Available at: <http://ghr.nlm.nih.gov/condition/klinefelter-syndrome>.

Genetic Home Reference. Turner syndrome. Available at: <http://ghr.nlm.nih.gov/condition/turner-syndrome>.

Hyett, J., Moscoso, G., Papapanagiotou, G., et al., 1996. Abnormalities of the heart and great arteries in chromosomally normal fetuses with increased nuchal translucency thickness at 11–13 weeks of gestation. Ultrasound Obstet. Gynecol. 7, 245–250.

Royal Australian and New Zealand College of Obstetricians and Gynaecologists, 2013. College statement: Prenatal screening and diagnosis of chromosomal and genetic abnormalities in the fetus in pregnancy (C-Obs 59); November. RANZCOG, East Melbourne.

Royal Australian and New Zealand College of Obstetricians and Gynaecologists, 2014. Mid-trimester fetal morphology ultrasound screening (C-Obs 57). March. RANZCOG, East Melbourne. Available at: <www.ranzcog.edu.au/document-library/fetal-morphology.htmlRANZCOG>.

Royal Australian and New Zealand College of Obstetricians and Gynaecologists, 2015. Prenatal assessment of fetal structural abnormalities (C-Obs 60). March. RANZCOG, East Melbourne. Available at: <www.ranzcog.edu.au/document-library/prenatal-assessment-of-fetal-structural-abnormalities.html>.

Royal Australian and New Zealand College of Obstetricians and Gynaecologists, 2015. Prenatal screening and diagnosis of chromosomal and genetic abnormalities in the fetus in pregnancy (C-Obs 59). March 2015. Available at: <www.ranzcog.edu.au/document-library/prenatal-screening-chromosomal-abnormalities.html>.

Chapter 27

Assessing fetal wellbeing

Jackie Chua

The method used in the assessment of fetal wellbeing depends on the level of risk to the fetus: low-risk or high-risk pregnancy. Monitoring can be antepartum or intrapartum.

In a fetus with low-risk status, screening only fetal movements has been shown to identify the fetus at risk of intrauterine death. Continuous monitoring has not decreased cerebral palsy rates. Asphyxia at birth still has a very strong association.

Tests available for assessing fetal wellbeing

- fetal movement, including kick charts
- cardiotocography (CTG)
- fetal scalp pH or lactate
- fetal pulse oximetry
- biophysical assessment
- amniotic fluid volume assessment
- growth
- Doppler flow studies

Fetal movement

Antepartum stillbirths account for 50% of the perinatal mortality rate. In late antepartum intrauterine fetal death, 60% occur at less than 37 weeks gestation and 2% at gestation over 42 weeks.

FETAL MOVEMENT IN LATE PREGNANCY

- Activity of individual fetuses varies, with only 1% of quiet phases lasting over 45 minutes.
- The perception of fetal movement varies between different women. There is reduced activity in fetuses with malformations.
- There appears to be no advantage to formal counting compared with informal inquiry at antenatal clinic.

- Fetal movement assessment should be used as a screening test to prompt other investigations.
- Less than 10 movements within 2 hours when the fetus is active is the current recommendation.
- High-risk pregnancies, including hypertensive disorders, vascular diseases, thyroid disease, diabetes, isoimmunisation, multiple pregnancies, as well as reduced fetal movements, vaginal bleeding and prolonged pregnancy, should have regular assessment, including umbilical artery Doppler recordings, fetal growth measurement, amniotic fluid volume, as well as CTG and biophysical profile score.

Cardiotocography (CTG)

A CTG is considered normal when the fetal baseline heart rate is between 110 and 160 beats/minute, the variability of heart rate is between 6 and 25 beats/minute, there are two or more accelerations in a 20-minute period and there are no baseline decelerations. An acceleration of fetal heart rate is a rise in heart rate of ≥ 15 beats/minute and lasting for 15 seconds or more.

Some factors that need to be taken into consideration when interpreting a CTG are the gestational age, drugs administered to the mother, the speed of the paper (usually at 1 cm/minute), maternal positioning and fetal abnormalities (e.g. complete heart block).

The variability represents fetal reserve and is an indicator of central, cerebral and myocardial oxygenation. If the period of unreactivity lasts longer than 40 minutes, this is considered a suspicious CTG. If the resting phase is over 120 minutes in duration, the positive predictive value for fetal morbidity/mortality is up to 85%.

False-positive rates of CTG in prediction of fetal hypoxia are up to 20%–40%. False-negative rates are 0.3/1000 for stillbirth and 7/1000 for hypoxia or acidosis. About 10%–15% of CTG recordings are unsatisfactory for interpretation.

CTG usage has resulted in an increased incidence of operative delivery. It does cause a reduction in neonatal seizures.

Fetal scalp pH or lactate

- Test in labour when the membranes have ruptured from the fetal scalp by sampling blood. The pH is proportional to $PaCO_2$ and lactic acid. This test has better specificity in comparison to CTG and there is no impact on operative delivery rates.
- In the first stage of labour, the mean fetal scalp pH is 7.33.
- A pH > 7.25 is regarded as normal.
- A pH of 7.20–7.25 is an equivocal result; repeat in 1 hour.
- A pH < 7.20 indicates acidosis; delivery should be undertaken immediately.
- Fetal scalp sampling for lactate testing: a lactate reading > 4.2 mmol/L may be more sensitive then scalp pH for adverse outcome. This is considered equivalent to scalp pH.

Fetal pulse oximetry

- Fetal oxygen saturation during labour has a normal range of 30%–65%.
- There is a reduction of fetal oxygenation during cord compression.

Biophysical assessment

Biophysical assessment involves the following five parameters with a score of 0 or 2 for each:
1. CTG
2. fetal breathing movement > 30 seconds in 30 minutes

3. fetal movements of at least three in 30 minutes
4. fetal tone considered normal if prompt return to flexion after extension of limbs/ trunk
5. amniotic fluid volume: more than one pool of > 2 cm in two planes

Table 27.1 lists perinatal mortality rates for biophysical assessment scores:
- false-positive rate 50%
- not shown to improve outcome in high-risk pregnancies
- however, normal biophysical assessment has a good negative predictive value and tends to be reflective of the normal Doppler readings

Table 27.1 Biophysical assessment: perinatal mortality rates	
SCORE	PERINATAL MORTALITY RATE
8–10/10	< 1 in 1000 (false-negative 0.9/1000)
6/10	> 90 in 1000
4/10	60–600 in 1000

Amniotic fluid volume assessment
- amniotic fluid volume is a reflection of fetal wellbeing or placental health
- different methods of measurement: amniotic fluid index (AFI), deepest vertical pocket (DVP)
- decreased liquor volume is associated with increased perinatal mortality and increased risk of operative delivery
- should be used in conjunction with other methods

Growth
- In high-risk pregnancies, estimated fetal weight can help identify small-for-gestational-age pregnancies.
- Customised growth charts for ethnicity have been proposed.

Doppler flow studies
- Low-risk pregnancies: not shown to reduce mortality or morbidity.
- High-risk pregnancies:
  - fetal umbilical artery Doppler monitoring reduces perinatal morbidity and mortality
  - can also decrease inductions
  - risk increases with increasing resistance measured through Doppler velocity
  - resistance index (RI) thought to be best predictor of outcome
  - other blood vessels have been investigated for prediction of adverse pregnancy outcomes, such as uterine artery Doppler, but not currently used routinely
  - mainly helpful in timing of delivery
- When middle cerebral artery Doppler pulsatility index is low, it can be associated with redistribution.
- Current research is looking at the cerebro-umbilical ration to identify brain blood flow redistribution.

Biochemical markers of placental function

Pregnancy-associated plasma protein A, PAPP-A, is commonly used in the first trimester screen. A low level has an association with adverse pregnancy outcome such as pre-eclampsia and growth restriction.

Further reading

East, C.E., Leader, L.R., Sheehan, P., et al., 2015. Intrapartum fetal scalp lactate sampling for fetal assessment in the presence of a non-reassuring fetal heart rate trace. Cochrane Database Syst. Rev. (5), CD006174, doi:10.1002/14651858.CD006174.pub3.

Prior, T., Kumar, S., 2015. Expert Review – identification of intra-partum compromise. Eur. J. Obstet. Gynecol. Reprod. Biol. 190, 1–6.

Regan, J., 2013. Reduced fetal movements. O&G Magazine 15 (4), 55–56. Available at: <www.ranzcog.edu.au/editions/doc_view/1606-55-reduced-fetal-movements.html>.

Royal Australian and New Zealand College of Obstetricians and Gynaecologists, 2014. Intrapartum Fetal Surveillance. Clinical Guideline, 3rd ed. RANZCOG, East Melbourne. Available at: <http://www.ranzcog.edu.au/college-statements-guidelines.html>.

Chapter 28

Drugs and drugs of abuse in pregnancy

Justin Nasser

The decision on whether to prescribe a drug to pregnant women must take into account the risk of the therapy and the risk of withholding the treatment. This requires a thorough up-to-date understanding of the drug and its risk/benefit ratio in pregnancy, as well as knowledge about the pharmacokinetics of the drug in pregnancy and the accurate assessment of the gestational age at the time of possible in utero exposure.

During the period from fertilisation to implantation, the pregnancy is relatively immune from teratogenic effects from medications, as the fetomaternal circulation has not developed. The period of organogenesis (17–70 days postconception) is when the embryo is most susceptible to teratogens. After this period, the risk of structural defects abates, but the fetus may be affected by anomalies in the functional development of organs and systems.

Teratogens

A teratogen is an agent that acts to irreversibly alter the growth, structure or function of a developing embryo or fetus. Recognised teratogens include:
- viruses (e.g. rubella, cytomegalovirus)
- environmental factors (e.g. hyperthermia, irradiation)
- chemicals (e.g. mercury)
- therapeutic/recreational drugs

Information on the teratogenic effect of specific medications is not always readily available, as few therapies have been specifically tested for safety and efficacy in human pregnancies. Current methods to assess teratogenic risk rely on pregnancy registries and case-control surveillance studies which have inherent shortcomings in design.

Information about the potential teratogenic risk of medications can be sourced from the Australian Government Therapeutic Goods Administration (see Box 28.1) and online databases (see Box 28.2).

Box 28.1 **Australian categorisation of drugs in pregnancy**

Category A
These are drugs which have been taken by a large number of pregnant women and women of childbearing age without any proven increase in the frequency of malformations or other direct or indirect harmful effects on the fetus having been observed.

Category B
These are drugs which have been taken by only a limited number of pregnant women and women of childbearing age without an increase in the frequency of malformations or other direct or indirect harmful effects on the human fetus having been observed.

- B1: studies in animals have not shown evidence of an increased occurrence of fetal damage.
- B2: studies in animals are inadequate or may be lacking, but available data show no evidence of an increased occurrence of fetal damage.
- B3: studies in animals have shown evidence of an increased occurrence of fetal damage, the significance of which is considered uncertain in humans.

Category C
These are drugs which, owing to their pharmacological effects, have caused or may be suspected of causing harmful effects on the human fetus or neonate without causing malformations. These effects may be reversible.

Category D
These are drugs that have caused, are suspected to have caused or may be expected to cause, an increased incidence of human fetal malformations or irreversible damage. These drugs may also have adverse pharmacological effects.

Category X
These are drugs which have such a high risk of causing permanent damage to the fetus that they should not be used in pregnancy or when there is a possibility of pregnancy.

From Prescribing medicines in pregnancy database, 2016, Therapeutic Goods Administration, used by permission of the Australian Government <www.tga.gov.au/prescribing-medicines-pregnancy-database>

Box 28.2 **Examples of databases on teratogenic information**

- MotherToBaby, a service of the Organization of Teratology Information Specialists (OTIS): http://mothertobaby.org
- Reproductive Toxicology Centre: www.reprotox.org
- European Network Teratology Information Services: www.entis-org.eu
- Teratogen Information System: http://depts.washington.edu/terisweb/

Drug pharmacokinetics and pregnancy

Drug pharmacokinetics is affected by the complex changes that occur in maternal, fetal and placental physiology during pregnancy.

Drug absorption

- Reduction in intestinal motility results in a 30%–50% increase in gastric and intestinal emptying time.
- Reduced gastric acid secretions result in an increase in gastric pH.

- Nausea and vomiting may affect the ability of a drug to be absorbed.
- Increased cardiac output, respiratory rate, tidal volumes and pulmonary blood flow influence absorption of inhalational agents.

Drug distribution

- Plasma volume increases by 50%, resulting in a decrease in peak serum concentration of many drugs.
- Body fat is increased in pregnancy, creating a larger volume of distribution for lipophilic substances.

Protein binding

- Plasma volume increases at a greater rate than albumin production, resulting in a physiologic dilutional hypoalbuminaemia.
- Maternal and placental hormones occupy available binding sites on proteins, thereby decreasing the ability to bind drugs.
- The net effect of a decreased binding capacity is an increase in the unbound ('free') pharmacologically active drug fraction.

Drug elimination

- Glomerular filtration rate increases by 50% in pregnancy, resulting in increased renal clearance of drugs.
- Pregnancy hormones have a variable effect on hepatic microsomal enzymes and biliary excretion, resulting in altered drug metabolism.

Placental–fetal compartment

- Unbound, non-ionised, lipid soluble molecules have a greater ability to cross the placental barrier.
- Fetal albumin concentrations increase as pregnancy advances, and fetal plasma proteins show variable binding affinities for different drugs.
- Fetal and placental drug metabolism occurs.

Subsequently, embryonic/fetal exposure to maternally ingested drugs is complex, and the effect is dependent on the specific drug properties and gestational age at the time of exposure.

Specific drugs in pregnancy

Anticonvulsants

- Aim for monotherapy (at higher dose if necessary) if possible.
- Supplemental folic acid reduces the risk of associated congenital abnormalities.

CARBAMAZEPINE

- often considered the drug of choice because of relatively low teratogenic effects
- associated with neural tube defects
- associated with haemorrhagic disease of the newborn, which can be prevented by maternal supplementation of vitamin K in the last 4 weeks of pregnancy

PHENYTOIN

- associated with fetal hydantoin syndrome: intrauterine growth restriction (IUGR), microcephaly, digital/nail hypoplasia, cleft lip/palate, low nasal bridge, rib/heart/genitourinary anomalies

VALPROIC ACID
- associated with neural tube defects (1%–2%), cleft palate and cardiac anomalies

Antibiotics
- the most commonly prescribed drugs in pregnancy

PENICILLINS/CEPHALOSPORINS
- clearance increased and, therefore, higher dose required to achieve similar antimicrobial concentrations
- reassuring large clinical experience

TETRACYCLINE
- may cause discolouration of adult teeth

NITROFURANTOIN
- little teratogenic risk
- associated with haemolytic reactions in those with glucose-6-phosphate dehydrogenase deficiency

SULFONAMIDES
- displaces bilirubin from carrier protein and may increase risk of neonatal jaundice if used late in third trimester

DOXYCYCLINE
- little teratogenic risk

METRONIDAZOLE
- little teratogenic risk

AZITHROMYCIN
- little teratogenic risk

Methotrexate
- Exposure in first trimester is associated with craniofacial, skeletal, cardiopulmonary and gastrointestinal abnormalities, and developmental delay.
- Exposure later in pregnancy appears to be safe.

Warfarin
- a recognised teratogen
- warfarin embryopathy: nasal hypoplasia, microphthalmia, limb hypoplasia, IUGR, central nervous system (CNS) abnormalities, deafness, developmental delay and neurologic dysfunction
- associated with intrauterine fetal death (IUFD) and stillbirth
- compatible with breastfeeding, as does not enter breast milk to significant degree

Lithium
- associated with small increased risk of cardiac anomalies
- associated with fetal and neonatal cardiac arrhythmias, hypoglycaemia, nephrogenic diabetes insipidus, polyhydramnios and preterm delivery

Retinoids

- can affect multiple organ systems, including CNS, cardiovascular and endocrine

Angiotensin-converting enzyme (ACE) inhibitors

- Exposure in first trimester is associated with risk of heart and CNS abnormalities.
- Exposure in later pregnancy is associated with renal failure, oligohydramnios, aortic arch obstructive malformations, patent ductus arteriosus and IUFD.

Selective serotonin reuptake inhibitors (SSRIs)

- There is a small increase in the risk of cardiac defects (especially paroxetine).
- Sertraline is associated with an increased risk of omphalocele.
- Paroxetine is associated with the risk of anencephaly, craniosynostosis and omphalocele.
- Exposure late in pregnancy is associated with transient neonatal complications, including jitteriness, transient tachypnoea of newborn, weak cry and poor tone.

Drugs of abuse in pregnancy

Alcohol

- Alcohol and its metabolites cross the placenta and are directly toxic to the fetus.
- Minimum safe exposure levels are uncertain.
- Fetal alcohol syndrome is associated with neurological impairment, microcephaly, long philtrum, thin upper lip, flattening of maxilla, microphthalmia, hypotonia and IUGR.

Cigarette smoking

- Smoking is associated with spontaneous abortion, IUGR, low birth weight, preterm delivery, premature rupture of membranes, placenta praevia and placental abruption.
- These complications contribute to an increased perinatal mortality rate in smokers.
- Effects are dose related.
- Mothers who smoke are more likely to use illicit drugs concurrently.

Cocaine

- Cocaine use results in vasoconstriction, tachycardia, hypertension and an increase in circulating catecholamines.
- It is associated with an increased risk of spontaneous abortion, IUGR, prematurity and placental abruption.
- Teratogenic effects are uncertain.
- Beta-blockers should not be used to control maternal blood pressure because the resultant unopposed alpha-adrenergic stimulation can lead to coronary vasoconstriction and end-organ ischaemia.

Cannabis

- Cannabis is the most common drug of abuse in pregnancy.
- Cannabis use does not appear to be an independent risk factor for adverse pregnancy outcomes.
- Cigarettes, alcohol and other illicit drug use are common.

Amphetamines
- High-quality information on the effect in pregnancy is lacking.
- Amphetamines are associated with abruption and preterm delivery.

Lysergic acid diethylamide (LSD)
- There are isolated reports of amniotic bands with LSD use in pregnancy.

Glue/petrol
- Long-term toluene inhalation is associated with cerebellar degeneration and cortical atrophy.
- Infants have an increased risk of neurodevelopmental problems, including spastic quadriplegia and lead poisoning.

Opiates
- Opiate abuse is associated with a two to five times increased risk of perinatal mortality.
- Many of the maternal risks are similar to those that occur in the non-pregnant state: infection, vasculitis, nutritional deficiencies and psychosocial difficulties. Pregnancy-specific complications include pre-eclampsia, antepartum haemorrhage and puerperal morbidity.
- Fetal problems include microcephaly, IUGR, prematurity, malpresentation and passage of meconium.
- Neonatal problems include those associated with prematurity, opiate withdrawal ('neonatal abstinence syndrome'), postnatal growth deficiency, microcephaly, neurobehavioural deficits and sudden infant death syndrome.
- The time of onset of neonatal opiate withdrawal depends on the half-life of the drug: heroine and morphine 48 hours; methadone 72 hours.

MANAGEMENT OF OPIATE ABUSE IN PREGNANCY
- methadone stabilisation preferred
- acute withdrawal avoided
- regular antenatal care, preferably at multidisciplinary specialised clinics
- screen for blood-borne viruses and sexually transmitted diseases
- serial ultrasound assessment of fetal growth and wellbeing
- antenatal paediatric assessment regarding neonatal withdrawal and social circumstances/safety
- avoid narcotics for pain relief if possible
- continuous cardiotocograph monitoring in labour (may show reduced variability)
- avoid opioid antagonists as may precipitate acute withdrawal

References
Buhimschi, C., Weiner, C., 2009. Medications in pregnancy and lactation. Part 1: teratology. Obstet. Gynecol. 113, 166–188.

Buhimschi, C., Weiner, C., 2009. Medications in pregnancy and lactation. Part 2: drugs with minimal or unknown human teratogenic effect. Obstet. Gynecol. 113, 417–432.

Kennedy, D., 2012. Medications in pregnancy and lactation. Aust. Doc. 17–24.

Kennedy, D., 2014. The safety of drugs in pregnancy and breastfeeding. O&G Magazine. 16;2, 47–49.

Loebstein, R., Koren, G., 2002. Clinical relevance of therapeutic drug monitoring during pregnancy. Ther. Drug Monit. 24, 15–22.

Chapter 29

Infections in pregnancy

Michael Flynn

Urinary tract infection

Asymptomatic bacteriuria
- Incidence is 2%–10% in pregnancy. This is similar prevalence to non-pregnant women.
- If untreated, 15%–45% will develop symptomatic infection.
- Treatment can prevent 70%–80% of urinary tract infections and pyelonephritis.
- Diagnosis: a single voided specimen urine culture can detect 80% of asymptomatic carriers.
- About 75%–90% of urinary tract infections in pregnancy are due to *Escherichia coli*.
- Treatment: amoxycillin or cephalosporin are safe in pregnancy.
- Prevention: screening mid-stream urine (MSU) is performed as first-visit screen.
- Bacteriuria is associated with increased risk of preterm birth, low birth weight and increased perinatal mortality, and treatment has been shown to decrease these risks.

Acute symptomatic urinary tract infection
- Acute cystitis occurs in about 1% of pregnancies, especially in the second trimester. Pyelonephritis occurs in 1%–2% of pregnancies, in which 7% of women will suffer from bacteraemia and 1% septic shock.
- Possible reasons for increased pyelonephritis in pregnancy include anatomic changes to the urinary tract, and possible immunosuppression.

MANAGEMENT
- Rehydrate.
- Diagnose from MSU specimens and blood cultures.
- Antibiotics are given intravenously if the patient is systemically unwell.
- Lower temperature (paracetamol).
- Assess the fetus.
- There is a recurrence of 10%–15%; therefore, test urine regularly.

Relapses and reinfection

- *Relapse* means recurrence of infection by the same organism, and *reinfection* is due to a different strain of bacteria after successful eradication.
- Relapse or reinfection occurs in 10%–15% of treated urinary tract infections.

MANAGEMENT

- Treat the current infection.
- Prophylaxis uses oral nitrofurantoin 50 mg daily or cephalothin 500 mg daily for duration of pregnancy.
- Intravenous pyelogram is required after delivery.

Syphilis

Incidence. Incidence in Australia is 2 in 1000.

Screening

- This should be performed with a specific *Treponema pallidum* assay such as *T. pallidum* haemagglutination assay (TPHA), *T. pallidum* particle assay or syphilis enzyme immunoassay (EIA).
- Syphilis may be transmitted to the fetus in the second trimester, with the following consequences:
  - premature delivery in 20%
  - intrauterine fetal death (IUFD) in 20%
  - subclinical infection in 20%
  - congenital infection in 40%

Clinical syndromes

PRIMARY SYPHILIS

- Incubation period is 10–90 days with an average of 21 days.
- It presents as a painless genital sore; then in the third to sixth week lymphadenopathy occurs, and serology is positive in 25% of cases.

SECONDARY SYPHILIS

- Bilateral symmetrical papulosquamous eruption appears 2 weeks to 6 months after primary lesion. *T. pallidum* is present in lymph nodes and condyloma lata.

LATENT SYPHILIS

- This covers early syphilis (duration < 4 years) and late syphilis (duration > 4 years). It is non-infectious except in pregnancy.

TERTIARY SYPHILIS

- Neurological and vascular lesions are present.

In pregnancy, the fetus is 'safe' under 18 weeks gestation because it cannot mount an immunological attack and cause tissue damage and inflammation. Congenital syphilis is associated with intrauterine growth restriction (IUGR), café-au-lait spots, bullous rash, saddle nose, nasal congestion, hepatosplenomegaly, notched teeth, osteochondritis and corneal scarring. Congenital syphilis may also be asymptomatic.

Management of syphilis

- Early syphilis (primary, secondary or latent of < 12 months): treat with benzathine penicillin 2.4 million units intramuscularly as a single dose, or procaine penicillin 1.5 g intramuscularly daily for 10 days, or erythromycin 500 mg four times a day for 15 days.
- Late syphilis (incubation > 12 months): treat with intramuscular benzathine penicillin 1.8 g (2.4 million units) weekly for 3 weeks, or procaine penicillin 1.5 g intramuscularly for 15 days, or erythromycin 500 mg four times a day for 30 days.
- Check for other sexually transmitted diseases and treat the partner.

Toxoplasmosis

- *Toxoplasma gondii* is an obligate intracellular organism. The birth prevalence is 0.23 in 1000 births to non-immune mothers. The rate of maternal infection is 1.6 in 1000.
- The risk of transmission rises with increasing gestational age. However, the fetus is more severely affected if infected before 20 weeks gestation, and is usually asymptomatic if infected in the third trimester.
- Congenital toxoplasmosis can result in microcephalus, hydrocephalus, seizures, reduced intellect, chorioretinitis, cataract, hepatitis and pneumonitis.
- Primary infection is rare in pregnancy in Australia.
- Antenatal screening is not recommended in Australia, with selective testing recommended only for those women at increased risk or those with symptoms of acute toxoplasmosis including malaise, fever and cervical lymphadenopathy. Advice for risk minimisation in pregnancy includes washing hands after gardening, washing vegetables, avoiding uncooked meat and minimising contact with young kittens and their litter.
- Immunoglobulin M (IgM) is not a reliable marker of recent infection.
- If IgG-positive and IgM-positive and symptoms suggestive of infection, then repeat and check IgG titres and IgG avidity (suggestive of infection within 3 months).
- If the above is suggestive of recent acute maternal toxoplasmosis, then treatment depends on gestational age.
- Consider treatment with sulfadoxine and pyrimethamine and folic acid or spiramycin if maternal diagnosis certain.
- Ultrasound and amniocentesis with *T. gondii* polymerase chain reaction (PCR) on amniotic fluid helps with diagnosis.

Rubella

- The incubation period is 14–21 days; then a rash develops which lasts 2–7 days.
- Fewer than 5% of women are not immune to rubella at antenatal clinic screening.

Possible outcomes of maternal rubella infection

- no effect on the fetus
- placental infection only
- placental/fetal infection causing asymptomatic infection but affecting organs
- death of fetus (abortion, IUFD)

- congenital rubella syndrome (bilateral cataracts, IUGR, congenital heart disease, especially patent ductus arteriosus, sensorineural deafness and microphthalmia)

Risk to fetus of maternal infection

- At < 8 weeks gestation, up to 85% of the fetuses are infected and all infected fetuses will develop complications such as cardiac, eye, ear and neurological defects.
- At < 12 weeks gestation, 50%–80% of fetuses are infected, and of these 65%–85% have clinical defects.
- Between 13 and 16 weeks gestation, 30% of fetuses are infected and one-third suffer sensorineural deafness.
- At > 16 weeks gestation, 10% of fetuses are infected, with rare clinical manifestations.

Diagnosis of maternal rubella

- four-fold rise in IgG titres
- rubella-specific IgM antibody (false-positives occur with rheumatic factor)
- reinfection: low IgM and rapid rise in IgG
- reinfection occurring more often with vaccination (80%) than with natural immunity (3.4%)

Diagnosis of intrauterine/congenital rubella

- rubella PCR, culture and fetal IgM can be performed following chorionic villus sampling, amniocentesis of fetal blood sampling
- virus isolated from infant's pharynx, urine and cerebrospinal fluid in the first 3 months of life
- IgM rubella-specific antibody present in cord blood
- persistence of rubella antibodies after 6 months

Vaccination

It is advisable not to vaccinate during or within 3 months of pregnancy. However, if vaccination occurs in pregnancy or 3 months before pregnancy, the risk to the fetus is negligible. Rubella vaccination affords protection in 95% of cases. The vaccine consists of attenuated virus given subcutaneously.

Hepatitis B

The incubation period ranges from 50 to 180 days.

Hepatitis B virus (HBV)

- The infective particle consists of two shells, the outer surface antigen (HBsAg) and the inner core (HBcAg).
- The organism cannot be cultured, and diagnosis is dependent on the presence of serological markers of antigen and antibody to the viral particle.
- The surface antigen (HBsAg) is the first to appear and is present throughout the acute infective stage until the presence of surface antibody (anti-HBs), which signals recovery and immunity.
- The hepatitis Be antigen (HBeAg) is a soluble protein derived from the core. It is detected in the acute phase of the infection and continues to be present as long as viral replication persists. This represents high infectivity.
- Chronic carriers of hepatitis B have HBsAg in their blood for more than 6 months.

Factors in perinatal transmission

The major risk to the neonate is vertical transmission, mostly at the time of delivery.

- About 85%–90% of infants will develop hepatitis B if their mothers are HBeAg-positive.
- Fewer than 5% of infants will be infected if the mother is anti-HBe-positive.
- Intrauterine transmission occurs in only 3%–8% of infants of HBeAg-positive mothers.

Prevention of hepatitis B

- Hepatitis B immunoglobulin and vaccine has 94% efficacy in preventing perinatal transmission.
- Hepatitis B immunoglobulin alone has an efficacy of 71%, while hepatitis B vaccine alone has 75% efficacy.
- Therefore, to prevent transmission to the newborn, it is necessary to give the baby 0.5 mL hepatitis B immunoglobulin (intramuscularly) and hepatitis B vaccine within 12 hours. Minimise invasive procedures.
- There is no evidence that caesarean section reduces the perinatal transmission of hepatitis B.
- With vaccine and immunoglobulin given, breastfeeding poses no additional risk of vertical transmission.

Hepatitis C

- Screen at first antenatal visit, especially if from high-risk group.
- Vertical transmission is 6% if the hepatitis C virus is ribonucleic acid (RNA)-positive. Risk is proportional to RNA load.
- Minimise invasive procedures.
- There is no clear evidence of mode of delivery and reduction of perinatal transmission.
- Decreased use of internal monitoring devices may reduce risk of vertical transmission.
- Hepatitis C virus has been found in breast milk, although studies have not shown a higher risk of vertical transmission during breastfeeding. Consider expressing and discarding milk if nipples cracked and bleeding.

Human immunodeficiency virus (HIV) and pregnancy

Maternal to child transmission (MTCT)

- The management of a mother who is HIV-positive in pregnancy will depend on a number of factors.
  - Whether the patient was known to be HIV-positive preconception and on highly active antiretroviral therapy (HAART).
  - HIV RNA viral load.
  - Other concurrent medical conditions.
  - Effective transplacental: data from termination of pregnancies at 16–24 weeks gestation show that up to 66% of fetuses are infected.
- Labour and delivery: transmission occurs when the neonate is exposed to infected blood.

- Postpartum transmission: occurs through breastfeeding. In industrialised countries, HIV-infected mothers are advised not to breastfeed.

Managing HIV in pregnancy

- Adopt an appropriate multidisciplinary approach with adequate counselling.
- At the first visit, perform the routine screening tests plus those for *Toxoplasma,* cytomegalovirus, tuberculosis, *Cryptococcus* and *Candida.*
- Cervical cytology and colposcopy are essential.
- Review immune status with CD4 lymphocyte count and viral RNA copy number.
- Check full blood count, liver function test, urea and electrolytes.
- Avoid invasive testing (amniocentesis, chorionic villus sampling, cordocentesis).
- If conceived while on HAART and viral load is undetectable, there is no contraindication to vaginal delivery. If the baby is formula fed, the MTCT is considered 2%.
- If viral load greater than 50 copies /mL at 36 weeks, strong consideration to intrapartum zidovudine, planned caesarean section and formula feeding should be employed.
- The neonate should undertake an antiretroviral post-exposure prophylaxis regimen individualised according to risk as the final strategy to minimise MTCT.

Cytomegalovirus

- Cytomegalovirus (CMV) is a herpes virus and the commonest cause of intrauterine infection. Primary infection occurs in 1 in 300 pregnancies, with fetal infection occurring in 40% of these, and 10% of infected fetuses having congenital problems.
- Most primary infections are asymptomatic, but suspect in viral illness with atypical lymphocytes which is monospot-negative. Antenatal testing is complex.
- At-risk women include those in prolonged contact with young children including day care workers.

Fetal complications

These include IUFD, IUGR, hepatosplenomegaly, central nervous system complications, ascites, abdominal calcification, intracranial calcification, hyperechogenic bowel and neonatal jaundice. The major long-term effect is neurosensory deafness.

Diagnosis

- Anti-CMV IgM is the screening tool but may remain positive for months after primary infection.
- If IgM-positive, then repeat 2–4 weeks later and check IgG avidity.
- Direct viral detection can be via CMV fluorescence antibody, CMV isolation or PCR of maternal fluids.
- Once primary infection is confirmed, fetal diagnosis can be via amniocentesis or fetal blood sampling. However, positive results do not predict any degree of fetal damage and sensitivity less than 20 weeks duration is less than 50%.

Pathogenesis of fetal complications

- This includes placental infection.
- Fetal infection causes cytolysis with areas of focal necrosis and healing by fibrosis and calcification. The risk of fetal infection from primary maternal infection is approximately 30%, but the severity of fetal damage is variable and unpredictable.

- Of infants exposed to CMV in utero, the overall risk of long-term sequelae of a congenitally infected child may be 15% with these sequelae including sensorineural deafness, epilepsy or learning disability.

Antenatal advice

- All pregnant women should be advised about simple infection control mechanisms to reduce transmission risk (e.g. hand-washing after nappy changes and contact with respiratory secretions in children under age 2).
- There is no therapy that alters the disease course; therefore, counselling and support are required.
- The risk of transmission is equal throughout the pregnancy; however, an adverse neurological outcome is more frequent in the first half of pregnancy.

Listeriosis

Listeria is a small, non-sporing, gram-positive rod-shaped bacterium. Those infected may present with malaise, headache, fever, diarrhoea and abdominal pain.

Bacteriological investigations include blood and urine cultures, and cervical swab culture. Amniocentesis with Gram stain and culture is definitive diagnosis.

Complications of listeriosis in pregnancy

- fetal: IUFD and premature labour; mortality rate if untreated is 40% in the second and third trimesters
- neonatal: microabscesses in liver, lungs, adrenals and central nervous system; treatment of maternal listeriosis is with amoxycillin, gentamicin and delivery dependent on gestation
- advise to avoid uncooked or unpasteurised foods, pâté and soft cheeses to decrease pregnancy risk

Varicella zoster

This is known as chickenpox in the primary infection and as shingles with reactivation of the infection. Up to 4% of pregnant women are not immune. The incubation period lasts 14–18 days. The contagious period lasts 7 days after the rash disappears.

Congenital varicella syndrome can show as skin scars, eye and limb abnormalities, IUGR, cortical atrophy or decreased sphincter control. It is gestational related with an incidence of 0.55% less than 12 weeks, 1.4% at 12–28 weeks and no cases reported after 28 weeks.

Infection in late pregnancy

In late pregnancy, the severity of perinatal infection is dependent on timing before delivery. Up to 7 days before delivery, maternal IgG is protective and neonatal infection is usually mild. If infection occurs 7 days before or 2 days after delivery, there is a risk of severe neonatal varicella infection.

Management

- Establish the diagnosis by serology.
- Isolate the woman.

- If zoster rash appears over 7 days before labour and the vesicles have crusted, the risk of transmission is negligible.
- If zoster rash appears within 7 days of delivery, then zoster immunoglobulin for the neonate should be considered.
- Prepregnancy screening should include zoster serology.

EXPOSURE IN PREGNANCY
- If seronegative and the exposure is < 96 hours, then passive immunisation with varicella zoster immunoglobulin.

Group B streptococcus

This is the leading cause of early-onset neonatal sepsis. Colonisation of the vagina occurs in up to 20% of women at some stage during pregnancy. The reservoir of group B streptococcus (GBS) also occurs in the gastrointestinal tract. This recolonises the genital tract after treatment, so there is no need to treat the asymptomatic woman unless in labour.

Neonatal sepsis occurs with an incidence of 1 in 1000, although 1%–2% of infants will be colonised at birth.

Management
- Antepartum treatment is relatively ineffective because the gastrointestinal tract is the primary reservoir.
- Intrapartum antibiotics are used in the prevention of neonatal sepsis and also to reduce maternal morbidity.
- Guidelines for prevention suggest either a risk-based or screening approach to identify those patients requiring intrapartum antibiotics. It is probable that screening has a more protective approach than the risk-based approach.
- Screening is via low vaginal and anorectal swab between 35 and 37 weeks.
- Clinical risk factors include < 37 weeks gestation, rupture of membranes > 18 hours, maternal fever > 38°C.
- All women with a previously affected GBS child or GBS bacteriuria in pregnancy should be treated intrapartum.
- Intrapartum treatment is with a benzylpenicillin 3 g intravenous loading dose followed by 1.8 g intravenously every 4 hours until delivery. If there is a penicillin allergy, then clindamycin 900 mg intravenously every 8 hours is appropriate.

Herpes simplex

- Incidence of newborn infection is rare (1 in 10 000 to 1 in 40 000).
- Up to 60% of neonates with herpes infection do not have associated maternal history or signs of herpes at the time of delivery. Primary genital herpes is more likely to cause severe infection and neonatal symptoms than recurrent infection.
- Congenital or transplacental spread is rare and is associated with primary infection.
- Vertical transmission at time of vaginal delivery may occur in up to 40%–50% of deliveries from women with primary infection, and in up to 1 to 3 % with recurrent infection.

Risk factors for intrapartum infection
- maternal primary infection
- multiple lesions
- premature delivery
- premature rupture of membranes

Management
- If lesions are present and membranes have been ruptured for < 4 hours, a caesarean section reduces the risk of transmission, particularly in primary infections in women who are herpes simplex antibody negative.
- Acyclovir shortens the duration of viral shedding, especially during the primary attack.
- If recurrent infections during pregnancy, consider antiviral therapy from 36 weeks gestation.

Further reading

Australasian Society for Infectious Diseases (ASID), 2014. Management of Perinatal Infections. ASID, Sydney.

Chapter 30

Red blood cell and platelet alloimmunisation in pregnancy

Glenn J Gardener

Red blood cell isoimmunisation

Background and pathophysiology

Maternal alloimmunisation against red blood cell (RBC) antigens leads to the formation of IgG-class antibodies that can cross the placenta and cause fetal RBC haemolysis, resulting in haemolytic disease of the fetus and newborn (HDFN). Approximately 1.2% of pregnancies will have RBC antibodies detected with clinically significant RBC antibodies occurring at a prevalence of 0.4%. Anti-D is the most commonly encountered RBC antibody in pregnancy followed by anti-K (Kell) and anti-c. In the fetus, haemolytic disease can cause severe anaemia, hydrops fetalis and perinatal death if levels of fetal haemoglobin are < 5 g/dL. In the neonate, haemolytic disease can cause severe anaemia, hyperbilirubinaemia and kernicterus.

Before the widespread introduction of anti-D immunoglobulin (Ig) prophylaxis, HDFN secondary to Rh alloimmunisation was a major cause of perinatal morbidity and mortality. HDFN due to Rh isoimmunisation is a preventable disease and anti-D immunoprophylaxis has been responsible for a 100-fold decrease in perinatal mortality from Rh alloimmunisation over the last four decades.

Anti-K antibodies cause anaemia secondary to euthyroid suppression, and severe fetal anaemia can occur at low antibody levels.

The management of RBC alloimmunisation in pregnancy requires collaborative care between obstetricians, maternal fetal medicine specialists, neonatologists and the blood transfusion laboratory. While fetal and neonatal risks are usually the main concern in pregnancies with RBC antibodies, the screening and provision of appropriately matched blood or blood products to the mother when required should not be overlooked.

Antibodies against the ABO blood group system can also cause mild to moderate anaemia and jaundice in the newborn and occasionally in the fetus.

Prevention of HDFN

- All pregnant women should have a blood group and antibody screen performed at first booking and repeated at 28 weeks gestation.
- Rh-negative pregnant women are at risk of Rh alloimmunisation due to fetomaternal haemorrhage and less frequently from needle sharing, receiving an incompatible Rh-positive RBC transfusion or following transplantation.
- Antenatal and postnatal anti-D immunoglobulin (anti-D Ig) prophylaxis significantly reduces the incidence of HDFN by reducing sensitisation of pregnant women to the Rh antigen.
- For anti-D to be effective, it must be given in sufficient dose and before alloimmunisation has occurred.

Current recommendations from Australia's National Blood Authority (2003) for anti-D immunoprophylaxis are as follows.

All Rh-negative women (who are not already alloimmunised to Rh factor) should be offered anti-D Ig.

- first trimester indications: anti-D 250 IU (50 µcg)
  - chorionic villus sampling
  - miscarriage from 12 weeks gestation (there is insufficient evidence to suggest that a threatened miscarriage before 12 weeks gestation necessitates anti-D administration)
  - miscarriage requiring curettage prior to 12 weeks gestation
  - termination of pregnancy
  - ectopic pregnancy
- second and third trimester indications: anti-D 625 IU (125 µcg)
  - obstetric haemorrhage
  - amniocentesis, cordocentesis
  - external cephalic version
  - abdominal trauma, or any other suspected intrauterine bleeding or sensitising event
- All Rh-negative women (who are not already alloimmunised to Rh) at 28 weeks gestation and again at 34 weeks gestation: 625 IU (125 µcg).
- Postnatally all Rh-negative women who deliver an Rh-positive baby should have quantification of fetomaternal haemorrhage by the Kleihaur–Betke test or by flow cytometry to guide the appropriate dose of anti-D to be administered within 72 hours of birth.

Prepregnancy management of RBC alloimmunisation

- Women with RBC antibodies should have prepregnancy counselling with a care provider who has knowledge and expertise with the condition (e.g. maternal fetal medicine specialist).
- Information regarding the possible implications to the fetus, neonate and mother as a result of maternal RBC alloimmunisation should be provided.

Antenatal management of RBC alloimmunisation

- When RBC alloimmunisation is identified during pregnancy, the particular antibody or antibodies should be specified and their levels reported by titre and/or quantitation.

- The paternal phenotype can be ascertained by serology while paternal genotyping can establish whether he is homozygous or heterozygous.
- If the paternal genotype is homozygous for the RBC antigen, then all offspring are potentially at risk of HDFN.

Determination of fetal Rh type

- Non-invasive fetal genotyping using cell-free fetal DNA from maternal blood can accurately determine fetal Rh type without imposing any risk to the pregnancy.
- Invasive testing by chorionic villus sampling or amniocentesis is no longer necessary to establish the fetal Rh genotype.
- Non-invasive testing of the fetal genotype is not available for RBC antigens other than Rh.
- Invasive testing may be considered if the benefits of the procedure outweigh the risks (miscarriage, worsening of alloimmunisation).
- The cause of alloimmunisation and previous pregnancy history (including neonatal outcomes) should be ascertained so as to gain an assessment of risk of HDFN.
- Paternal RBC antigen phenotype or genotype testing should be established where appropriate but the results should not be relied on alone for important clinical decisions in case of non-paternity.

Antibody quantification

- When a clinically significant antibody is detected in pregnancy, antibody levels should be assessed monthly until 28 weeks gestation and then every 2 weeks thereafter until delivery.
- An anti-D level < 4 IU/mL (or anti-c level < 7.5 IU/mL) correlates with a low risk of fetal anaemia. For antibody levels above these thresholds, referral to a maternal fetal medicine (MFM) specialist is indicated.
- Referral to an MFM specialist should also be considered with any level of anti-K antibodies detected as fetal anaemia can occur even with low titres.

Non-invasive assessment of fetal anaemia

- Pregnancies at risk of HDFN should be monitored by weekly ultrasound measurement of the fetal middle cerebral artery peak systolic velocity (MCA PSV).
- MCA PSV monitoring of fetal anaemia has 100% sensitivity and a false-positive rate of 12% for predicting moderate or severe fetal anaemia.
- Referral to an MFM specialist is recommended when the MCA PSV rises above 1.5 multiples of the median (MoM) or there are other signs of fetal anaemia (e.g. fetal skin oedema, polyhydramnios, fetal cardiomegaly, ascites or hydrops).
- If the MCA PSV is > 1.5 MoM, fetal blood sampling (FBS) and intrauterine transfusion (IUT) are indicated. The risk of fetal loss associated with FBS and IUT is 1%–3% per procedure.

Intrauterine transfusion

- Ultrasound-guided IUT is undertaken in a tertiary healthcare facility when FBS confirms fetal anaemia.

- RBC preparations for IUT should be type O negative for the corresponding maternal RBC antibodies.
- In cases of severe fetal anaemia, IUT with RBCs can prevent hydrops and fetal death and promote prolongation of the pregnancy.
- Repeat fetal transfusions may be needed, with timing based on empiric time intervals or on MCA PSV values.

RBCs for intrauterine transfusion should be:

- leucodepleted
- CMV negative
- irradiated to prevent graft versus host disease
- plasma reduced (haematocrit 0.75–0.85)
- < 5 days old
- group O with low-titre haemolysins (or ABO identical with the fetus)
- Rh and Kell negative, and RBC antigen negative for maternal alloantibodies
- indirect antiglobulin test crossmatch compatible with the mother's plasma

Platelet isoimmunisation

- Alloimmune thrombocytopenia occurs with destruction of fetal platelets by maternal allo-antibodies directed against paternally inherited fetal platelet antigens.
- This leads to fetal and neonatal thrombocytopenia and affects 1 in 1000 births.
- Fetal and neonatal alloimmune thrombocytopenia (FNAIT) is the leading cause of severe thrombocytopenia in the fetus and neonate and of intracranial haemorrhage (ICH) in term infants.
- In infants with FNAIT, up to 75% of haemorrhages occur prenatally.
- The risk of recurrence of FNAIT is very high if there has been a previous affected infant.
- FNAIT should also be suspected in cases of intrauterine fetal death attributed to intracranial haemorrhage, even if confirmatory investigations were not performed.

Pathophysiology

- Human platelet antigens (HPA) are epitopes on platelet surface glycoproteins which are inherited in an autosomal co-dominant manner.
- HPA-1a is the most common antigen incompatibility in and approximately 2% of Caucasians are HPA-1a negative. HPA-4a incompatibility is more common in Asians.
- A pregnant mother who is HPA negative can become sensitised to HPA-positive fetal platelets and produce IgG class antibodies that can cross the placenta and cause fetal platelet destruction and thrombocytopenia.
- In contrast to Rh alloimmunisation, FNAIT often affects a first pregnancy and anti-platelet antibody levels are not predictive of fetal or neonatal thrombocytopenia.
- The severity of FNAIT is affected by pregnancy order, previous history and the particular HPA antigen involved.
- In FNAIT, the mother remains asymptomatic and maternal platelet levels are normal.

Diagnosis

- All of the following features are required for a diagnosis of FNAIT:
  - fetal or neonatal thrombocytopenia

- identification of a fetal/paternal and maternal platelet antigen incompatibility
- identification of maternal antibodies against that antigen

Parental and fetal/neonatal platelet antigen typing

- Parental platelet antigen typing is recommended in the following situations:
  - a previous proven or suggested history of FNAIT
  - fetal cerebral ventriculomegaly or intracranial haemorrhage
  - a newborn with severe thrombocytopenia (platelet count is $< 50 \times 109$/L)
  - a maternal sister with a previous proven or suggested history of FNAIT
- Routine prenatal screening by maternal HPA-1a typing is not cost-effective due to the low prevalence of FNAIT and inability to predict the risk of intracranial haemorrhage in pregnancies at risk.
- If the father is heterozygous for the platelet antigen, fetal platelet antigen genotyping can be performed by amniocentesis which carries a risk of miscarriage of 0.5%–1%. If the fetus does not carry the platelet antigen that caused the maternal alloimmunisation, then it is not at risk of FNAIT.

Management of pregnancies at risk of FNAIT

- FNAIT should be managed in an experienced multidisciplinary environment lead by an MFM specialist and involving haematology, neonatology and blood transfusion services.
- Intravenous immunoglobulin (IVIG) and glucocorticoid therapy can reduce the severity of FNAIT, thereby reducing the need for FBS and platelet IUT.
- IUT with platelets can prevent fetal or neonatal haemorrhage from severe thrombocytopenia, regardless of cause.
- FBS and platelet IUT should be considered in FNAIT cases where there is recent intracranial haemorrhage, in cases that are shown to be refractory to IVIG therapy and glucocorticoid therapy.
- Caesarean delivery is usually undertaken at 36–37 weeks gestation and if planning vaginal delivery, FBS should be undertaken to ensure that the fetal platelet count is $> 100 \times 10^9$/L.
- Instrumental delivery, fetal scalp sampling and fetal scalp electrode monitoring should be avoided.
- Pregnancies at risk of FNAIT should be monitored by ultrasound every 4 weeks from 16 weeks gestation until delivery for evidence of fetal intracranial haemorrhage.
- In severe cases of FNAIT with intracranial haemorrhage in the second trimester and where the partner is heterozygous for the platelet antigen, then in vitro fertilisation with preimplantation genetic diagnosis can be used or alternatively a platelet antigen compatible sperm donor.

Further reading

Liley, H.G., Gardener, G.J., 2014. Immune hemolytic disease. In: Nathan and Oski's Hematology and Oncology of Infancy and Childhood, 8th ed. Elsevier, Philadelphia, pp. 76–100.

National Blood Authority, 2003. Guidelines on the prophylactic use of Rh D immunoglobulin (anti-D) in obstetrics. National Health and Medical Research Council.

Norfolk, D., 2013. Handbook of Transfusion Medicine, 5th ed. United Kingdom Blood Services, London.

Royal College of Obstetricians and Gynaecologists, 2014. The management of women with red cell antibodies during pregnancy. Green-top Guideline No. 65. RCOG, London.

Soothill, P.W., Finning, K., Latham, T., et al., 2014. Use of cffDNA to avoid administration of anti-D to pregnant women when the fetus is RhD-negative: implementation in the NHS. Br. J. Obstet. Gynaecol. 122 (12), 1682–1686.

Society for Maternal-Fetal Medicine (SMFM), Berry, S.M., Stone, J., Norton, M.E., et al., 2013. Fetal blood sampling. Am. J. Obstet. Gynecol. 209 (3), 170–180.

Spencer, J.A., Burrows, R.F., 2001. Feto-maternal allo-immune thrombocytopenia: a literature review and statistical analysis. Aust. N. Z. J. Obstet. Gynaecol. 41 (1), 45–55.

Chapter 31

Antepartum haemorrhage

Michael Flynn

Definition. Antepartum haemorrhage is bleeding from the genital tract in the period from 20 weeks gestation to the birth of the baby.

Incidence. It occurs in 3% of pregnancies of > 28 weeks gestation and 5% of pregnancies of > 20 weeks gestation.

Significance. Up to 20% of very preterm babies are born in association with antepartum haemorrhage (APH) so is associated with significant perinatal and maternal morbidity and mortality.

Aetiology

- placenta praevia
- placental abruption
- marginal bleed
- vasa praevia
- uterine rupture
- local causes: cervix, vagina
  The source is almost entirely maternal in origin.

Placenta praevia

Incidence. Incidence is about 1%, rising with frequency of previous caesarean section.

Presentation. The placenta is attached to the lower segment of the uterus and/or covering the cervix. The presentation is usually that of a painless APH with a high presenting part. The absence of contractions and pain makes diagnosis more likely.

Routine second-trimester ultrasound will diagnose low-lying and placenta praevia.

Classification

- major praevia: placenta lies over the internal cervical os
- minor praevia: if the leading edge of the placenta is in the lower uterine segment but not covering the cervical os

Risk factors

- previous caesarean increasing in relative risk with each caesarean
- previous placenta praevia
- previous termination of pregnancy
- advanced maternal age
- multiple pregnancy
- previous deficient endometrium
- assisted conception
- increased parity

Management

- Suspect possible praevia in any bleeding after 20 weeks with high mobile presenting part.
- If asymptomatic and suspected at morphology scan, management is confirmation of diagnosis in the early third trimester (approximately 32 weeks.) For persistent placenta praevia, a planned caesarean section is indicated.
- When presenting symptomatically, management depends on gestational age and both maternal and fetal wellbeing.
- Assessment will involve:
  - resuscitation of the mother, with insertion of intravenous line as well as full blood count and cross-match of blood
  - fetal assessment with fetal heart rate monitoring and possible steroid prophylaxis for prematurity
- If stable, perform ultrasound to confirm diagnosis and confirm fetal wellbeing and growth. The patient would be admitted until blood loss ceases or delivery. Use anti-D prophylaxis if the mother is Rh-negative. Avoid digital examination and intercourse in the third trimester.
- The decision to deliver will combine assessment of maternal risks and stability, fetal risks and stability, and gestational age. This can be a high-risk delivery and local massive transfusion protocols should be in place. Preoperative counselling regarding possible hysterectomy due to risk of persistent postpartum haemorrhage is appropriate. Cell salvage will decrease the risk of transfusion.
- Tocolysis and cervical cerclage is not appropriate in this clinical situation.

Placenta accreta

- Invasion of the placenta through the decidua basalis then into and through the myometrium are known as placenta accreta, increta and percreta; however, all are generally termed placenta accreta. This will clinically present as a morbidly adherent placenta but clinical suspicion should commence at morphology scan with placenta located in the anterior lower segment in the presence of a previous caesarean section.
- Placenta percreta is defined when the placenta breaches the uterine serosa.
- More definitive diagnosis of accreta should occur at 32 weeks gestation where Doppler ultrasound and magnetic resonance imaging (MRI) assessment of more ambiguous cases can occur.
- Management in the third trimester should be close to or in hospital.
- Delivery is aimed at before 36–37 weeks and should be well planned as a high-risk delivery. Interventional radiology with prophylactic catheter placement should be considered.
- The risk of hysterectomy increases with the number of previous caesareans.

Placental abruption

Incidence. Incidence is 1%.

Definition. Abruption is haemorrhage from decidual detachment of a normally situated placenta. The woman presents with abdominal pain, tense and tender uterus, which is large for dates, and hypovolaemic shock that may be out of proportion with visible bleeding.

Risk factors

- hypertension
- increased parity
- poor nutrition
- previous abruption (after one abruption the recurrence risk is 5%–15% and after two the risk is 25%)
- trauma, external cephalic version
- sudden reduction in uterine volume (e.g. after delivery of the first twin)
- polyhydramnios
- smoking
- substance abuse: cocaine

Differential diagnosis

- placenta praevia
- uterine rupture
- degeneration of fibroid
- rectus sheath haematoma
- acute polyhydramnios
- acute surgical conditions

Complications of placental abruption

- coagulopathy—abruption is the commonest obstetric cause of coagulopathy: 10% of abruptions demonstrate significant changes in coagulation profiles; there is a reduction in platelets and fibrinogen, increased fibrin degradation products and prothrombin time; fibrin degradation products inhibit myometrial activity, increase the risk of postpartum haemorrhage and may have cardiotoxic effects
- postpartum haemorrhage
- renal failure
- acute tubular necrosis from hypovolaemia and disseminated intravascular coagulopathy
- increased perinatal mortality

Management

- Resuscitate and restore circulatory volume to prevent renal shutdown and to clear fibrin degradation products.
- Cross-match for blood and, if indicated, platelets and fresh frozen plasma. Check full blood count, coagulation profile, renal function and electrolytes and liver biochemistry.
- Monitor urine output.
- Perform fetal assessment and delivery.
- Kleihauer test to quantify fetomaternal haemorrhage.

Vasa praevia

This diagnosis is the presence of fetal vessels within the membranes travelling in close association to the internal cervical os. It is either associated with a velamentous (lateral non-central) insertion of the cord, or a placenta with more than one lobe and communicating vessels traversing through the membranes.

If these vessels are ruptured, the subsequent blood loss is fetal not maternal and as such has significant fetal mortality.

Diagnosis

Accurate diagnosis of vasa praevia can be made via transvaginal colour Doppler ultrasound. Screening should occur on those patients with a low-lying placenta or those with bilobed placenta diagnosed at time of morphology scan. The optimal time for assessment would be 32 weeks gestation.

Vasa praevia must be included in the differential diagnosis of intrapartum vaginal bleeding, and is associated with an ominous cardiotocography pattern. In the presence of blood loss and ominous fetal heart rate, although theoretical tests (Apt tests for alkali denaturation that make it possible to differentiate fetal and maternal bloods) are available, vasa praevia may result in fetal anaemia and death. Hence, emergency delivery is indicated.

In the case of asymptomatic second-trimester diagnosis, consideration to admission at 30 weeks gestation and delivery by caesarean section from 35 weeks after maturation of fetal lungs is indicated.

Local causes

- These include cervicitis, polyps, ectropion and cervical cancer.
- Speculum examination should be routine assessment within APH.

Further reading

Royal College of Obstetricians and Gynaecologists, 2011. Antepartum haemorrhage. Green-top Guideline No.63. RCOG, London.

Royal College of Obstetricians and Gynaecologists, 2011. Placenta praevia, placenta praevia accreta and vasa praevia: diagnosis and management. Green-top Guideline No. 27. RCOG, London.

Chapter 32

Fetal complications in later pregnancy

Jackie Chua
Michael Flynn

Intrauterine fetal death (IUFD)

Definition. IUFD is the delivery of a live fetus with no signs of life after 20 weeks. The intrauterine diagnosis is via the absence of fetal heart sounds and fetal movements confirmed by detailed ultrasound assessment. Signs of longer duration demise include Spalding's sign (overlapping skull bones on ultrasound) or Robert's sign (gas in the fetal cardiovascular system). About 50% of all IUFDs occur at over 37 weeks gestation.

Aetiology

Aetiology varies with gestational age and between developed and non-developed countries. Within developed countries, near-term the aetiologies include:

- unexplained
- fetal growth restriction (FGR)
- placental abruption
- infection
- chromosomal and congenital anomalies

Complications

- infections, especially with rupture of membranes
- maternal distress
- coagulopathy and disseminated intravascular coagulopathy

COAGULOPATHY AND DISSEMINATED INTRAVASCULAR COAGULOPATHY

This can occur when gestation is over 14 weeks, and generally when the fetus has been dead for over 4 weeks. There is a slow reduction in fibrinogen of about 500 mg/L per week, which is unlikely to be associated with bleeding tendency until levels are lower than 1 g/L. The coagulopathy is due to fibrinogen consumption with release of thromboplastins from retained products of conception. There may also be raised fibrin degradation products, prothrombin time and activated partial thromboplastin time with a reduction in platelets. Disseminated intravascular coagulopathy occurs in one-third of patients with IUFD for over 4 weeks. Spontaneous labour occurs in 80% of cases within 2 weeks, with only 10% undelivered after 3 weeks.

Investigations

- photograph of the fetus
- X-ray/magnetic resonance imaging (MRI)
- cytogenetics: blood, skin, placenta/amnion
- autopsy
- bacteriology: swabs of the fetus and placenta
- maternal: blood group and antibodies, full blood count, Kleihauer test, antiphospholipid antibodies, HbA1c, *Toxoplasma,* cytomegalovirus and rubella serology, thyroid function

Delivery of the dead fetus

PROSTAGLANDINS

Prostaglandin pessaries or gel

- Give prostaglandin E_2 analogue 1–2 mg via gel or sustained release, as in term induction of labour.
- Contraindications include hypersensitivity to prostaglandin and induction of labour at term.
- Cautious use is required with the concomitant use of oxytocin after previous uterine surgery and in patients with obstructive airways disease.

VAGINAL

Misoprostol (prostaglandin E_1 analogue)

- This appears to be effective in induction of IUFD. The possibility of uterine rupture with previous caesarean section is noted.
- It is the method of choice with dose decreasing from mid-trimester to late-third trimester.

Oxytocin

- If the cervix is favourable, artificial rupture of membranes may be performed to reduce induction to delivery interval without a significant rise in infection rates.

CAESAREAN SECTION

- Indications include major placenta praevia, severe cephalopelvic disproportion, previous classical caesarean section or more than two previous caesarean sections, the presence of uterine rupture or transverse lie and unsuccessful version.

Fetal growth restriction (FGR)

Definition. FGR is where the estimated birth weight is less than the tenth percentile for gestational age (but some neonates with FGR will be heavier). The clinical relevance of FGR is a four-fold rise in intrauterine fetal death, greater risk of birth hypoxia, neonatal complications and impaired neurodevelopment. The majority of term FGR has no morbidity or mortality.

Causes
- idiopathic, racial
- uteroplacental insufficiency as a result of pre-eclampsia, or abruption
- chromosomal abnormalities
- structural/anatomical abnormalities
- infections
- maternal causes (e.g. smoking, drugs, alcohol, nutrition)
- multiple pregnancies

Screening
- Clinical assessment alone detects fewer than 50% of cases. This includes abdominal palpation and symphysial fundal height, which has a sensitivity of 60%–74% and a false-positive rate of 55%.

Diagnosis
- Abdominal circumference and estimated fetal weight by ultrasound are the most accurate diagnostic measurements to predict growth restriction. Ultrasound scan measuring abdominal circumference in the third trimester can detect 85% of FGR.
- There used to be differentiation between symmetrical and asymmetrical FGR, but it is not generally used any more as an indicator for chromosome type of growth restriction.
- FGR and polyhydramnios can be an indication for chromosome abnormality.

Management
- ultrasound
  - biometry and estimated fetal weight +/–10%
  - Doppler: monitoring umbilical artery Doppler for brain sparing then decompensation type of parameters
    — other blood vessels looked at include middle cerebral artery, ductus venosus and umbilical vein
    — uterine artery for presence or absence of a notch in the waveform may indicate high risk for placental insufficiency in first and second trimester
  - amniotic fluid index: decreases
- biophysical profile: late signs
- cardiotocography (CTG): late signs
- delivery
  - timing difficult
  - Growth Restriction Intervention Trial (GRIT) trial: no difference in total perinatal deaths between immediate versus delayed delivery group and both had similar 2-year neurological outcomes
  - Doppler best indicator for delivery after 29 weeks with ductus venosus a good predictor of intact survival
  - Cochrane for high-risk and low-risk pregnancies and Doppler surveillance found no benefit with an increased intervention rate

Disorders of amniotic fluid volume

- amniotic fluid homeostasis: fetal urine production and swallowing, secretions and transfer across membranes

Screening

- abdominal palpation
- increased abdominal girth and difficulty feeling fetal parts
- smaller than expected

Diagnosis

- ultrasound
- subjective assessment
- objective assessment
- amniotic fluid index
- deepest vertical pocket (twins)

Polyhydramnios

RISK FACTORS

- fetal abnormalities (neural tube defects, gastrointestinal defects limiting swallowing of liquor)
- hydrops fetalis
- multiple pregnancy, especially monozygotic twins
- maternal diabetes
- idiopathic

COMPLICATIONS OF POLYHYDRAMNIOS

- preterm rupture of membranes
- premature labour
- unstable lie and fetal malpresentation
- cord prolapse
- postpartum haemorrhage, placental abruption
- maternal discomfort

MANAGEMENT

- ultrasound examination of fetus and assessment of amount of liquor
- glucose tolerance test
- indomethacin: risk of premature closure of ductus arteriosus
- close monitoring in high-risk unit with possible amnio reduction

Oligohydramnios

FACTORS ASSOCIATED WITH REDUCED AMNIOTIC FLUID VOLUME

- placental insufficiency and FGR
- iatrogenic
- fetal abnormalities (renal or renal tract abnormalities)
- premature rupture of membranes
- post-term pregnancy

COMPLICATIONS OF OLIGOHYDRAMNIOS

- cord compression and fetal distress
- increased perinatal morbidity and mortality
- postural/musculoskeletal deformities
- pulmonary hypoplasia, especially if early onset or prolonged

MANAGEMENT

- ultrasound examination of fetus for anomalies
- assessment of fetal wellbeing
- assessment for rupture of membranes

Further reading

Baschat, A.A., Galan, H.L., Bhides, A., et al., 2006. Doppler and biophysical assessment in growth restricted fetuses: distribution of test results. Ultrasound Obstet. Gynecol. 27, 41–47.

Bricker, I., Neilson, J.P., Dowswell, T., 2008. Routine ultrasound in late pregnancy (after 24 weeks' gestation). Cochrane Database Syst. Rev. (4), Art. No. CD001451, doi: 10.1002/14651858.

GRIT Study Group, 2004. Wellbeing at 2 years of age in the Growth Restriction Intervention Trial (GRIT): multicentre randomized controlled trial. Lancet 364, 513–520.

Grivell, R.M., Wong, L., Bhatia, V., 2009. Regimens of fetal surveillance for impaired fetal growth. Cochrane Database Syst. Rev. (1), Art. No. CD007113, doi: 10.1002/14651858.

Kinzler, W.L., Vintzileos, A.M., 2008. Fetal growth restriction: a modern approach. Curr. Opin. Obstet. Gynecol. 20, 125–131.

Lalor, J.G., Fawole, B., Alfirevic, Z., et al., 2008. Biophysical profile for fetal assessment in high risk pregnancies. Cochrane Database Syst. Rev. (1), Art. No.: CD000038, doi: 10.1002/14651858.

Chapter 33

Breech presentation

Michael Flynn

Incidence. There is an increase in incidence with decreasing gestation. At 20–25 weeks gestation, 30%–40% of fetuses are breech, and at 32 weeks gestation the incidence is 15%, while at term 2%–4% of fetuses are in the breech presentation.

Types

- frank/extended at knee: 65% of breech presentations
- complete/flexed at knee: 10% of breech presentations
- footling: 25% of breech presentations

Risk factors

Fetal and maternal risk factors are listed in Table 33.1.

External cephalic version

Spontaneous changes in fetal polarity are reduced with increasing gestation. The likelihood of spontaneous version at 32 weeks is about 55%, compared with 25% at 36 weeks. The risks of external cephalic version include tocolytic side effects, placental abruption, cord accidents and premature labour and is not appropriate where caesarean section is indicated on other grounds.

The absolute contraindications to external cephalic version include multiple pregnancy (except after the delivery of the first twin), antepartum haemorrhage, placenta praevia, rupture of membranes, labour and fetal abnormalities. Relative contraindications include previous caesarean section, fetal growth restriction (FGR) and oligohydramnios. Tocolysis improves success of external version. Anti-D is required in women who are Rh-negative. The success rate is 50%–90% of version; however, the decrease in overall caesarean section rates is more variable.

Table 33.1 Risk factors for breech presentation	
FETAL	**MATERNAL**
prematurity	past history
multiple pregnancy	primigravida
abnormality	uterine abnormalities
intrauterine fetal death	pelvic tumour
raised or lowered amniotic fluid volume	contracted pelvis
placenta praevia	drugs: anticonvulsants, drugs of abuse
reduced growth or activity	idiopathic

Management of breech presentation

Diagnosis
- Perform a clinical examination.
- If remote from term, document and observe.
- If after 36 weeks gestation, perform an ultrasound scan to confirm diagnosis; assess fetal anatomy, position of legs and estimated weight; assess amniotic fluid volume.

Term breech trial
This randomised multicentre trial compared the policy of elective caesarean section with vaginal birth for selected breech deliveries. The results were:
- no difference in maternal morbidity or mortality in both treatment arms
- statistically significant increase in perinatal/neonatal morbidity in planned vaginal birth group compared with elective caesarean section

This study has changed practice with at least 90% breech presentations now delivered by caesarean section. Some expert groups consider breech vaginal delivery an option with adherence to strict selection and labour criteria.

Delivery of the breech presentation diagnosed in late labour
- If possible, rapid assessment via ultrasound to exclude absolute contraindications even if at advanced stage.
- The common method is assisted breech delivery.
- Lithotomy position: clean the perineum and drape.
- Catheterise the bladder.
- Employ analgesia.
- Perform episiotomy.

BREECH BORN BY MATERNAL EXPULSIVE EFFORTS UP TO THE UMBILICUS
After the knees have delivered, flex the knees by pressing on the popliteal fossa to deliver the legs. Place a warm cloth over the breech and with the next contraction place hands on the baby's pelvis and pull down towards the floor until the anterior shoulder is delivered. The anterior arm is delivered by hooking a finger onto the cubital fossa and pulling the arm down over the baby's abdomen.

LÖVSET'S MANOEUVRE

Rotating the posterior shoulder to the anterior allows the other arm to be delivered in the same manner as the first. The head is delivered by various ways, including forceps, suprapubic pressure and lateral rotation of head in pelvis, or grasping feet and placing the body onto the maternal abdomen with the symphysis acting as fulcrum.

Possible hazards in vaginal delivery

- occipital bone trauma during vaginal breech delivery from the impact on the maternal pubis
- intra/periventricular injury, secondary haemorrhage or ischaemia (avoiding vaginal delivery does not necessarily prevent intracranial haemorrhage)
- bruising resulting in jaundice
- trauma to internal organs, with the accoucheur placing hands over the baby's abdomen rather than the pelvis
- entrapment of the head, especially in the woman who commences active pushing before the second stage or with a footling breech

Preterm breech presentation

- If not in labour, there is no benefit from external version prior to 37 weeks gestation.
- Term Breech Trial findings may not be applicable to preterm.
- Studies published are all retrospective, and individual decision-making is therefore appropriate.
- Preterm breech presentation is mostly handled by caesarean section.

Further reading

Hannah, M.E., Hannah, W.J., Hewson, S.A., et al., for the Term Breech Trial Collaborative Group, 2000. Planned caesarean section versus planned vaginal birth for breech presentation at term: a randomised multicenter trial. Lancet 356, 1375–1383.

Royal Australian and New Zealand College of Obstetricians and Gynaecologists (RACOG), 2016. Management of breech presentation at term. College Statement C-Obs 11. RANZCOG, St Leonards.

Chapter 34

Multiple pregnancy

Jackie Chua
Michael Flynn

This is considered a high-risk pregnancy because of the increased maternal and perinatal risks.

Incidence. Incidence varies with geographical location. The incidence from spontaneous conception is about 1.25% of births, from clomiphene-induced ovulation 7%, and from assisted reproductive techniques up to 10%–20%. Monozygotic twinning has an incidence of 3.5 in 1000 deliveries.

Mechanism of twinning

Dizygotic twins

- Dizygotic twins are always DCDA (dichorionic diamniotic) and account for 70% of twin pregnancies. This occurs as a result of duplication of the normal process of conception, with separate chorions, amnions and placental circulations.
- The geographic variation in the incidence of twin pregnancies is due to differences in dizygotic twinning.
- The risks for dizygotic twinning include older maternal age (> 35 years), past history and family history of twinning.

Monozygotic twins

- Monozygotic twins account for 30% of twin pregnancies.
- Monozygotic twinning is determined by the timing at which splitting of the blastocyst occurs:
  - before 3 days after fertilisation (about 30%): DCDA
    — results in separate chorion, amnion and placental circulation

- between 4 and 8 days after fertilisation (about 70%): MCDA (monochorionic diamniotic)
  — results in a single common placenta but two amnions and one chorionic membrane
- after 8 days (about 1%): MCMA (monochorionic monoamniotic)
  — common amnion, chorion and placenta
- after 13 days (rare): conjoined twins

Diagnosis of chorionicity and amnionicity

- in first trimester, high accuracy rates for chorionicity and amnionicity: determined by number of gestational sacs present, number of fetal heart beats or crown rump length (CRL) seen, or number of yolk sacs or amnions seen
- in second trimester, less accurate: determined by gender, number of placentas, dividing membrane, membrane thickness, presence or absence of the 'twin peak sign'

Prenatal diagnosis

- must know chorionicity
- monozygotic pregnancies have similar risk to singleton pregnancies: one risk for the pregnancy
  - rare: postzygotic non-disjunction
- dizygotic pregnancies
  - each fetus has individual risk
- first trimester screening applicable with or without the biochemistry
- second trimester screening inaccurate as analytes are increased due to number of fetuses
- invasive testing: chorionic villus sampling and amniocentesis
- multifetal reduction in specialised centres for anomalies or reduction of fetal numbers

Complications of twin pregnancy

General
- increased miscarriage rate: vanishing twin
- increased perinatal mortality rate: five to seven times of singleton pregnancies
  - death of one DCDA twin associated with preterm delivery
  - death of one MC twin has risk of hypotensive blood transfusion and 25% risk of neurological damage to the surviving twin
- fetal abnormalities: higher incidence of cardiac and central nervous system malformations
- intrauterine growth restriction (IUGR)
- premature delivery: in up to 45% of twins, compared with 5%–6% of singleton births
- postpartum haemorrhage
- pre-eclampsia: three to five times the risk associated with singleton births; tends to be more severe

Specific: monochorionic twinning

TWIN-TO-TWIN TRANSFUSION SYNDROME (TTTS)
- 15% incidence
- requires arterial to venous anastomosis, which is unbalanced, and one of the fetuses, the donor, starts to transfuse the other twin, the recipient
- associated with velamentous cord insertion

Staging (Quintero)
- stage 1: polyhydramnios (deepest vertical pocket of amniotic fluid > 8 cm) in one twin and oligohydramnios (deepest vertical pocket of amniotic fluid < 2 cm) in the other with bladder seen in the donor
- stage 2: polyhydramnios and oligohydramnios present with no bladder seen in the donor
- stage 3: abnormal Dopplers
  - donor: absent end diastolic flow or reversed in the umbilical artery
  - recipient: abnormal venous Dopplers
- stage 4: fetal hydrops
- stage 5: fetal demise of one or both twins

Management
- termination of pregnancy
- conservative: 90% mortality rate
- cord occlusion/ligation
- serial amnioreduction
- laser coagulopathy: best treatment outcome with decreased morbidity

SELECTIVE INTRAUTERINE GROWTH RESTRICTION (sIUGR)
- 15% incidence
- one twin is small for gestational age where the other twin is growing normally
- associated with increased risk of fetal demise and risk of neurological sequelae
- three classifications

TWIN REVERSED ARTERIAL PERFUSION SEQUENCE (TRAP) OR ACARDIAC TWINNING
- 1% of monozygotic pregnancies
- associated with chromosomal abnormalities, arterial to arterial anastomosis
- leads to major deformities/fetal demise in the recipient twin and possible heart failure in the donor twin

Antenatal management of twin pregnancy

Diagnosis
- Multiple pregnancy is a differential diagnosis if the fundal height is greater than dates and is associated with hyperemesis.
- Diagnosis is confirmed by ultrasound scan.

Antenatal care

- More frequent visits are advisable because of raised maternal and fetal risks.
- Weekly visits between antenatal visits and ultrasound assessment from about 30 weeks gestation are appropriate. Advise regarding employment, rest and iron supplementation.

Ultrasound role

- determining zygosity
- look for fetal abnormality
- assess growth and wellbeing: increased fetal surveillance with serial scans
- treatment: laser therapy

Prevention of premature labour

- Twins are five times more likely to be preterm than singletons.
- Delivery prior to 32 weeks is more likely with monochorionic twins.
- No studies have shown that routine hospitalisation, cervical suture or tocolysis increase pregnancy length.

Delivery of twins

- In 70% of cases, the first twin is a cephalic presentation, and both twins are cephalic in 40%.
- Common practice is delivery at 37–38 weeks, as there is increased risk of stillbirth.

Indications for elective caesarean section

- malpresentation of the first twin
- monoamniotic twins
- other obstetric indications, such as placenta praevia

Vaginal delivery

- Vaginal delivery is probably appropriate for cephalic/cephalic presentation with normal growth and wellbeing.
- Evidence is unclear on method of delivery when the second twin is breech.
- Both twins are continuously monitored during labour.
- Epidural anaesthesia is recommended.
- Augmentation and induction of labour is acceptable in the absence of any obstetric contraindications.
- The third stage requires active management because of the risk of postpartum haemorrhage.

Twin with single intrauterine fetal death

The incidence of antepartum death of one twin is 3%–4%. The outcome of the surviving twin is related to whether the twins are monochorionic or dichorionic. In monochorionic twins there is a high rate of vascular communication between the twins and a risk of significant twin-to-twin transfusion. Neurological abnormalities in the surviving twin result from thromboplastins released from the dead fetus, which can cause thrombotic occlusion of cerebral vessels. Fetal magnetic resonance imaging (MRI) is helpful.

Triplet pregnancy

Incidence. Triplet pregnancies have a wide geographical variation, with an increased incidence in Africa. In Western countries, the incidence is 1 in 6400. For clomiphene-induced pregnancies, the incidence is 5 in 1000 and for assisted reproductive techniques 3%–4%.

Complications of triplet pregnancy

- maternal: anaemia, pre-eclampsia, antepartum haemorrhage
- fetal: premature labour, with up to 80% delivering before 37 weeks gestation; IUGR; malpresentation; increased perinatal mortality rate (five times that of singleton)
- reduction to twin or singleton pregnancy reduces morbidity and mortality rates

Delivery

The perinatal mortality rate rises as the time interval between deliveries lengthens. This may be due to progressive fetal anoxia with changes in uteroplacental haemodynamics. As a result, caesarean section is indicated. The risk of postpartum haemorrhage is heightened.

Further reading

Evans, M.I., Ciorica, D., Britt, D.W., et al., 2005. Update on selective reduction. Prenat. Diagn. 25, 807–813.

Gratacos, E., Lewi, L., Munoz, B., et al., 2007. A classification system for selective intrauterine growth restriction in monochorionic pregnancies according to umbilical artery Doppler flow in the smaller twin. Ultrasound Obstet. Gynecol. 30, 28–34.

Pharoah, P.O.D., Adi, Y., 2000. Consequences of in utero death in a twin pregnancy. Lancet 355, 1597–1602.

Quintero, R.A., Morales, W.J., Allen, M.H., et al., 1999. Staging of twin–twin transfusion syndrome. J. Perinatol. 19 (8), 550–555.

Roberts, D., Gates, S., Kilby, M., et al., 2008. Interventions for twin–twin transfusion syndrome: a Cochrane review. Ultrasound Obstet. Gynecol. 31, 701–711.

Senat, M.-V., Deprest, J., Boulvain, M., et al., 2004. Endoscopic laser surgery versus serial amnioreduction for severe twin-to-twin transfusion syndrome. NEJM 351, 136–144.

Wald, N.J., Rish, S., 2005. Prenatal screening for Down syndrome and neural tube defects in twin pregnancies. Prenat. Diagn. 25, 740–745.

Chapter 35

Preterm prelabour rupture of membranes

Justin Nasser

Definitions. Prelabour (premature) rupture of membranes (PROM) refers to membrane rupture before the onset of uterine contractions irrespective of gestational age. Preterm prelabour rupture of membranes (PPROM) refers to membrane rupture before the onset of uterine contractions in a pregnancy that is < 37 completed weeks of gestation.

Incidence. PROM occurs in 10% of all pregnancies. PPROM occurs in 3% of pregnancies and is responsible for, or associated with, approximately one-third of preterm births.

Aetiology of PPROM

- The pathogenesis of PPROM is poorly understood and in the majority of cases the exact aetiology is unknown.
- There are multiple possible aetiologies that probably share a common final pathway leading to membrane rupture. Such factors include those leading to membrane stretch, membrane degradation, uterine contractility, local inflammation and increased susceptibility to ascending genital tract infection.

Risk factors of PPROM

- past history of PPROM/preterm delivery
- urogenital tract infection/colonisation
- antepartum haemorrhage
- cigarette smoking
- past history of cervical surgery

- amniocentesis in current pregnancy
- cervical length ≤ 25 mm
- positive fetal fibronectin (fFN)
- connective tissue disorders
- nutritional deficiencies
- lean maternal body mass
- multiple pregnancy/polyhydramnios

Most cases of PPROM occur in women without risk factors and there is currently no reliable way of predicting and preventing PPROM.

Clinical significance of PPROM

Both mother and fetus are at risk from complications associated with PPROM.

Maternal risks

- those associated with infection, including chorioamnionitis, endometritis and septicaemia
  - risk of intrauterine infection increases with duration of membrane rupture
  - clinical signs indicating chorioamnionitis include maternal pyrexia, tachycardia, leucocytosis, uterine tenderness, offensive vaginal discharge and fetal tachycardia
- those associated with operative delivery, which is more likely in the setting of PPROM

Fetal risks

- preterm delivery
  - most cases of PPROM will deliver within 1 week after membrane rupture; however, latency increases with decreasing gestational age
  - morbidities associated with preterm delivery: hyaline membrane disease, intraventricular haemorrhage, periventricular leukomalacia and other neurologic sequelae, infection (e.g. sepsis, pneumonia, meningitis), necrotising enterocolitis and retinopathy of prematurity; rates vary with gestational age and are increased by the presence of chorioamnionitis
- pulmonary hypoplasia: hydrostatic pressure from amniotic fluid is essential to lung development and maturation in the mid-second trimester; loss of amniotic fluid at this stage of development can irreversibly arrest lung development and result in pulmonary hypoplasia; associated with significant neonatal mortality regardless of gestational age at birth
- musculoskeletal/facial deformities: due to the reduction in amniotic fluid and restriction of fetal movement
- malpresentation
- placental abruption
- umbilical cord complications (e.g. compression, prolapse)

Diagnosis

In the majority of cases, the diagnosis can be confidently made based on a history of fluid loss per vagina and direct visualisation of amniotic fluid in the posterior fornix by sterile speculum examination. If amniotic fluid is not immediately visible, fluid leakage through the internal os can be provoked by the Valsalva manoeuvre or coughing. Repeat speculum examination after a period of recumbency may assist the diagnosis.

A number of ancillary tests with varying degrees of sensitivity/specificity and false-positive/false-negative rates can be used to assist in the diagnosis. These include:

- nitrazine test
- ferning/arborisation
- AmniSure test
- other biochemical tests: fFN, alpha-fetoprotein (AFP), diamine-oxidase, prolactin, human chorionic gonadotrophin (hCG)
- ultrasound assessment of amniotic fluid volume
- intra-amniotic indigo carmine with passage of blue fluid per vagina

Other causes of fluid loss include leucorrhoea, urinary incontinence, vaginitis, cervicitis, mucus show, semen and vaginal douches.

Management of PPROM

The management of PPROM is determined by several factors, including:

- gestational age
- available obstetric and neonatal services
- presence/absence of maternal/fetal infection
- presence/absence of labour and/or cervical changes
- fetal presentation
- assessments of fetal wellbeing

These factors need to be considered in each case and a decision made as to whether conservative or aggressive management is most appropriate.

Delivery is indicated when the risk to the fetus of complications of prematurity are outweighed by the risks to the mother/fetus of complications of PPROM.

Initial management

- The initial management involves confirming the diagnosis by history and clinical examination. At the time of sterile speculum examination, endocervical swabs (*Chlamydia*, gonorrhoea) and ano-vaginal swabs (group B streptococcus) should be collected.
- Mid-stream urine (MSU) for microscopy, culture and sensitivities (M/C/S) should be collected.
- Digital examinations should be avoided unless delivery is anticipated.
- Generally, expeditious delivery is indicated if labour is advanced, or in the presence of non-reassuring fetal status and/or infective complications, regardless of gestational age. In the absence of these conditions, subsequent management is dependent on the gestational age at time of PPROM and the subsequent presence or absence of conditions necessitating delivery.

PPROM: 34–37 weeks

- The risk of serious neonatal complications with delivery after 34 weeks is low.
- There is no significant differences in neonatal sepsis or composite neonatal morbidity/mortality when expectant management is compared to immediate delivery.
- Respiratory complications appear higher in the immediate delivery group.
- Maternal haemorrhagic and infective complications appear higher in the expectant management group.

- Current evidence suggests that either immediate delivery or, in the absence of signs of infection or fetal compromise, a policy of expectant management with appropriate surveillance of maternal and fetal wellbeing are reasonable in pregnant women who present with PPROM close to term.
- Both oxytocin and misoprostol have been shown to be effective agents for labour induction.
- There is no significant improvement in neonatal outcomes and an apparent increased risk of chorioamnionitis with expectant management in PPROM after 34 weeks.
- Current evidence suggests that delivery should be expedited to reduce the risk of associated complications when PPROM occurs near term.

PPROM: 24–33 weeks

- PPROM remote from term is generally managed in hospital due to a short latency period and high complication rate/intervention rate.
- Some studies have demonstrated favourable outcomes and cost savings with home management of selected cases after an initial period (48–72 hours) of hospital admission.
- In the absence of complications, ongoing observation, administration of corticosteroids and adjuvant antibiotics (see below), and serial monitoring is indicated, with consideration for delivery occurring at 34 weeks.

PPROM: < 23 completed weeks

- Good quality data to guide management in pre-viable PPROM are sparse.
- Perinatal mortality is high and decreases with advancing gestation.
- More than half are delivered within 1 week of PPROM, either as a result of spontaneous labour or induced labour due to maternal/fetal indications.
- Induction of labour is achieved with either high-dose oxytocin or by vaginal/oral prostaglandins.
- After conservative management, approximately one-quarter will remain pregnant 1 month after membrane rupture. These women should be monitored for signs necessitating delivery.
- Depending on specific circumstances, outpatient management may be appropriate.
- Serial ultrasound assessments should occur to evaluate liquor volume and fetal growth. Ultrasound assessment of lung volumes (direct and indirect) is useful in predicting pulmonary hypoplasia.
- Persistent oligohydramnios following PPROM is associated with poorer outcomes regardless of gestational age at delivery.
- PPROM following amniocentesis is associated with more favourable outcomes.
- If the pregnancy reaches a stage where resuscitation of the newborn is planned, consideration should be given for in utero transfer to an institution with appropriate facilities for emergency delivery and neonatal intensive care.

Antenatal corticosteroids

- Antenatal corticosteroids significantly reduce the risks of respiratory distress syndrome, intraventricular haemorrhage and necrotising enterocolitis, without increasing the risks of maternal or neonatal infections in women with PPROM.
- The maximum benefit is in those fetuses between 28 and 32 weeks gestation.
- Data on the benefit of repeat weekly doses of corticosteroids, or administration of rescue steroids remote from initial course in women with PPROM who remain undelivered, are conflicting.

Adjuvant antibiotics

- Antibiotic therapy in women with PPROM is used in an attempt to treat/prevent ascending infection in order to prolong the latency period and reduce gestational-age-dependent morbidity and neonatal infections.
- Antibiotic use is associated with an increase in latency times and reductions in chorioamnionitis, neonatal infection, use of surfactant, neonatal oxygen therapy and abnormal neonatal cerebral ultrasound scans.
- Current data support erythromycin 250 mg orally four times daily for 10 days or until delivery following diagnosis of PPROM.
- The use of extended spectrum amoxycillin-clavulanic acid is associated with an increased risk of necrotising enterocolitis and is not recommended.
- Intrapartum antibiotics for group B streptococcus prophylaxis, and antibiotic therapy for chorioamnionitis/sepsis, should be considered in addition to the above regimen.

Magnesium sulfate

- The neuroprotective benefits to preterm neonates from exposure to magnesium sulfate have been demonstrated in many clinical trials.

Progesterone

- Progesterone provides no benefit in the current pregnancy affected by PPROM.
- Progesterone supplementation in future pregnancies can reduce the risk of recurrent preterm birth.

Tocolysis

- The benefit of tocolytic therapy in the setting of PPROM is unclear and is not routinely recommended.
- Tocolysis is associated with an increased risk of chorioamnionitis without significant benefit to the neonate.
- It is contraindicated in the presence of chorioamnionitis.
- As in the setting of preterm labour with intact membranes, tocolysis may have a role in delaying delivery in order to obtain maximum benefit of corticosteroids and allow in utero transfer to an appropriate facility for delivery.

Emerging therapies

- Various agents (gelatine sponge, platelets, cryoprecipitate, fibrin) have been used to form a cervical plug/act as a membrane sealant.
- Amnioinfusion has been used in an attempt to replace amniotic fluid.
- Current data are insufficient to recommend their implementation into routine practice.

Further reading

American College of Obstetricians and Gynecologists, 2016. ACOG Practice Bulletin No. 160: Premature Rupture of Membranes. Obstet. Gynecol. 127 (1), e39–e51.

Canavan, T., Simhan, H., Caratis, S., 2004. An evidence-based approach to the evaluation and treatment of premature rupture of membranes: Part I. Obstet. Gynecol. Surv. 59 (9), 669–677.

Canavan, T., Simhan, H., Caratis, S., 2004. An evidence-based approach to the evaluation and treatment of premature rupture of membranes: Part II. Obstet. Gynecol. Surv. 59 (9), 678–689.

Kenyon, S., Boulvain, M., Neilson, J.P., 2003. Antibiotics for preterm rupture of membranes. Cochrane Database Syst. Rev. (2), Art. No.: CD001058, doi:10.1002/14651858.

Lin, M.G., Nuthalapaty, F.S., Carver, A.R., et al., 2005. Misoprostol for labor induction in women with term premature rupture of membranes: a meta-analysis. Obstet. Gynecol. 106 (3), 593.

Mackeen, A.D., Seibel-Seamon, J., Muhammad, J., et al., 2014. Tocolytics for preterm premature rupture of membranes. Cochrane Database Syst. Rev. (2), CD007062.

Mercer, B.M., 2004. Preterm premature rupture of membranes: Diagnosis and management. Clin. Perinatol. 31, 765–782.

Morris, J.M., Roberts, C.L., Bowen, J.R., et al., 2015. Immediate delivery compared with expectant management after preterm pre-labour rupture of the membranes close to term (PPROMT trial): a randomised controlled trial. Lancet.

Morris, J., Roberts, C., Crowther, C., et al., 2006. Protocol for immediate delivery versus expectant care of women with preterm prelabour rupture of membranes close to term (PPROMT) Trial [ISRCTN44485060]. BMC Pregnancy Childbirth 6, 9.

Royal Australian and New Zealand College of Obstetricians and Gynaecologists (RANZCOG), 2006. Preterm premature rupture of membranes. RANZCOG: Melbourne. Guideline No. 44, November.

Waters, T.P., Mercer, B., 2011. Preterm PROM: Prediction, prevention, principles. Clin. Obstet. Gynecol. 54 (2), 307–312.

Waters, T.P., Mercer, B.M., 2009. The management of preterm premature rupture of membranes near the limit of fetal viability. Am. J. Obstet. Gynecol. 201 (3), 230–240.

Chapter 36

Preterm labour

Justin Nasser

Definition. Preterm or premature labour is the onset of regular painful uterine contractions accompanied by effacement and dilatation of the cervix after 20 weeks and before 37 completed weeks of pregnancy.

Incidence. Preterm labour occurs in 5%–10% of all deliveries.

Common complications in premature infants include respiratory distress syndrome, intraventricular haemorrhage, bronchopulmonary dysplasia, patent ductus arteriosus, necrotising enterocolitis, sepsis, apnoea and retinopathy of prematurity.

The frequency of major morbidity rises as gestational age decreases.

Ongoing advances in neonatal medicine have resulted in dramatically improved outcomes for preterm infants; however, there remains significant risk of long-term morbidity, such as cerebral palsy, developmental delay, visual and hearing impairment, and chronic lung disease.

Significance

- Prematurity is the cause of 75% of perinatal deaths and a major determinant of short-term and long-term morbidity in infants and children.
- Two-thirds of the perinatal deaths occur in the 30%–40% of preterm infants who are delivered prior to 32 weeks gestation.

Aetiology

Preterm labour may be classified as *spontaneous* or *indicated*.

Spontaneous preterm labour

- Spontaneous preterm labour occurs in the absence of overt maternal or fetal conditions necessitating delivery. It commonly occurs in the absence of an obvious cause,

or may follow preterm premature rupture of the membranes or related diagnoses such as incompetent cervix.
- Risk factors associated with spontaneous preterm labour include a history of previous preterm birth, multiple pregnancy, polyhydramnios, urogenital tract infection, previous cervical surgery, uterine anomalies, periodontal disease, bleeding in the second trimester, extremes of age, smoking, low prepregnancy weight and pregnancies achieved through assisted reproductive technologies.
- Most women who deliver preterm have no apparent risk factors.

Indicated preterm labour
- Indicated preterm labour occurs when conditions exist that create undue risk to the mother, the fetus or both, should the pregnancy continue, and a clinical decision is made to expedite delivery. In these situations, the labour may be induced or the delivery achieved by caesarean section.
- The most common diagnoses that precede an indicated preterm birth are pre-eclampsia, fetal distress, intrauterine growth restriction, placental abruption and fetal demise.

Prevention of preterm labour

Many interventions aimed at reducing the incidence of preterm labour have been implemented and assessed, including:
- cervical length assessment
  - cervical length is most accurately measured by transvaginal ultrasound
  - the median cervical length at 20 weeks is 42 mm, and the 1st percentile is 23 mm.
  - a short cervical length is associated with an increased risk of preterm delivery, and the shorter the cervical length the greater the risk
  - therapeutic interventions should be considered when the cervical length measures less than 25 mm in the second trimester
- supplemental progesterone
  - progesterone therapy may reduce the risk of preterm delivery in women with a short cervix (10–20 mm) detected by transvaginal ultrasound
  - the optimal timing, dose and route of delivery of progesterone has not been established
- cervical cerclage
  - women with a history of cervical incompetence may benefit from a cervical cerclage
  - cervical cerclage reduces the risk of preterm birth in women with a history of preterm delivery and a cervical length less than 25 mm before 24 weeks

Other measures such as detection and treatment of asymptomatic bacteriuria, detection and treatment of bacterial vaginosis, smoking cessation and nutritional supplementation have not shown consistent benefit in reducing preterm labour.

In fact, the incidence of preterm labour appears to be rising. The lack of success in preventing preterm labour can be attributed to:
- the current incomplete understanding of the physiology of normal parturition
- the current incomplete understanding of the pathogenesis of preterm labour
- the poor sensitivity and positive predictive value of currently available screening tests

Because of the difficulties of predicting and preventing preterm labour, the main goal of management is in early diagnosis of those at true risk of delivery, and implementation of therapies aimed at optimising perinatal outcomes.

Diagnosis of preterm labour

The clinical diagnosis of preterm labour is often unreliable, with up to 50% of women with signs and symptoms suggestive of preterm labour not progressing to preterm delivery.

A number of ancillary tests have been developed in an attempt to identify both asymptomatic and symptomatic women who are truly likely to deliver prematurely. The most clinically useful of these tests are:
- cervical length and morphology assessment by transvaginal ultrasound
- fetal fibronectin (fFN) detection in cervicovaginal secretions

Cervical length and morphology
- Well-defined, reproducible changes in the appearance of the cervix by transvaginal ultrasound occur as labour progresses.
- The cervix undergoes progressive shortening and widening along the endocervical canal commencing at the internal os ('funnelling').
- The initial changes are almost always asymptomatic and not identified by digital vaginal examination.
- In symptomatic women, a cervical length of > 3 cm is likely to exclude the diagnosis of preterm labour.
- Cervical length of < 2.5 cm at 16–24 weeks gestation is a strong predictor of preterm birth when used as a screening test in both low-risk and high-risk women. The shorter the cervical length and the earlier in pregnancy that the shortening occurs, the greater the likelihood of preterm birth.

Fetal fibronectin (fFN)
- fFN is a glycoprotein 'glue' that binds chorion to decidua.
- Disruption of the maternal fetal interface causes release of fFN into the cervicovaginal secretions.
- In a normal pregnancy, fFN should be almost undetectable in vaginal secretions from 22–35 weeks.
- The presence of fFN in the cervicovaginal secretions is a predictor of preterm birth.
- Quantitative measurement of fFN appears to improve predictive value compared with use of the qualitative test using a 50 ng/mL threshold.
- The presence of fFN in the cervicovaginal secretions is a predictor of preterm birth; however, its clinical utility is in its negative predictive value, as < 1% of women with a negative test will deliver within 1 week.

The use of both fFN and cervical sonography may increase the utility of these tests in assessing at-risk women.

Management of preterm labour

Because of the lack of success in predicting and preventing preterm labour, the aim of management is largely to reduce the likelihood and impact of prematurity-related sequelae.

Interventions shown to reduce perinatal morbidity and mortality in women who deliver preterm include:

- in utero transfer to a facility with appropriate neonatal facilities
- administration of corticosteroids to the mother to facilitate fetal lung maturation and reduce complications of prematurity
- administration of antibiotics to prevent neonatal group B streptococcus infection
- administration of magnesium sulfate to mothers with imminent preterm birth between 24 and 30 weeks; this has been shown to reduce the risk of cerebral palsy and protect gross motor function in their infants
- tocolytic therapy to delay delivery and facilitate corticosteroid administration and in utero transfer to an appropriate facility for delivery; nifedipine is the tocolytic of choice

In the absence of GBS prophylaxis or chorioamnionitis, there is no evidence to support the routine use of antibiotics for women in spontaneous preterm labour.

Women in acute preterm labour do not benefit from progesterone supplementation.

There are a number of therapeutic agents that can suppress uterine muscle activity, but all have potential adverse side effects. Current evidence suggests that:

- calcium channel blockers (e.g. nifedipine) or an oxytocin antagonist (atosiban) can delay delivery for 2–7 days with minimal side effects
- beta-agonists (e.g. ritodrine, terbutaline, salbutamol) are effective at delaying delivery for 48 hours, but are associated with greater side effects
- magnesium sulfate is an ineffective tocolytic
- the benefit of cyclo-oxygenase inhibitors (e.g. indomethacin) is uncertain.

Much of the improvement in perinatal morbidity and mortality associated with prematurity is due to the advances in neonatal management.

Further reading

American College of Obstetricians and Gynecologists, Committee on Practice Bulletins-Obstetrics, 2016. Practice Bulletin No. 159: Management of Preterm Labor. Obstet. Gynecol. 127, e29.

Dodd, J.M., Jones, L., Flenady, V., et al., 2013. Prenatal administration of progesterone for preventing preterm birth in women considered to be at risk of preterm birth. Cochrane Database Syst. Rev. (7), Art. No.: CD004947, doi:10.1002/14651858.CD004947.pub3.

Grimes-Dennis, J., Berghella, V., 2007. Cervical length and prediction of preterm delivery. Curr. Opin. Obstet. Gynecol. 19, 191–195.

Goldenberg, R.L., Culhane, J.F., Iams, J.D., et al., 2008. Preterm birth 1. Epidemiology and causes of preterm birth. Lancet 371, 75–84.

Iams, J., 2003. Prediction and early detection of preterm labour. Obstet. Gynecol. 101, 402–412.

Iams, J.D., 2014. Prevention of preterm parturition. N. Engl. J. Med. 370 (19), 1861.

Iams, J.D., Romero, R., Culhane, J.F., et al., 2008. Preterm birth 2. Primary, secondary, and tertiary interventions to reduce the morbidity and mortality of preterm birth. Lancet 371, 164–175.

Queensland Clinical Guidelines, 2015. Preterm labour and birth. Queensland Health. Available from: <http://www.health.qld.gov.au/qcg/>.

Royal Australian and New Zealand College of Obstetricians (RANZCOG), 2013. RANZCOG College Statement C-Obs 29. Progesterone: Use in the Second and Third Trimester of Pregnancy for the Prevention of Preterm Birth. Available at: <http://www.ranzcog .edu.au/the-ranzcog/policies-and-guidelines/college-statements/422-progesterone-use-in-the

-second-and-third-trimester-of-pregnancy-for-the-prevention-of-preterm- birth-c-obs-29b .html>.

Vidaeff, A.C., Ramin, S.M., 2009. Management strategies for the prevention of preterm birth. Part I: Update on progesterone supplementation. Curr. Opin. Obstet. Gynecol. 21, 480–484.

Vidaeff, A.C., Ramin, S.M., 2009. Management strategies for the prevention of preterm birth. Part II: Update on cervical cerclage. Curr. Opin. Obstet. Gynecol. 21, 485–490.

Chapter 37

Induction of labour

Thea Bowler

Induction of labour refers to techniques that stimulate uterine activity to achieve delivery prior to the onset of spontaneous labour.

Mechanism of labour

The exact mechanism of labour is still unknown, although it is thought that the release of fetal cortisol increases placental oestrogen and prostaglandin production. Oestrogen is thought to sensitise the myometrium to oxytocin. Prostaglandin E_2 and F_2-alpha are synthesised by the decidua and amnion, and may promote cervical ripening and sensitisation of the myometrium to oxytocin. Other factors such as progesterone, relaxin and prostacyclin dominate early in pregnancy to inhibit uterine contractility.

Induction of labour

The sensitivity of the myometrium to prostaglandin and oxytocin rises as gestation increases. However, the myometrium is relatively insensitive to oxytocin before term.

Induction of labour generally involves cervical ripening, amniotomy and stimulation of uterine contractions using oxytocin. Cervical favourability (Bishop's score) is an indicator of the myometrial sensitivity to oxytocin and therefore likelihood of successful induction.

Indications
Examples of common indications for induction of labour include:
- prolonged pregnancy (induction of labour for post-term pregnancy results in lower caesarean section rates and perinatal mortality)
- premature rupture of membranes
- hypertensive disorders of pregnancy
- maternal diabetes

- maternal medical conditions
- intrauterine fetal death
- intrauterine growth restriction
- oligohydramnios
- twin pregnancy
- antepartum haemorrhage
- isoimmunisation
- unstable lie
- chorioamnionitis
- intrahepatic cholestasis of pregnancy

Contraindications

Table 37.1 lists contraindications for induction of labour.

Table 37.1 Contraindications for induction of labour	
ABSOLUTE	**RELATIVE**
absolute cephalopelvic disproportion	antepartum haemorrhage
presumed fetal distress	grand multiparity
placenta praevia	previous caesarean section
vasa praevia	overdistended uterus
abnormal presentation	face or breech presentation
previous classical caesarean section	history of rapid labour
invasive carcinoma of cervix	
cord presentation	

Likelihood of successful induction

Prognostic factors for successful induction include:
- parity
- previous vaginal delivery
- gestational age
- membrane status (intact or ruptured)
- indication for induction
- maternal body mass index (BMI)
- fetal size
- cervical favourability

Pre-induction cervical assessment

The cervix remains closed because of its rigidity due to the collagen fibres that make up the bulk of cervical stroma. Cervical connective tissue consists mainly of collagen and a matrix of large proteoglycan molecules.

Cervical changes are due to:
- changes in proteoglycan
- collagen degradation
- increased vascularity
- accumulation of interstitial fluid.

A uniform means of assessing the cervix is the Bishop's score (see Table 37.2). The Bishop's score assesses the favourability of the cervix for induction of labour by assigning points to each of the five cervical features and adding these points. With a low score (0–3), there is a high risk of a failed induction, resulting in caesarean section (> 20%), compared with a score of 8 or more, where the failed induction rate is < 3%. With a high score, the cervix is said to be 'ripe'.

Techniques of induction

Mechanical

'SWEEPING' OF THE MEMBRANES
- Membrane sweeping involves insertion of a finger beyond the internal cervical os and rotating it to circumferentially separate the membranes from decidua.
- Compared to conservative management, membrane sweeping:
  - increases likelihood of spontaneous delivery within 48 hours
  - reduces frequency of prolongation of pregnancy beyond 41 and 42 weeks
  - reduces frequency of formal induction
  - needs to be performed to eight women to prevent one formal induction of labour

BALLOON CATHETERS
A single or double balloon catheter can be placed transcervically to mechanically dilate the cervix in patients in whom there is a contraindication to prostaglandin.

Compared with vaginal prostaglandin, balloon catheters result in:
- no difference in caesarean section rate
- no difference in rate of delivery within 24 hours
- no difference in neonatal morbidity or mortality
- lower risk of uterine hyperstimulation

AMNIOTOMY
- Surgical rupture of the forewaters with an AmniHook or other instrument is often performed prior to administration of oxytocin.

Table 37.2 **The Bishop's score**				
CERVICAL FEATURE	**BISHOP'S SCORE**			
	0	**1**	**2**	**3**
dilatation	< 1 cm	1–2 cm	3–4 cm	> 4 cm
length	4 cm	2–4 cm	1–2 cm	< 1 cm
consistency	firm	medium	soft	
position	posterior	central	anterior	
station	3	2	1, 0	> +1

- Risks include cord prolapse, intrauterine infection (especially with an increased induction-to-delivery interval) and an increased incidence of cardiotocograph abnormalities.

Medical

Uterine rupture can occur with any agent that enhances uterine tone. Administration of oxytocin requires continuous electronic fetal monitoring and assessment of uterine contractions.

PROSTAGLANDIN

The favourability of the cervix is the best available predictor of a successful induction of labour. At present, the most effective method of cervical ripening is the use of local prostaglandins. When comparing local prostaglandin induction with amniotomy/oxytocin induction, prostaglandin is associated with a decrease in length of labour, lower caesarean section rates (by reducing the number of failed inductions) and fewer Apgar scores (at 1 minute) below 4.

Types of prostaglandin agents

Prostaglandin E_2 is used for cervical ripening for induction of labour. It is manufactured in a triacetin-based gel with 1 or 2 mg dinoprostone in each unit dose of 3 g (2.5 mL). A slow-release delivery system vaginal insert is also available.

Actions of prostaglandins

These soften and efface the cervix by a combination of reducing the collagen concentration and changing the glycosaminoglycan composition and hydration.

Other effects

Prostaglandin E_2 produces vasodilatation and 30% increased cardiac output. It relaxes bronchial and gastrointestinal smooth muscle.

Contraindications to prostaglandin E_2

These include grand multiparity, rupture of membranes, high presenting part, previous uterine surgery, cephalopelvic disproportion, abnormal cardiotocograph, malpresentation and unexplained vaginal bleeding.

Side effects of prostaglandins

These include uterine hyperstimulation with fetal heart rate changes (4%), irritation of the vagina, nausea, vomiting, diarrhoea, pyrexia, bronchoconstriction, hypertension, blurred vision, facial flush and vasovagal reaction.

OXYTOCIN

- In vivo, oxytocin is synthesised in the paraventricular nucleus of the hypothalamus and is transported to the posterior pituitary gland. It is released as a free peptide in response to suckling/nipple stimulation, genital stimulation and stretching of the cervix. Increased sensitivity of the myometrium occurs with increasing gestational age.
- Although regimens vary, the required oxytocin dose to provide adequate uterine contractility is usually between 4 and 16 milliunits per minute. As the physiological dose is individualised, low doses are used initially and are titrated according to strength and frequency of contractions, uterine relaxation and progress of labour.

- Complications include water retention, hyponatraemia, uterine hyperstimulation and rupture and neonatal hyperbilirubinaemia.

Augmentation of labour

Aims
- accelerate progress of labour
- reduce operative vaginal delivery rates
- lower caesarean section rates
- lower the need for analgesia
- reduce the psychological impact associated with slow labour
- primary role of augmentation is to reduce the rate of labour dystocia in primigravid women, which may occur in up to 40% of cases

Methods
- Environment. The presence of a support person may reduce the length of labour.
- Ambulation. This reduces the need for oxytocic augmentation.
- Amniotomy. For a labour that has become prolonged, amniotomy may increase the strength and frequency of contractions. Amniotomy alone for prolonged labour does not alter the caesarean section rate.
- Oxytocin: This increases the strength and frequency of contractions. When performed with amniotomy at an early stage in delayed labour, oxytocin administration reduces time to delivery and the caesarean section rate.

Considerations in augmentation
The differential diagnosis of slow progress in labour includes:
- reduced uterine contractility
- increased resistance in soft tissues (relative disproportion, including malpresentation)
- absolute cephalopelvic disproportion

To differentiate between these mechanisms, adequate uterine contractility is required and oxytocics are suggested.

Care must be taken with oxytocin use in obstructed labour to avoid increasing the risk of uterine rupture.

Further reading

Bishop, E.H., 1964. Pelvic scoring for elective induction. Obstet. Gynecol. 24, 266.

Grant, J.M., 1993. Sweeping the membranes in prolonged pregnancy. Br. J. Obstet. Gynaecol. 100, 889–890.

Hannah, M., Hannah, W.J., Hellmann, J., et al., 1992. Induction of labor as compared with serial antenatal monitoring in post-term pregnancy: a randomized controlled trial. Canadian Multicenter Post-Term Pregnancy Trial Group. NEJM 326 (24), 1587–1592.

Gulmezoglu, A., Crowther, C., Middleton, P., et al., 2012. Induction of labour for improving birth outcomes for women at or beyond term. Cochrane Database Syst. Rev. doi:10.1002/14651858.CD004945.pub3.

Chapter 38

Malpresentation and malposition

Michael Flynn
Thea Bowler

Stages of labour

Labour is divided into three stages.

1. The **first stage** commences with painful contractions, which dilate and efface the cervix. This stage ends with full dilatation of the cervix, and is further divided into the latent and active phases. The latent phase is characterised by gradual cervical change and the active phase by more rapid cervical dilatation.
2. The **second stage** begins at full dilatation and ends with the delivery of the baby.
3. The **third stage** ends when the placenta is delivered.

At term, about 95% of fetuses are cephalic in presentation. Of these, up to 95% will deliver in the occipito-anterior position. Malpresentations and malpositions increase the maternal risks of prolonged labour, infection, obstructed labour, tissue necrosis resulting in vesico/rectovaginal fistulas, and deep venous thrombosis. Fetal risks of malpresentation and malposition are cord prolapse, traumatic delivery and hypoxia.

Occipito-posterior position

The fetal head usually engages in the lateral position, and in 80% of cases it rotates anteriorly. About 20% of fetuses are in the occipito-posterior position in early labour (usually occiput to the right). With increasing flexion in labour, there is a tendency for the fetal head to rotate when it reaches the pelvic floor. Approximately 5% of fetuses deliver in the occipito-posterior position.

Risk factors for persistent occipito-posterior position
- anterior placenta
- anthropoid or android pelvis, where the pelvic brim is longer in the anterior–posterior diameter than in the transverse
- inefficient uterine contractions
- maternal obesity
- nulliparity
- previous occipito-posterior delivery
- gestational age ≥ 41 weeks
- birthweight ≥ 4000 g

The effect of epidural anaesthesia on occipito-posterior position is controversial.

Diagnosis

The occipital bone is the only bone that is overridden by its neighbours. When the diamond-shaped anterior fontanelle can be palpated on vaginal examination, this indicates deflexion of the fetal head.

The maternal abdomen appears flat below the umbilicus, and fetal limbs can be palpated anteriorly on the maternal abdomen.

Ultrasound can be used to visualise the fetal orbits facing anteriorly within the pelvis.

Characteristics of labour
- The woman complains of backache.
- There is a tendency for incoordinate uterine action and prolonged labour.
- There is early distension of the perineum and dilatation of the anus, while the fetal head is high in the birth canal.

Management
- Slow progress in the first stage of labour often requires oxytocin augmentation.
- In the second stage, adequate uterine contractions are required for rotation of the fetal head on the pelvic floor. Occasionally, the fetus will spontaneously deliver in the occipito-posterior position.
- An instrumental delivery may be indicated for a prolonged second stage. Vacuum extraction, using the posterior cup position, will encourage flexion and rotation of the fetal head to correct the relative disproportion. Kielland's rotational forceps may also be used.
- Delivery by caesarean section is indicated if the station of the head is above the ischial spines.

Face presentation

Risk factors
- Fetal factors include anencephaly, cystic hygroma, goitre, prematurity and multiple pregnancy.
- Maternal factors include bicornuate uterus and pelvic tumours.

Diagnosis

Most are diagnosed in labour just before delivery. Up to 60% are in the mento-anterior position, 26% mento-posterior and 15% mento-transverse (right or left). The landmarks at vaginal examination are the mouth, jaw, nose, malar and orbits. The mouth and maxilla form a triangle.

Management

Aim for a vaginal delivery, especially if the baby is in the mento-anterior position. However, if the baby is in the mento-posterior position and there is failure to rotate, the baby cannot be delivered vaginally and caesarean section is required.

Instrumental delivery should be approached with caution. Engagement occurs when the mento-anterior face is at +2 station; therefore, forceps should only be applied when the face has caused the perineum to bulge.

Brow presentation

Incidence. Incidence is about 1 in 1000 deliveries.

Risk factors
- fetal: as with face presentation
- maternal: contracted pelvis

Diagnosis
- Vaginal examination: this includes palpation of the anterior fontanelle, orbital ridges and saddle of the nose.
- Labour in the brow presentation is often prolonged and obstructed, with low likelihood of spontaneous vaginal delivery.

Management
- No treatment is necessary if diagnosed in early labour and progress of labour is adequate. The baby may deflex to a face presentation (30%) or flex to a vertex presentation (20%).
- Spontaneous vaginal delivery of brow presentation is rare.
- Perform caesarean section if there is failure to progress in the first or second stage.
- Instrumental vaginal delivery is contraindicated due to significant risk of maternal and perinatal morbidity.

Transverse and oblique lie

Incidence. 1 in 300 deliveries. More common at earlier gestations.

Risk factors
- fetal: prematurity, multiple pregnancy, polyhydramnios, fetal death and placenta praevia
- maternal: multiparity, contracted pelvis, pelvic tumours and abnormal uterine shape

Diagnosis
- Uterus is small for dates; there is no fetal pole in fundus or pelvis.
- Confirm the diagnosis by ultrasound examination. Additionally, a survey of maternal and fetal anatomy should be performed if diagnosed prior to labour.

Labour

- Labour is often incoordinate and obstructed with high risk of maternal and perinatal morbidity and mortality.
- Uterine rupture may occur and there is a risk of cord prolapse in 10%–15% of cases.

Management

- If the unstable lie persists over 37 weeks management options include admission to hospital to await labour with caesarean section if the fetus remains transverse, or active management with external version of the fetus followed by induction. If the woman has immediate access to hospital and is informed of the risks of expectant management, outpatient management may be considered. If the unstable lie persists after 38 weeks, external version is unsuccessful or labour commences, caesarean section is indicated.
- Internal version of the fetus may result in uterine rupture, and this is indicated only for a second twin.

Cord prolapse and presentation

Incidence. Incidence is about 1 in 200–300 deliveries.

Risk factors

- poorly applied presenting part
- fetal: non-vertex presentation, prematurity, low birthweight, multiple gestation
- maternal: multiparity, polyhydramnios, rupture of membranes
- iatrogenic: operative manoeuvres, including artificial rupture of membranes and forceps delivery

Management

- Advise the woman to present as soon as possible when membranes rupture, especially women with risk factors.
- When a cord prolapse is diagnosed, the presenting part must be pushed away from the cord to avoid cord compression, and immediate delivery of the baby is required.

Diameters of presenting parts

- occipito-anterior = suboccipito-bregmatic = 9.5 cm
- occipito-posterior = occipito-frontal = 11 cm
- face presentation = submento-bregmatic = 9.5 cm
- brow presentation = mento-vertical = 14 cm

Further reading

Ritchie, J.K., 1998. Malpositions of the occiput and malpresentations. In: Dewhurst's Textbook of Obstetrics and Gynaecology for Postgraduates. Blackwell Scientific, Oxford.

Chapter 39

Operative delivery

Thea Bowler

Caesarean section

Caesarean delivery constitutes approximately one-third of births in many countries. Although now a relatively safe procedure, emergency caesarean section carries an increased risk of maternal mortality and morbidity.

The most commonly performed uterine incision is a lower segment transverse incision however a classical caesarean section with a vertical uterine incision is occasionally indicated.

Indications for caesarean section

ELECTIVE

- repeat caesarean section
- malpresentation
- multiple pregnancy
- placenta praevia
- morbidly adherent placenta
- maternal medical conditions including certain infections, cardiovascular disease, neurological disease
- maternal request

EMERGENCY

- presumed fetal distress
- failure to progress
- failed instrumental delivery

Complications of caesarean section

HAEMORRHAGE

- Haemorrhage accounts for 6% of maternal deaths associated with caesarean section.
- There is a 2%–4% risk of blood transfusion following elective caesarean section.
- There are higher risks of postpartum haemorrhage (PPH) with placenta praevia, morbidly adherent placenta, placental abruption, atonic uterus, multiparity, second-stage caesarean and prolonged labour.

URINARY TRACT INJURY

- The risk of bladder injury at caesarean section is less than 1%.
- This is higher in emergency caesarean sections for prolonged obstructed labour or repeat caesarean section with the bladder adherent to the lower segment.
- Ureteric injuries are very uncommon.

ANAESTHETIC COMPLICATIONS

- Regional anaesthesia is a safer alternative to general anaesthesia.
- Risks of general anaesthesia include aspiration, failed intubation and greater maternal blood loss.
- Risks of regional anaesthesia include hypotension, inadequate block, high block, epidural haematoma with neurological sequelae, epidural abscess, headache and local anaesthetic toxicity.

INFECTIONS

- Wound infections occur in 1%–9% of caesarean sections. There is a higher risk of infection with premature rupture of membranes and prolonged labour.
- Endometritis occurs in 6% of elective and up to 11% of emergency caesarean sections. There is a 10–20 times higher risk of endometritis after caesarean section compared with vaginal delivery. The risk increases with duration of labour and presence of chorioamnionitis. Common pathogens include group B streptococcus, *Escherichia coli* and anaerobes.
- Chest infections are complications for 10% of patients after abdominal surgery. High-risk factors for chest infection include obesity, general anaesthetic, smoking and upper respiratory tract infection.
- There is a 2% risk of urinary tract infection with single catheterisation.
- Antibiotic prophylaxis, given prior to skin incision, has been shown to decrease the risk of postoperative febrile morbidity. This is irrespective of whether the caesarean section was emergency or elective.

VENOUS THROMBOEMBOLISM

- Thromboembolism accounts for 17% of deaths after caesarean section. The recurrence risk after one episode of deep venous thrombosis is 12%.
- Pharmacological and mechanical thromboprophylaxis reduce the risk of venous thromboembolism (VTE) after caesarean section.

Indications for classical caesarean section

- absence of the lower uterine segment (this may occur with extreme prematurity, placenta praevia, or fibroids obscuring the lower segment)
- transverse lie or shoulder presentation
- presence of a uterine constriction ring
- caesarean hysterectomy (commonly for morbidly adherent placenta, tumours of the cervix)
- conjoint twins

Trial of labour after caesarean section

A woman with a previous caesarean section has the option in a subsequent pregnancy to undergo either an elective repeat caesarean section or to attempt vaginal delivery.

The likelihood of successful vaginal delivery following caesarean section is 60%–80%.

Prognostic factors for vaginal delivery after caesarean section include:
- previous vaginal delivery: if the woman has had a previous vaginal delivery, there is a greater likelihood of delivering vaginally again
- indication for the first caesarean section: the vaginal delivery rates are lowest when the initial indication was for failure to progress
- spontaneous onset of labour
- maternal body mass index (BMI): likelihood of successful vaginal birth after caesarean (VBAC) is lower with BMI > 30

Up to 40% of women undergo a repeat caesarean section after one lower segment caesarean section for a non-recurring cause. The risks and benefits of repeat caesarean section and trial of vaginal delivery require consideration when deciding on the mode of delivery.

RISKS OF TRIAL OF LABOUR

Uterine rupture
- Risk of uterine rupture is 0.5%–0.7% after one lower segment caesarean section with associated complications:
  - blood transfusion   1.8/1000
  - urinary tract injury   0.8/1000
  - hysterectomy   0.9/1000
  - maternal death   0.02/1000
  - fetal acidosis   1.5/1000
  - perinatal death   0.4/1000
- The overall risk of rupture after a classical caesarean section is 6%, with 2% scar dehiscence before labour; therefore, a trial of labour is contraindicated.
- The risk of rupture after two caesarean sections is approximately 1.3%.

Risks of caesarean section

MATERNAL RISKS
- higher overall maternal mortality rate compared with vaginal delivery, although comparable rates with elective caesarean section
- higher febrile morbidity
- increased blood loss
- anaesthetic risks
- risk of organ injury
- increased risk of deep venous thrombosis
- longer hospital stay
- increasing risk of morbidly adherent placenta with each caesarean section

NEONATAL RISKS
- increased risk of respiratory distress secondary to retained lung fluid
- increased risk nursery admission

Contraindications/relative contraindications to trial of labour after caesarean section
- previous classical or vertical lower uterine segment incision
- previous uterine rupture
- more than one previous caesarean section
- less than 18 months since the previous caesarean section

- morbid maternal obesity
- estimated fetal weight > 4 kg

Instrumental delivery

This includes the forceps and vacuum extractor. The indications and prerequisites are similar for both.

Indications
- failure to progress in the second stage
- malposition of the fetal head
- fetal distress during the second stage
- maternal conditions, including pre-eclampsia, neurological conditions and cardiorespiratory diseases requiring iatrogenic shortening of the second stage of labour
- maternal fatigue/exhaustion

Prerequisites for instrumental delivery
- an indication for the use of instruments
- suitable presenting part
- fully dilated cervix
- membranes ruptured
- clinical assessment not suggestive of absolute cephalopelvic disproportion
- station of presenting part below the ischial spines
- no fetal head palpable abdominally
- position of fetal head (must be known)
- adequate uterine contractions
- empty bladder
- adequate analgesia
- verbal consent

Forceps

TYPES OF FORCEPS
- outlet forceps: Wrigley's forceps
- non-rotational: Neville Barnes' forceps
- rotational: Kielland's forceps

COMPLICATIONS
- maternal: genital tract soft tissue injury, increased incidence of episiotomy and major perineal trauma, bladder and rectal injury
- fetal: facial soft tissue damage, intracranial haemorrhage, skull fractures, facial nerve palsy, corneal abrasion

Vacuum extractor

COMPLICATIONS
- higher failure rate than forceps delivery; more likely sequential use of instruments
- maternal: genital tract injury (lower incidence than forceps)
- fetal: swelling on the scalp produced by the vacuum cup (the chignon), which disappears over 1–2 days; scalp markings and abrasions; cephalohaematoma (a collection

of blood under the periosteum) in up to 6% of babies delivered with vacuum extraction; subgaleal haemorrhage in 1 in 300 deliveries, retinal haemorrhage

Perineal lacerations

Lacerations can occur anywhere along the birth canal, including the uterus, cervix, vagina and perineum.
- **first-degree tear**: injury to the skin of the perineum and vaginal mucosa
- **second-degree tear**: injury to the skin and musculature of the perineum, not involving the anal sphincter
- **third-degree tear**: injury to the perineum involving the anal sphincter
  - *grade 3a tear:* < 50% external anal sphincter torn
  - *grade 3b tear:* > 50% external sphincter torn
  - *grade 3c tear:* both external and internal sphincters torn
- **fourth-degree tear**: injury involving the anal sphincter and anorectal mucosa

The centre point of the perineum is the perineal body. The muscles that blend into this point are the external anal sphincter, levator ani, transverse perineal muscles and bulbocavernosus. The anal sphincter consists of the internal and external layers. The internal sphincter is circular and is situated in the upper two-thirds of the anal canal. The external sphincter consists of three layers. In perineal lacerations, the deep layer is important, as it plays a major role in the continence of flatus and faeces.

Repair of perineal trauma
Up to 70% of women are likely to require perineal repair.

TECHNIQUE
- The vaginal skin may be repaired with continuous or interrupted sutures.
- The perineal skin closure may be subcuticular or interrupted.
- Comparing the two techniques, studies have shown no difference in the long-term complaints of pain or dyspareunia. However, there appears to be a significant advantage in the reduction of pain, in the short term, when using subcuticular sutures.

CHOICE OF SUTURE
Reports comparing polyglycolic acid and chromic catgut show a definite reduction of pain in the short term when using polyglycolic acid, although no long-term differences were found. Therefore, it appears that the optimal choice in the repair of perineal trauma is the use of polyglycolic acid sutures and subcuticular sutures to the skin.

REPAIR OF THIRD OR FOURTH-DEGREE TEAR
- Repair should take place in the operating theatre.
- The anal mucosa should be repaired with interrupted or continuous sutures. Polyglactin causes less discomfort than monofilament sutures.
- The internal anal sphincter should be repaired with mattress or interrupted sutures.
- A full thickness external sphincter laceration should be repaired using an overlapping technique.
- A partial thickness external sphincter laceration should be repaired using an end-to-end anastomosis.
- Polyglactin and monofilament sutures are equivalent for the repair or internal and external sphincters.

Episiotomy

Tissues cut by an episiotomy include:
- vaginal epithelium and perineal skin
- bulbocavernosus muscle
- transverse perineal muscles (superficial and deep)
- occasionally, the external anal sphincter and levator ani
  Therefore, an episiotomy is at least a second-degree perineal laceration.

INDICATIONS FOR EPISIOTOMY

- vaginal breech deliveries
- in fetal distress, to expedite delivery
- past history of pelvic floor repair or third-degree tear
- imminent perineal tear
- instrumental delivery

TYPES OF EPISIOTOMY

- mid-line
- mediolateral; lowest risk of anal sphincter injury
- J-shaped

REPAIR OF AN EPISIOTOMY

This has three stages:
1. The initial stage of repair commences at the apex of the vaginal laceration. The vaginal mucosa is repaired down towards the fourchette.
2. The second stage consists of repairing the deep muscles of the pelvic floor.
3. The final stage is to repair the superficial perineal muscles and skin.

Further reading

Chauhan, S.P., Martin, J.N., Henrichs, C.E., et al., 2003. Maternal and perinatal complications with uterine rupture in 142 075 patients who attempted vaginal birth after caesarean delivery: a review of the literature. Am. J. Obstet. Gynecol. 189 (2), 408–417.

Enkin, M., Keirse, M., Chalmers, I., 2000. A Guide to Effective Care in Pregnancy and Childbirth. Oxford University Press, Oxford.

O'Grady, J.P., Gimovsky, M., 1992. Instrumental Delivery: A Lost Art? Progress in Obstetrics and Gynaecology, vol. 10. Churchill Livingstone, London, pp. 183–211.

Royal College of Obstetricians and Gynaecologists, 2015. The management of third- and fourth-degree perineal tears. Green-top guideline No. 29, June. RCOG, London.

Spong, C.Y., Landon, M.B., Gilbert, S., et al., 2007. Risk of uterine rupture and adverse perinatal outcome at term after caesarean delivery. Obstet. Gynecol. 110, 801–807.

Vacca, A., 2003. Handbook of Vacuum Extraction in Obstetric Practice. Edward Arnold, London.

Chapter 40

Pain relief in labour

Thea Bowler

About two-thirds of women in labour rate the pain as severe or intolerable. There is a need for antenatal preparation, with balanced information and opportunity to discuss expectations and options for analgesia.

Pain in labour

Causes
- dilatation of the cervix
- contraction and distension of uterus
- distension of the vagina and perineum
- pressure on other organs and lumbosacral plexus

Sensory pathways
- Pain during the first stage of labour is visceral, originating in the uterus and cervix. This pain is caused by ischemia of uterine and cervical tissue and distension of uterine and cervical mechanoreceptors and is conducted through T10 – L1.
- Mild pain of early uterine contractions is conducted through T11–T12.
- When the pain becomes more intense, the pathway is T10–L1.
- Pain in the second stage is predominantly caused by somatic pain from distension of the vagina, perineum and pelvic floor conducted via sacral segment S2–S4 (pudendal nerve).

Analgesia in labour

Non-pharmacological methods
- position/postural changes/mobilisation
- warm or cold packs

- massage
- hydrotherapy
- hypnotherapy
- breathing techniques
- transcutaneous electrical nerve stimulation (TENS): electrodes placed paravertebrally at T10–L1 and S2–S4 (uses the gate control theory of pain)
- sterile water injections: intradermal injection into the sacral region, effective for reducing lower back pain associated with labour

Pharmacological methods

- Inhalational agents: nitrous oxide acts quickly and is simple and safe. Side effects include nausea, vomiting, dizziness, euphoria, disorientation and sedation.
- Systemic opioid analgesia: morphine administered intramuscularly has a duration of action of 3–4 hours with a maternal half-life of 1 hour and a neonatal half-life of 6 hours (most infants delivered 3 hours after a dose will have undetectable cord levels). It has a similar analgesic effect to pethidine; however, the metabolite of pethidine has a longer half-life in the newborn so therefore morphine is used preferentially for intrapartum analgesia. Side effects include nausea, vomiting, reduced gastric motility and neonatal respiratory depression.
- Pudendal block: transvaginal injection of 10 mL local anaesthetic into the region of each pudendal nerve produces anaesthesia of the vagina and perineum that is useful for instrumental deliveries where there is no regional anaesthesia.
- Regional anaesthesia: lumbar epidural is the most effective and reliable form of pain relief in labour. The local anaesthetic may be delivered by intermittent boluses or constant infusion.
- General anaesthesia is associated with increased neonatal respiratory depression, maternal blood loss and post-operative pain. Physiological changes of pregnancy (such as increased oxygen consumption, airway oedema and vascularity; increased breast tissue; and reduced lower oesophageal tone) make intubation and ventilation more difficult with higher risk of failed or difficult intubation and gastric acid aspiration.

ADVANTAGES OF EPIDURAL

- The mother remains conscious, is able to maintain airways and can participate in the birth.
- There is minimal or no fetal/neonatal depression, with higher Apgar scores than those associated with narcotic analgesia.
- It can be continued for intrapartum or postpartum surgical procedures.
- Epidural anaesthesia does not affect the overall caesarean section rate; however, it is associated with greater numbers of caesarean sections for fetal distress. It is also associated with a prolongation of the second stage of labour and more instrumental deliveries.

DISADVANTAGES OF EPIDURAL

- It is not always successful in providing analgesia. There is a 5% chance of having to resite the catheter due to ineffective block.
- There may be hypotension from reduced peripheral vascular resistance. This is a result of sympathetic blockade with decreased vasoconstriction and increased venous pooling. The blockade also produces a secondary tachycardia. A corresponding decrease in uteroplacental blood flow may result in fetal heart rate abnormalities.

Hypotension is managed with intravenous fluids and metaraminol administered by the anaesthetist.
- There is the potential for rare but serious drug-related and neurological complications.

COMPLICATIONS OF LUMBAR EPIDURAL

- **Local anaesthesia toxicity.** Central nervous system effects of circumoral numbness, restlessness, visual changes, confusion and convulsion, and arrhythmia and hypotension, are managed by ensuring adequate airway/ventilation, assessing cardiorespiratory status and treating convulsions.
- **Massive subarachnoid injection of local anaesthetic or total spinal.** This is avoided by applying a small test dose. The complications, including hypotension, nausea, coma, fixed dilated pupils, phrenic nerve paralysis and ventilatory failure, are managed by providing ventilatory support, assessing cardiovascular status and giving intravenous fluids (maintain these until the anaesthetic wears off).
- **Dural puncture.** This occurs in about 1% of patients. The majority of these develop symptoms, especially positional headache. The most effective treatment is autologous blood patch, but there is a risk of infection.
- **Anaphylactic reactions.** Allergic and anaphylaxis reaction may occur as with any other pharmacological agents.
- **Epidural haematoma.** Very rarely a small bleed in the epidural space may compress the spinal cord and result in permanent neurological damage. Treatment is with emergency decompression.
- **Infection.** This is very rare but may include meningitis or epidural abscess.
- **Neurological injury.** There is a 1 in 1000 risk of temporary nerve damage, a 1 in 13 000 chance of persistent symptoms beyond 6 months and a 1 in 250 000 risk of severe neurological injury including paralysis.

SPINAL ANALGESIA

- intrathecal administration of anaesthetic via a single injection
- advantages: rapid onset, a dense block, less anaesthetic required with lower risk of toxicity; compared with epidural, there is less need for conversion to general anaesthesia during surgical procedures
- disadvantages: hypotension, limited duration of anaesthesia (90–120 minutes)

Chapter 41

Labour ward emergencies

Thea Bowler

Up to 5% of deliveries have postpartum complications.

Maternal collapse

Significant causes
- vasovagal syncope and postural hypotension
- haemorrhage: postpartum/antepartum haemorrhage, splenic artery aneurysm rupture, hepatic rupture
- thromboembolism
- amniotic fluid embolism
- epilepsy
- eclampsia
- intracranial haemorrhage
- cardiac disease: myocardial infarction, aortic dissection, cardiomyopathy, arrhythmia
- sepsis
- drug toxicity/overdose: magnesium sulfate, local anaesthetic, illicit drugs
- anaphylaxis

Management
Prompt resuscitation while considering the differential diagnosis.
- tilt: left lateral tilt of 15 degrees to relieve aortocaval compression and improve venous return
- airway: clear airway, early intubation
- breathing: supplemental high-flow oxygen, bag-mask ventilation until intubation can be performed
- circulation: chest compressions, attach defibrillator and check rhythm, two large-bore cannulae, volume replacement
- drugs: administration of drugs according to the advanced life support algorithm
- defibrillate if required

Throughout resuscitation, consider the cause of collapse and investigate/treat accordingly.

- investigations: collecting blood for full blood count, electrolytes, blood sugar level, blood group and hold, coagulation profile, liver and renal function tests
- monitoring: electrocardiograph, pulse, blood pressure, oxygen saturation, fluid balance, fetal heart rate
- treatment of the cause
- recourse to perimortem caesarean section

Perimortem caesarean section

- In maternal cardiopulmonary arrest, irreversible brain injury can occur within 4–6 minutes due to the gravid uterus impairing venous return and cardiac output.
- Perimortem caesarean section should be performed if there is no response after 4 minutes of correctly performed cardiopulmonary resuscitation in a woman beyond 20 weeks gestation.
- Delivery of the fetus and placenta aids maternal resuscitation by increasing venous return and cardiac output, reducing oxygen consumption, facilitating chest compressions and improving ventilation.

Postpartum haemorrhage

Primary postpartum haemorrhage

Primary postpartum haemorrhage is the loss of more than 500 mL blood within 24 hours of delivery. The incidence is 1%–5%.

In maternal mortality statistics in Australia, haemorrhage has been a major factor of direct maternal deaths. In these, postpartum haemorrhage was a significant contributor.

CAUSES

- uterine atony (most common cause)
- retained products of conception, retained placenta
- soft-tissue laceration
- coagulation defect
- uterine rupture

RISK FACTORS

- retained placenta
- grand multiparity with increased fibrous tissue and reduced muscular tissue in the uterus
- antepartum haemorrhage
- overdistension of the uterus with conditions such as polyhydramnios and multiple pregnancy
- large placental site (associated with multiple pregnancy, molar pregnancy)
- past history of postpartum haemorrhage
- fibroid uterus (especially intramural)
- prolonged labour
- chorioamnionitis
- tocolytic agents, halogenated anaesthetic agents
- coagulopathy
- 20% occurring in the absence of risk factors

MANAGEMENT
- Prevention: routine use of oxytocin and an active management of the third stage can reduce postpartum haemorrhage by 40%.
- Resuscitation: the immediate danger is inadequate circulation, not reduced oxygen-carrying capacity. Therefore, restore circulatory volume with intravenous fluids and cross-match blood. Insert two large-bore IV cannulae and consider indwelling catheter to monitor fluid balance.
- Reverse or prevent coagulopathy: if coagulation or platelet count are abnormal, treat with fresh frozen plasma and platelets.
- Treat the cause of haemorrhage.
- Non-pharmacological management: bimanual uterine compression, application of pressure to genital tract lacerations.

Medical treatment for atonic uterus

This involves an intravenous oxytocin bolus of initially 10 IU or ergometrine 250–500 µg. If haemorrhage is not controlled by simple methods, the woman requires a formal examination and exploration under anaesthesia. The genital tract is assessed for tears, retained products of conception and uterine rupture. If uterine atony continues after these causes are excluded, further medical treatment includes the use of rectal misoprostol, which may be effective in increasing uterine tone. Doses of up to 800 µg are used and maternal pyrexia should be monitored. Prostaglandin F2-alpha is a potent uterotonic and is administered via injection into the myometrium. Doses of up to 3 mg can be used.

Surgical management of continuing postpartum haemorrhage

Uterine artery ligation has minimal complications and reduces the pulse pressure by 60%–70% to allow endogenous haemostatic mechanisms to control bleeding.

Internal iliac artery ligation

This is usually bilateral.

Uterine compression sutures

B-Lynch sutures used to compress the uterus are often effective.

Balloon tamponade via Bakri balloon

An intrauterine balloon can be inserted vaginally or at caesarean section to limit ongoing uterine blood loss.

Recombinant activated factor VIIa

This has been used effectively in uncontrolled bleeding.

Hysterectomy

Hysterectomy may be needed for persistent atony, morbidly adherent placenta or uterine rupture. If it is not due to placenta praevia, a subtotal hysterectomy may be the operation of choice, as there is a higher maternal mortality with total hysterectomy.

Arterial embolisation

This can be performed by an interventional radiologist if the woman is haemodynamically and haemostatically stable.

Secondary postpartum haemorrhage

Definition. Secondary postpartum haemorrhage is fresh bleeding from the genital tract after the first 24 hours but before 6 weeks postpartum. It is most common in the second week.

CAUSES

- infection
- retained products of conception
- placental site subinvolution

INVESTIGATION

- This includes abdominal and vaginal examination to confirm involution of the uterus and closed external cervical os.
- Vaginal microbiological specimens should be collected.
- Pelvic ultrasound should be used to evaluate for retained products of conception.

MANAGEMENT

- antibiotics: suitable empirical cover for mixed genital flora
- evacuation of retained products
- uterotonic agents, including oxytocin and misoprostol

Summary of management of severe obstetric haemorrhage

- prompt restoration of circulatory volume
- accurate diagnosis of cause
- appropriate treatment to stop bleeding early

Amniotic fluid embolism

Incidence. Incidence is about 2 in 100 000. Previously, maternal mortality was 85%. Overall mortality rates are now thought to be 20%, accounting for 10% of maternal deaths internationally. Up to 85% of survivors suffer neurological injury due to cerebral hypoxia. The neonatal mortality rate is approximately 40%.

It presents with respiratory distress and cardiovascular collapse. Of those who survive the first hour, 40% will develop a coagulopathy.

Pathophysiology

Amniotic fluid embolism can occur in any trimester and is due to changes in the normal anatomical relationship between the membranes, placenta and uterine wall, with disruption of the integrity of the uterine blood vessels.

In the maternal circulation, the amniotic fluid/debris is deposited in the lungs and causes pulmonary vasoconstriction, which is probably due to an anaphylactic-type reaction to the amniotic fluid/debris. Severe hypoxia occurs with respiratory failure and cardiogenic shock; disseminated intravascular coagulopathy may also occur.

Risk factors

- hypertonic uterine activity
- caesarean section and instrumental delivery
- induction of labour
- precipitate labour

- polyhydramnios
- advanced maternal age
- grand multiparity

Presentation and diagnosis

- Most commonly, there is sudden collapse during labour/delivery or the immediate postpartum period with dyspnoea, pink frothy sputum and cyanosis, leading to cardiorespiratory failure. Convulsions occur in 10%–20% of cases.
- The major clinical findings include hypotension due to cardiogenic shock, hypoxia with respiratory failure, disseminated intravascular coagulation and coma or seizures.
- The diagnosis is confirmed by finding fetal squames in the sputum or blood from central venous line, or at postmortem during examination of the maternal lungs when fetal squames and debris are present.

Management

There is no specific treatment for amniotic fluid embolism and therapy is supportive.
- urgent delivery of the fetus
- securing airways and ventilating
- treating cardiovascular collapse: vasopressins (dopamine/dobutamine), intravenous (IV) fluids, blood products
- central venous line, arterial line
- correcting coagulopathy
- treating metabolic/electrolyte abnormalities
- watching for infection
- intensive care

Thromboembolism and pulmonary embolism

(*See Ch 46 for further details.*)

Clinical presentation of pulmonary embolism

- anxiety, tachycardia
- shortness of breath, apnoea, cyanosis
- possible retrosternal chest pain, haemoptysis, pleural friction rub and a split-second heart sound
- maternal collapse

Emergency management

- resuscitate
- secure airway, oxygen, ventilate if necessary
- anticoagulate with standard or low-molecular-weight heparin (IV heparin infusion for massive pulmonary embolism with cardiovascular compromise)
- investigate: ECG, chest X-ray, ventilation–perfusion (VQ) scan or computed tomography
- pulmonary angiogram (CTPA)
- surgery: employ embolectomy if the embolus is in the proximal part of the main pulmonary artery; if in inferior vena cava, insert umbrella filter

Prophylaxis

- early mobilisation in the postpartum period
- maintenance of adequate hydration
- mechanical thromboprophylaxis: graded compression stockings, sequential compression devices
- pharmacological thromboprophylaxis according to risk factors for venous thromboembolism (*see Ch 47*)

Regional anaesthesia toxicity

Incidence. Incidence is up to 1 in 1000. Increased susceptibility in the pregnant woman is due to:

- increased blood flow to the spinal cord
- reduced epidural space because of distended vessels
- a rise in pressure in the epidural space with uterine contractions

Presentation

- Signs and symptoms may occur almost immediately and within up to 20 minutes of administering local anaesthesia.
- Patient complains of metallic taste, tinnitus, confusion and disorientation.
- Respiratory muscle paralysis and cardiac arrest may occur.

Management

- prevention
- intubation and ventilation
- fluid resuscitation

Eclampsia

(*See Ch 44 for further details on eclampsia/pre-eclampsia.*)
    Incidence. Incidence is up to 1 in 1500.

Presentation

- Presentation includes hypertension, hyperreflexia and clonus, headache, visual changes and seizures.
- Twenty per cent of patients with eclampsia have diastolic blood pressure < 90 mmHg, urine dipstick test results of < 2+ protein and normal reflexes.
- Up to 40% have no significant oedema.
- Seventy per cent of deaths are due to intracerebral haemorrhage.
- Three serious complications of eclampsia are cerebrovascular injury, pulmonary oedema and coagulopathy.

Management

- secure airway; ventilate if necessary
- stop seizure and prevent recurrence: magnesium sulfate bolus and infusion
- control blood pressure
- diagnose and correct coagulopathy
- prevent pulmonary oedema; maintain strict fluid balance
- delivery of fetus

Inverted uterus

An inverted uterus occurs when the fundus of the uterus descends through the uterine body, cervix and vagina.

Presentation
- includes pain, bleeding
- a vaginal lump after placental delivery
- suspect uterine inversion if the cardiovascular shock is out of proportion to blood loss after delivery (due to a vasovagal response to visceral stimulation)

Risk factors
- overzealous cord traction
- fundal implantation site
- uterine atony
- short cord
- previous inversion: recurrence rate of up to 33%

Management
- resuscitation
- digital replacement, leaving placenta attached
- manual replacement with the aid of tocolytic agents
- O'Sullivan hydrostatic method
- operative procedures: manual removal of placenta and uterine exploration

Shoulder dystocia

Incidence. Incidence is 0.5%–0.7%.

Risk factors
- previous shoulder dystocia: recurrence rate approximately 10%
- excess maternal weight gain, maternal body mass index (BMI) > 30 kg/m^2
- maternal diabetes
- macrosomia > 4500 g
- induction of labour
- postdates pregnancy: a 20% incidence of macrosomia with infants delivered at 42 weeks compared with 12% delivered at 40 weeks
- intrapartum risks: prolonged first or second stage, oxytocin augmentation, assisted vaginal delivery

Complications
- fetal acidemia and hypoxic brain injury
- brachial plexus injury (90% spontaneous resolution)
- fractures of humerus or clavicle
- pneumothorax
- maternal: postpartum haemorrhage, third- and fourth-degree tears

Management
- Observe for signs of shoulder dystocia: difficult delivery of face and chin, retraction of the fetal head (turtle-neck sign), failure of restitution of fetal head.

- Do not apply excessive traction, as this will increase impaction. Advise woman not to push.
- Obtain assistance, including an anaesthetist, paediatrician and nursing staff.
- Consider episiotomy.
- McRoberts manoeuvre: flexion of maternal hips with thighs on abdomen. Increases anterior-posterior dimension of pelvis.
- Suprapubic pressure: rotation of anterior shoulder into the oblique pelvic diameter.
- Internal manoeuvres: Woods and Rubin manoeuvres attempt to rotate the fetal shoulders obliquely by application of pressure to the anterior or posterior shoulder. Delivery of the posterior arm reduces the diameter of the fetal shoulders by the width of the arm.
- Roll patient into all fours and attempt delivery.
- Manoeuvres of last resort (rarely required): Zavanelli manoeuvre, symphysiotomy.

Uterine rupture

This is the complete disruption of all uterine layers including serosa.

Risk factors
- previous caesarean delivery (classical caesarean > lower segment caesarean)
- previous uterine surgery (e.g. myomectomy with breach of cavity)
- prolonged obstructed labour
- medical induction or augmentation of labour
- macrosomia
- multiple gestation
- grand multiparity
- abnormal uterine architecture (e.g. uterus didelphus, bicornuate uteri)
- connective tissue disorders

SYMPTOMS AND SIGNS OF UTERINE RUPTURE
- acute fetal distress
- acute continuous abdominal pain
- reduction in contractions
- vaginal bleeding
- loss of station of presenting part

Management
- resuscitation of haemodynamically unstable patient
- notify anaesthetic and paediatric staff
- urgent caesarean section
- hysterectomy may be indicated if there is uncontrollable haemorrhage or an irreparable uterine defect

Chapter 42

Maternal mortality

Vivienne O'Connor

Maternal death in Australia is a rare event in the context of worldwide maternal deaths. In 2008–2012, there were 105 maternal deaths in Australia that occurred within 42 days of the end of pregnancy, representing a maternal mortality ratio (MMR) of 7.1 deaths per 100 000 women who gave birth. The women who died were aged between 17 and 50. Women aged 40 and over, women who are obese with a body mass index (BMI) of 30 or more, and women of Aboriginal and Torres Strait Islander origin, were among those at increased risk of maternal death. Maternal mortality for Aboriginal and Torres Strait Islander women is double that of other Australian women, with an Aboriginal and Torres Strait Islander MMR of 13.8 deaths per 100 000 women who gave birth compared with 6.6 deaths per 100 000 for other Australian women who gave birth. Cardiovascular conditions, sepsis and psychosocial conditions were the leading causes of maternal deaths among Aboriginal and Torres Strait Islander women.

Background facts

Between 1990 and 2015, maternal mortality worldwide dropped by about 44%. However, by the end of 2015, roughly 303 000 women will have died during and following pregnancy and childbirth. Every day, approximately 830 women die from preventable causes related to pregnancy and childbirth, with 99% of all maternal deaths occurring in developing countries. Maternal mortality is higher in women living in rural areas and among poorer communities. Young adolescents face a higher risk of complications and death as a result of pregnancy than other women. Most (62%) maternal deaths occurred in sub-Saharan Africa (179 000 deaths). Nearly a third of maternal deaths worldwide in 2013 occurred in two countries: 17% in India (50 000 deaths) and 14% in Nigeria (40 000 deaths).

Skilled care before, during and after childbirth can save the lives of women and newborn babies. Between 2016 and 2030, as part of the Sustainable Development Agenda, the target is to reduce the global MMR to less than 70 per 100 000 live births.

Definitions

The World Health Organization definition of maternal mortality is the death of a woman while pregnant or within 42 days of the termination of pregnancy, irrespective of the duration and site of the pregnancy, from any cause related to or aggravated by pregnancy or its management, but not from accidental or incidental causes. It also includes deaths from assisted reproduction technologies where pregnancy has not occurred, but not from incidental causes. In most Australian states and territories, incidental deaths are included in the definition.

Classifications

Direct maternal deaths

These result from obstetric complications of pregnancy, labour and puerperium (i.e. as a direct complication of pregnancy itself), from interventions, omissions, incorrect treatment or from a chain of events resulting from any of these. There were 49 maternal deaths directly related to the pregnancy in 2008–2012. The leading causes of direct maternal death were obstetric haemorrhage (11), thromboembolism (10) and hypertensive disorders (9) and, when combined, these accounted for more than 61% of all direct maternal deaths. Five of the direct deaths due to obstetric haemorrhage were related to the presence of pathological placentation (placenta accreta and/or percreta), and five were due to postpartum haemorrhage. Five non-obstetric haemorrhage deaths resulted from rupture of a splenic artery aneurysm and five were due to intracranial haemorrhage.

Indirect obstetric deaths

These result from preexisting disease or disease that develops during pregnancy that is not due to a direct obstetric cause, but may have been aggravated by physiological changes in pregnancy. The leading cause of indirect maternal death was cardiovascular disease (15).

Incidental deaths

These are due to conditions during pregnancy where the pregnancy is unlikely to have contributed significantly to death. Examples include road accidents, homicide and malignancies.

Maternal mortality ratio

This means deaths per 100 000 confinements (including both live and stillbirths). This compares to international standards of deaths per 100 000 live births. The total MMR has fallen from 12.7 deaths per 100 000 women who gave birth in 1973–1975 to 7.2 deaths per 100 000 women who gave birth in 2009–2011.

Contributing factors in those who died from haemorrhage were the failure to recognise the continuation and/or extent of the haemorrhage, delay in undertaking surgical treatment to arrest haemorrhage, and delay in blood transfusion.

In those with pre-eclampsia, intracerebral bleeding was the major cause of death. The reporting data in Australia can be improved. This includes variation in reporting, in referral for coronial investigation and quality of data on Indigenous status.

Reducing maternal mortality and morbidity

The 'three delays' model has been used in the global context to identify problems that could lead to change: delay in decision to seek care; delay in arrival to an appropriate care facility; and delay in receiving adequate care once reaching a facility.

Increasing use of modern contraceptives—in particular long-acting reversible contraception (LARC)—have made and can continue to make an important contribution to reducing maternal mortality in the developing world by spacing pregnancies, allowing the woman to improve her nutrition and preventing high-risk, high-parity births.

It is estimated that for every maternal death in Australia, there are other incidences of severe maternal morbidity, including haemorrhage, uterine rupture, renal failure and eclampsia. Identifying near-miss maternal morbidity from specific criteria provides meaningful information on the quality of care and can identify factors for system, group or individual improvement.

There is a plan to reduce the rate of stillbirths, neonatal and maternal deaths in England by 50% by 2030.

Further reading

Australian Institute of Health and Welfare, Humphrey, M.D., Bonello, M.R., et al., 2015. Maternal deaths in Australia 2008–2012. Maternal deaths series no. 5. Cat. no. PER 70. AIHW, Canberra.

Department of Health, Hunt, J., 2015. New ambition to halve rate of stillbirths and infant deaths. GOV.UK 2015 Nov 13. Available at: <www.gov.uk/government/news/new-ambition-to-halve-rate-of-stillbirths-and-infant-deaths>.

World Health Organization. Maternal mortality. Global Health Observatory (GHO) data. Geneva: WHO. Available at: <www.who.int/gho/maternal_health/mortality/maternal/en/>.

Chapter 43

Perinatal mortality, birth asphyxia and cerebral palsy

Vivienne O'Connor
Michael Flynn

Background facts for live-born babies

Perinatal data collection and reporting are one of the most sensitive reflections of the health of a society. In Australia, the differential perinatal rates can reflect the general health of different communities (e.g. Indigenous) and health resources.

Generally, approximately 8% of live-born babies are preterm (< 37 weeks gestation) and less than 1% are born postterm (> 42 weeks) with mean gestation age at birth being 39 weeks. Males live-born at term on average weigh 110 g more than females, with the average birthweight approximately 3360 g.

Definitions

- **Birth rate.** This is the number of live births per 1000 of the estimated mean population.
- **Intrauterine fetal death (IUFD).** This is death of a fetus in utero after 20 weeks gestation or at birth weighing at least 400 g.
- **Intrapartum death.** This is fetal death during labour. If a baby is born without signs of life, but also without maceration, there is a strong presumption that death occurred during labour. There are exceptions in both directions, which require judgment on the timing of death in relation to the presumed onset of labour.
- **Stillbirth (fetal death).** This is the death of a fetus before delivery when the gestation has reached at least 20 weeks or the weight is over 400 g. This Australian definition differs from the World Health Organization (WHO) definition, which requires the stillborn infant to weigh at least 1000 g or to have reached at least 28 weeks gestation. Therefore, caution is required in comparing international rates. The stillbirth rate is approximately 7.1 per 1000 births in Australia. Low birthweight occurred in

79% of stillborn babies, with 28% of these unexplained. The mean gestational age of stillborn babies is approximately 27 weeks compared with 39 weeks for live-born babies. Preterm birth occurred in 80% of stillborn babies, compared with 7.6% of live-born babies. Still birth is higher in first-time mothers and women with greater than four previous deliveries than in those with one previous delivery. It is often seen in the lower gestations and birth weights.

- **Neonatal death.** This is the death of a live-born baby of at least 20 weeks gestation or 400 g in weight within 28 days of delivery. In comparison, the WHO definition is the death of an infant of at least 1000 g or 28 weeks gestation that occurs within 7 days of birth. In Australia, the neonatal death rate (NDR) is generally around 2.5 per 1000 live births. Congenital abnormality occurs in a higher proportion of neonatal deaths (31.3%) than fetal deaths (20.8%). Spontaneous preterm birth was a common cause of neonatal death for babies born at 20–27 and 28–31 weeks. Twins and higher order multiples are prominent in this category.
- **Perinatal mortality rate (PMR).** This is the total number of stillbirths and neonatal deaths per 1000 total births. In Australia it has been stable at 10 per 1000 births. Of these, 72% were fetal deaths. The PMR of babies born to Aboriginal or Torres Strait Islander mothers remains almost twice that of babies born to other mothers. PMR varied by sociodemographic, maternal and pregnancy risk factors. Young maternal age, maternal Indigenous status and multiple gestation were associated with higher rates of perinatal deaths.

Perinatal mortality aetiology

The main categories of stillbirth, according to the Perinatal Society of Australia Perinatal Death Classification (PSANZ–PDC), system are:
- for singleton pregnancies (> 70% of stillbirths):
  - unexplained antepartum death (28%)
  - congenital abnormality (20%)
  - maternal conditions (13%)
  - spontaneous preterm (10%)
- in multiple pregnancy:
  - twin–twin transfusion (35%)
  - spontaneous preterm (24%)
  - unexplained antepartum death (15%)
  - congenital abnormality (11%)

Investigation
- full blood examination and biochemistry screen and bile salts
- coagulation profile and fibrinogen
- Kleihauer
- maternal bacteriology including blood cultures, vaginal and cervical swabs
- viral serology
- glucose assessment including HbA1c
- thyroid function
- maternal thrombophilia and antibody screen
- fetal microbiology including placental and fetal swabs
- fetal karyotype
- autopsy and placental histology

Unexplained stillbirth

- The presence of fetal growth restriction in approximately 40%–50% of unexplained stillbirths is an important consideration for future prevention strategies.
- Some risk factors are modifiable. Risk factors include maternal overweight and obesity, age > 35 years, smoking, primiparity, prolonged pregnancy and socioeconomic disadvantage.

Birth asphyxia

There is no general agreement on the definition of birth asphyxia. The Australian and New Zealand Perinatal Society defines perinatal asphyxia as an event or condition during the perinatal period that is likely to severely reduce oxygen delivery and lead to acidosis, together with a failure of at least two organs consistent with the effects of asphyxia.

Asphyxia may be *long-term chronic partial* asphyxia due to poor placental function or *severe acute* asphyxia due to such conditions as placental abruption, cord prolapse or uterine rupture.

Indicators

- Obstetric indicators of asphyxia may include an abnormal cardiotocograph (CTG), fetal acidosis and the presence of meconium liquor. The latter occurs in 0.5%–20% of all births and alone is an inadequate marker of perinatal asphyxia.
- CTG is a poor predictor of birth asphyxia. Although the false-negative CTG as a predictor of fetal acidosis is below 2%, the false-positive rate may be as high as 50%.
- Neonatal indicators are the Apgar score, delay in breathing, and hypoxic ischaemic encephalopathy. Apgar scores are poor predictors of birth asphyxia. Long-term studies on babies and children have shown that, although babies with very low Apgar scores (a score < 3 at 5 minutes) have an increased risk of cerebral palsy, most infants with low Apgar scores do not develop cerebral palsy. Conversely, 75% of children with cerebral palsy have Apgar scores ≥ 7 at 5 minutes.

Cerebral palsy

Definition. Cerebral palsy covers a range of neurological impairments, characterised by abnormal control of movement or posture resulting from abnormalities in brain development or an acquired non-progressive cerebral lesion.

Incidence. In Australia, it is estimated that a child is born with cerebral palsy every 18 hours. Worldwide, the incidence is the same (1 in 400 births). There is no prebirth test and no known cure. For most, the cause is unknown.

Aetiology

- Major associations of cerebral palsy are intrauterine growth restriction and extreme prematurity.
- Although the patterns of pathological response to brain injury are similar in all cases, it is usually impossible to determine the exact time of brain injury.
- Studies have claimed that at least 90%–94% of cerebral palsy cannot be related to intrapartum hypoxia.

- Other associated factors include fetal vascular events, intrauterine infective causes (rubella, cytomegalovirus, toxoplasmosis, listeriosis), genetic causes (chromosomal abnormalities, X-linked disorders), metabolic disorders (iodine deficiency), and lead and mercury toxicity. Postnatal cerebral palsy may be caused by meningitis, near-drowning episodes or complications of prematurity.
- In cases of cerebral palsy where intrapartum hypoxia was evident, many were found to have a preexisting neurological incident contributing to hypoxia.
- Less than 2% of cerebral palsy is caused by obstetric care alone.

Obstetric aspects of cerebral palsy

The Australian and New Zealand Perinatal Society suggests that to define the relationship of intrapartum events and cerebral palsy, the following are essential:
- evidence of metabolic acidosis in intrapartum fetal or umbilical arterial cord samples
- early onset of severe or moderate encephalopathy in infants of > 34 weeks gestation
- cerebral palsy of the spastic quadriplegic or dystonic type, as well as:
  - a hypoxic event noted immediately before or during labour
  - a sudden rapid and sustained deterioration of the fetal heart rate pattern
  - Apgar scores of 0–6 for longer than 5 minutes
  - evidence of multisystem involvement
  - early imaging evidence of acute cerebral abnormality

References and further reading

Australian Institute of Health and Welfare (AIHW), National Perinatal Statistics Unit: <www.npsu.unsw.edu.au>.

Headley, E., Gordon, A., Jeffery, H., 2009. Reclassification of unexplained stillbirths using clinical practice guidelines. Aust. N. Z. J. Obstet. Gynaecol. 49 (3), 285–289.

Hilder, L., Zhichao, Z., Parker, M., et al., 2014. Australia's mothers and babies 2012. AIHW National Perinatal Statistics Unit: Perinatal Statistics Series No. 30. Cat. No. PER 69. AIHW, Canberra. Available at: <www.aihw.gov.au/publications>.

MacLennan, A., 1999. A template for defining causal relationship between acute intrapartum events and cerebral palsy: international consensus statement. Br. Med. J. 319, 1054–1059.

Perinatal Society of Australia and New Zealand, 2009. Clinical practice guideline for perinatal mortality. Available at: <www.psanz.com.au>.

Royal College of Obstetricians and Gynaecologists, October 2010. Late intrauterine fetal death and stillbirth. Green-top Guideline No. 55. RCOG, London.

Chapter 44

Hypertension in pregnancy

Nikki Whelan

Cardiovascular changes in pregnancy

There are significant physiological adaptations of the cardiovascular system due to pregnancy. Plasma volume rises from an average non-pregnant 2600 mL to 3800 mL at about 32 weeks gestation. The total red cell volume grows constantly until term from 1400 mL to 1700 mL, so there is a fall in haemoglobin concentration as gestation progresses. Cardiac output rises from 5 L/minute to 7.5 L/minute, mostly during the first trimester, and the heart rate rises by 10% with an average resting rate of 88 beats/minute. The peripheral resistance is lowered by a combination of increased vasodilatory substances during pregnancy and decreased sensitivity to vasopressor substances.

Blood pressure falls in the first trimester and is at its lowest in the second trimester. The reduction in diastolic blood pressure is about 10 mmHg by mid-pregnancy. Blood pressure rises to non-pregnant levels towards the end of the third trimester.

Uterine blood flow increases steeply from 24 weeks gestation.

Other factors affecting blood pressure in pregnancy include posture (via the supine hypotension syndrome) and uterine contractions, which raise blood pressure.

Definitions. *Hypertension* in pregnancy is defined as:
- systolic blood pressure ≥ 140 mmHg, and/or (K1 first sound heard)
- diastolic blood pressure ≥ 90 mmHg (Korotkoff disappearance of sounds completely, where K5 is absent, K4 [muffling] should be accepted)
- correct cuff size is important

These measurements should be confirmed by repeated readings over several hours. Elevations of both systolic and diastolic blood pressure have both been associated with adverse fetal outcome and therefore both are important.

Severe hypertension in pregnancy is defined as:
- a systolic blood pressure ≥ 170 mmHg, and/or
- diastolic blood pressure ≥ 110 mmHg

This represents a level of blood pressure above which cerebral autoregulation is overcome in normotensive individuals. It is generally acknowledged that severe hypertension should be lowered promptly, albeit carefully, to avoid cerebral haemorrhage and hypertensive encephalopathy.

Classification

Classifications of hypertensive disorders in pregnancy are:
- pre-eclampsia/eclampsia
- gestational hypertension
- chronic hypertension
  - essential
  - secondary
  - white coat
- pre-eclampsia superimposed on chronic hypertension

Pre-eclampsia

Incidence. While 20% of women are hypertensive at some stage of their pregnancy (blood pressure ≥ 140/90 mmHg), about 5%–10% of primigravid women and 2% of multiparous women fulfil a diagnosis of pre-eclampsia.

Definition. Pre-eclampsia is a multisystem disorder unique to human pregnancy, characterised by hypertension and involvement of one or more other organ systems and/or the fetus. Proteinuria is the most commonly recognised additional feature after hypertension, but should not be considered mandatory to make the diagnosis.

A diagnosis of pre-eclampsia can be made when hypertension arises after 20 weeks gestation and is accompanied by one or more of the following:
- renal involvement
  - significant proteinuria: dipstick proteinuria, subsequently confirmed by spot urine protein/creatinine ratio ≥ 30 mg/mmol
  - serum or plasma creatinine > 90 µmol/L
  - oliguria < 80 mL/4 hours
- haematological involvement
  - thrombocytopenia < 100 000/µL
  - haemolysis schistocytes, red cell fragments on blood film, raised bilirubin, raised LDH > 600 mIU/L, decreased haptoglobin
  - disseminated intravascular coagulation
- liver involvement
  - raised serum transaminases
  - severe epigastric or right upper quadrant pain
- neurological involvement
  - convulsions (eclampsia) (rare in Australia with 4 per 10 000 pregnancies or 1 per 200 women with pre-eclampsia)
  - hyperreflexia with sustained clonus
  - persistent new headache
  - persistent visual disturbances (photopsia, scotomata, cortical blindness, posterior reversible encephalopathy syndrome, retinal vasospasm)
  - stroke
- pulmonary oedema
- intrauterine growth restriction
- placental abruption

Pathophysiology

Two placental conditions predispose to the development of pre-eclampsia. Ischaemia results from the failure of the normal development of the uteroplacental circulation with the presence of small defective spiral arteries, which then may become blocked by acute atherosis or thrombosis. Excessive placental size also predisposes to pre-eclampsia, as seen in multiple pregnancy, hydatidiform mole, fetal triploidy and placental hydrops.

Maternal contribution to pre-eclampsia occurs when endothelial activation results in acceleration of the normal systemic inflammatory response, which is present in all pregnancies. Activation of leucocytes and the coagulation process, and subsequent metabolic changes, result in the clinical features which are typically seen in pre-eclampsia: hypertension, oedema, proteinuria, platelet dysfunction, clotting derangements and possibly eclampsia.

The specific placental factor or factors that generate the systemic inflammatory response of pre-eclampsia remain unknown, but recent research has highlighted the contribution of three circulating placental products: soluble fms-like tyrosine kinase 1 (sFlt-1), endoglin and placental growth factor.

Placentation also depends on the invasion of the placental bed by cytotrophoblasts. Immune tolerance must occur in this setting to allow a continued relationship between the mother and the fetus.

Hence, at least four factors are likely to contribute to the development of pre-eclampsia: placental, endothelial, inflammatory and immunological.

Risk factors associated with pre-eclampsia

Risk factors are listed in Table 44.1. Other factors associated with pre-eclampsia include chronic hypertension, preexisting renal disease, autoimmune disease, more than 10 years since a previous pregnancy, a short sexual relationship prior to conception, and other thrombophilias (e.g. Factor V Leiden and possibly periodontal disease).

Table 44.1 Pre-eclampsia risk factors	
RISK FACTOR	**RELATIVE RISK**
previous history of pre-eclampsia	7.2
antiphospholipid syndrome	9.7
preexisting diabetes	3.6
multiple pregnancy	2.9
nulliparity	2.9
family history of pre-eclampsia	2.9
overweight (BMI) > 25-29.9	1.7
obese BMI > 30	2.7
maternal age > 40	2.0
systolic blood pressure > 130 mmHg before 20 weeks	2.4
diastolic blood pressure > 80 mmHg before 20 weeks	1.4

Source: SOMANZ. 2014. Guidelines for the management of hypertensive disorders of pregnancy. Sydney: Society of Obstetric Medicine of Australia and New Zealand. Available at: www.somanz.org

Recurrence risk

Studies of the risk of recurrent pre-eclampsia in women with a history of a hypertensive disorder in a prior pregnancy show variable results. Recurrence rates vary from 6%–55%, with the greatest risk in women with early-onset pre-eclampsia and chronic hypertension. An Australian study suggests a 14% risk of developing pre-eclampsia, and also a 14% risk of developing gestational hypertension in their next pregnancy.

Clinical spectrum

Pre-eclampsia is a multisystem disorder with both maternal and fetal consequences.

HYPERTENSION

Hypertension may be labile, often with flattened or the reverse of normal diurnal rhythm. This is thought to be due to decreased responsiveness to angiotensin II. Many of the complications of pre-eclampsia are due to arterial damage and loss of vascular autoregulation.

RENAL SYSTEM

Glomerular swelling of endothelial cells and intracapillary cells known as endotheliosis is the main response to pre-eclampsia. This causes a reduced glomerular filtration rate, which slows urate clearance and raises serum creatinine levels. In uncomplicated pregnancy, glomerular filtration normally increases. A serum creatinine level of 0.09 μmol/L in pregnancy may predict renal involvement.

Proteinuria is often a late sign of pre-eclampsia and indicates poorer prognosis for the mother and fetus.

The commonest cause of nephrotic syndrome in pregnancy is pre-eclampsia. There is a reduced maternal plasma volume due to increased leakiness of capillaries, and hypoalbuminaemia predisposing to reduction in colloid oncotic pressure and raised fluid in interstitial spaces. The complications of fluid changes include pulmonary and laryngeal oedema, and acute renal failure.

PLATELETS

The reduction of platelets in pre-eclampsia is due to increased consumption and lowered platelet lifespan. However, this is an inconsistent feature of pre-eclampsia.

COAGULATION

There is increased factor VIII consumption in early pre-eclampsia, and anti-thrombin III is lowered. Disseminated intravascular coagulation is a late and inconsistent feature of pre-eclampsia. The complications of coagulation/clotting changes include disseminated intravascular coagulation with widespread fibrin deposition, haemorrhage and necrosis.

HEPATIC CHANGES

- Liver dysfunction with elevated hepatic enzymes is often evident. Raised alkaline phosphatase is normal, due to the placental production, although raised transaminase levels reflect hepatic ischaemia of pre-eclampsia.
- Epigastric pain from the rare complication of subcapsular haematoma has associated mortality.
- The syndrome of haemolysis, elevated liver enzymes and low platelets is associated with microangiopathic haemolysis and is a variant of severe pre-eclampsia: HELLP.

CENTRAL NERVOUS SYSTEM INVOLVEMENT

- Eclampsia has an incidence of < 0.1%, with 50% occurring before labour. Most postpartum fits occur within 24 hours of delivery. Proteinuria increases the risk by seven to eight times.
- Hypertensive encephalopathy may be acute or subacute, with diffuse cerebral dysfunction, which improves with the lowering of blood pressure. The clinical presentation includes headache, nausea, vomiting and convulsions.
- Stroke in pre-eclampsia and or eclampsia is usually preceded by severe hypertension. In women who had experienced a stroke, 96% had a systolic blood pressure > 160 mmHg, 21% had a diastolic blood pressure > 105 mmHg and 13% had a diastolic blood pressure > 110 mmHg; mean arterial pressure was > 125 mmHg in 46% and > 130 mmHg in 21% of women who had experienced a stroke.
- Only 11% of women who experienced a stroke had a complete recovery without significant morbidity.
- Visual disturbance with cortical blindness occurs in 1%–3% of eclamptics and recovers with reduction in blood pressure.
- The cerebral pathology of eclampsia resembles hypertensive encephalopathy, with evidence of thrombosis, fibrinoid necrosis and microinfarction.
- Cerebral autoregulation is altered in hypertensive pregnant women, making them more sensitive to severe changes in blood pressure. Acute arterial hypertension can lead to damage to the blood–brain barrier with extravasation of fluid into the parenchyma resulting in cerebral haemorrhage and infarction. A mean arterial pressure of 140 mmHg (blood pressure 180/120) is an obstetric emergency and requires immediate treatment.

PLACENTAL AND FETAL INVOLVEMENT

Abnormal placentation reduces uteroplacental blood flow by changing the uteroplacental circulation from a low-resistance system to one of high resistance and underperfusion. The complications of this to fetuses are intrauterine growth restriction, death and complications of prematurity, when delivery is indicated.

Offspring of pregnancies affected by pre-eclampsia have higher blood pressures and body mass index (BMI) in childhood which may put them on a trajectory for cardiovascular disease later in life.

Management of pre-eclampsia

Pre-eclampsia is a progressive disease that will inevitably worsen if pregnancy continues. Current therapy does not ameliorate the placental pathology, nor alter the pathophysiology or natural history of pre-eclampsia. Delivery is the definitive management and is followed by resolution, generally over a few days but sometimes over a much longer course. At a mature gestational age, delivery should not be delayed.

PREVENTION

- Prophylactic therapy with aspirin is associated with a reduction in the recurrence rate of pre-eclampsia, delivery prior to 34 weeks gestation, preterm birth and perinatal death. Risk reduction is greatest if therapy is commenced prior to 20 weeks gestation and if doses > 75 mg are taken.
- The use of calcium supplementation has been demonstrated to reduce the risk of pre-eclampsia, especially in women with a low calcium intake. Calcium supplementation (1.5 g/day) should be offered to women at increased risk of pre-eclampsia, particularly those with a low dietary calcium intake.

- Randomised trials of antioxidants vitamins C and E have failed to show any significant benefit, and there was an increased risk of stillbirth and birthweight < 2.5 kg in the treatment arm of the study. Hence, prophylactic treatment with vitamins C and E is not recommended.
- Heparin with and without aspirin has not been assessed using large randomised trials. At present, therefore, there is no evidence for this treatment in the absence of a thrombophilia or antiphospholipid antibody syndrome.
- Observational studies have suggested that multivitamin supplementation containing folic acid may reduce the risk of pre-eclampsia, perhaps by improving placental and systemic endothelial function or by lowering blood homocysteine levels.
- Preconception counselling should be offered to all women at increased risk of pre-eclampsia, and particularly to women with preexisting disorders that may need to be stabilised prior to pregnancy.
- Potential novel therapies:
  - pravastatin
  - melatonin
  - proton pump inhibitors

INVESTIGATIONS

- initial assessment may be in a day assessment unit, unless severe hypertension, headache, epigastric pain or nausea and vomiting are present, which necessitate urgent admission
- urine dipstick testing for proteinuria, with spot protein/creatinine ratio if > 1+ (30 mg/dL)
- full blood count
- urea, creatinine, electrolytes
- liver function tests
- ultrasound assessment of fetal growth, amniotic fluid volume and umbilical blood flow

Additional investigations that may be useful in certain women include urine microscopy on a mid-stream specimen, coagulation studies, blood film, lactate dehydrogenase, fibrinogen, investigations for underlying systemic lupus erythematosus, renal disease, antiphospholipid syndrome, thrombophilias, fasting plasma free metanephrines/normetanephrines and 24-hour urinary catecholamines.

INDICATIONS FOR DELIVERY IN PRE-ECLAMPSIA OR GESTATIONAL HYPERTENSION
For indications for delivery in pre-eclampsia or gestational hypertension, see Table 44.2.

ANTIHYPERTENSIVE THERAPY
Severe hypertension
Antihypertensive treatment (see Table 44.3) should be started in all women with a systolic blood pressure > 160 mmHg or a diastolic blood pressure > 110 mmHg because of the risk of intracerebral haemorrhage and eclampsia. A Cochrane review has concluded that there is no good evidence to support the use of any short-acting agent over any other and practice should therefore be guided by local experience and familiarity.

Mild to moderate hypertension
There is controversy regarding the treatment of mild to moderate hypertension in women with pre-eclampsia. Antihypertensive treatment does not prevent pre-eclampsia

Table 44.2 Indications for delivery in pre-eclampsia or gestational hypertension

MATERNAL	FETAL
gestational age > 37 weeks	placental abruption
inability to control hypertension	severe intrauterine growth restriction
deteriorating platelet count	non-reassuring fetal status
deteriorating liver function tests	
deteriorating renal function tests	
persistent neurological symptoms	
eclampsia	
persistent epigastric pain, nausea or vomiting with abnormal liver function tests	
acute pulmonary oedema	

Source: SOMANZ. 2014. Guidelines for the management of hypertensive disorders of pregnancy. Sydney: Society of Obstetric Medicine of Australia and New Zealand. Available at: www.somanz.org

Table 44.3 Antihypertensive agents for treatment of severe hypertension

DRUG	DOSE	ROUTE	ONSET OF ACTION
labetalol	20–80 mg; maximum 80 mg	intravenous (IV) bolus over 2 minutes, repeat every 10 minutes as needed	5 minutes
nifedipine	10–20 mg; maximum 40 mg	oral	30–45 minutes; repeat in 45 minutes
hydralazine	10 mg; maximum 40 mg	IV bolus, repeat every 20 minutes	20 minutes
diazoxide	15–45 mg; maximum 300 mg	IV rapid bolus	3–5 minutes; repeat in 5 minutes

Source: SOMANZ. 2014. Guidelines for the management of hypertensive disorders of pregnancy. Sydney: Society of Obstetric Medicine of Australia and New Zealand. Available at: www.somanz.org

or the associated adverse perinatal outcomes, but it decreases by half the incidence of development of severe hypertension among women with mild hypertension.

In the absence of compelling evidence, treatment of mild to moderate hypertension in the range 140–160/90–100 mmHg should be considered an option and will reflect local practice (see Table 44.4). Above these levels, treatment should be considered mandatory.

- First-line drugs include methyldopa, labetalol and oxprenolol.
- Second-line drugs are hydralazine, nifedipine and prazosin.
- Angiotensin-converting enzyme (ACE) and angiotensin receptor blockers are contraindicated.
- All first-line and second-line drugs, plus enalapril, captopril and quinapril, are compatible with breastfeeding.

Intravenous fluids

Although maternal plasma volume is often reduced in women with pre-eclampsia, there is no maternal or fetal benefit to maintenance fluid therapy. As vascular permeability is

Table 44.4 Oral antihypertensives for moderate hypertension				
DRUG	**DOSE**	**ACTION**	**CONTRAINDICATIONS**	**PRACTICE POINTS**
methyl dopa	250–750 mg three times a day	central	depression	slow onset of action over 24 hours; dry mouth, sedation, depression, blurred vision
clonidine	75–300 µg three times a day	central		prompt onset of action; withdrawal effect; reduce over 7 days
labetalol	100–400 mg every 8 hours	beta-blocker, alpha-vasodilator		asthma, chronic airways limitation, bradycardia, bronchospasm, headache, nausea, tingling scalp
oxprenolol	20–160 mg three every 8 hours	beta-blocker with intrinsic sympathomimetic activity (ISA)		
nifedipine	20–60 mg slow release twice daily	calcium channel antagonist	aortic stenosis	severe headache, flushing, tachycardia, peripheral oedema, constipation
prazosin	0.5–5 mg every 8 hours	alpha-blocker		first dose effect orthostatic hypotension
hydralazine	25–50 mg every 8 hours	vasodilator		flushing headache, nausea, lupus-like syndrome

Source: SOMANZ. 2014. Guidelines for the management of hypertensive disorders of pregnancy. Sydney: Society of Obstetric Medicine of Australia and New Zealand. Available at: www.somanz.org

increased in women with pre-eclampsia, administration of large volumes of intravenous fluids may cause pulmonary oedema and worsen peripheral oedema.

Management of eclampsia

The drug of choice for the prevention of eclampsia is magnesium sulfate. However, the case for its routine use in women with pre-eclampsia in countries with low maternal and perinatal mortality rates is controversial and is perhaps best determined by individual units monitoring their outcomes. In some units, the presence of severe headache, hyperreflexia with clonus, epigastric pain or severe hypertension are considered indications for prophylaxis.

Trial data suggest the use of magnesium does not appear to affect rates of caesarean section, infectious morbidity, haemorrhage or neonatal depression, nor the duration of labour (although necessitated higher doses of oxytocin).

RESUSCITATION

- **Usually self-limiting.** Intravenous diazepam (2 mg/minute to maximum of 10 mg) or clonazepam (1–2 mg over 2–5 minutes) can be used while $MgSO_4$ is being prepared.
- **Magnesium sulfate.** The possible mechanisms of action include cerebral vasodilatation, thereby decreasing cerebral ischaemia or perhaps blocking neuronal damage associated with ischaemia. It prevents but does not terminate seizures. The dose

includes an intravenous loading dose of 4 g over 10–15 minutes followed by an infusion of 1–2 g/hour for 24 hours. Side effects are hypocalcaemia, hyporeflexia and cardiac arrest. The Eclampsia Trial Collaborative Group found magnesium sulfate to be superior to phenytoin or diazepam in decreasing recurrent seizures, maternal mortality and intensive care admission.

CONTROL HYPERTENSION

Stabilise blood pressure (see above).

DELIVERY

In the presence of eclampsia, there is no role for continuation of the pregnancy once the woman is stable.

When delivery is indicated, the mode of delivery depends on favourability of the cervix, the speed required for delivery and the fetal condition. In many cases, induction of labour and vaginal delivery is appropriate. In severe pre-eclampsia, prophylactic antihypertensive and anticonvulsant therapy are continued. Lumbar epidural is favoured for analgesia due to its ability to lower blood pressure and possibly increase uterine blood flow. Caution with epidural, with strict investigation of platelet levels, coagulation profile and clotting times, is important to avoid complications of bleeding and spinal haematoma. The use of general anaesthesia for caesarean section is associated with a marked hypertensive response to laryngoscopy and intubation.

Oxytocin in doses over 2 mU/minute intravenously acts as an antidiuretic and, although it is not contraindicated in severe pre-eclampsia, strict fluid balance must be adhered to.

Fetal wellbeing is monitored by continuous cardiotocography. The maternal pushing in the second stage should be shortened.

The use of ergometrine in the third stage is contraindicated, and the immediate postpartum period requires intensive monitoring of blood pressure, renal function and fluid balance.

Chronic hypertension in pregnancy

This is a major predisposing factor to pre-eclampsia, although alone it may not be associated with the maternal and fetal risks of pre-eclampsia. If superimposed on chronic hypertension, pre-eclampsia tends to recur in subsequent pregnancies, and it is therefore often difficult to differentiate between the two. A diagnostic guide includes decreasing platelet count, serum urate level (< 0.30 mmol/L is unlikely to be pre-eclampsia), a 24-hour urinary protein concentration (except if hypertension is due to chronic renal failure) and liver biochemistry.

Management
- Cease therapy if hypertension is mild to moderate before pregnancy.
- Use a first-line drug where possible for controlling the hypertension.
- Watch closely for the development of pre-eclampsia, using the tests described above.
- Fetal monitoring should include an early dating ultrasound scan and 4-weekly growth scans in the third trimester, tracking growth, liquor volume and umbilical artery blood flow.
- Manage jointly with obstetric physicians.

Unusual causes of hypertension in pregnancy

Phaeochromocytoma

This is a tumour of the adrenal medulla associated with significant maternal and fetal mortality.

- Clinical presentation: sustained or paroxysmal hypertension; the patient complains of headache, palpitation, sweating, chest and abdominal pain, and visual symptoms.
- It may be familial or associated with other syndromes, such as multiple endocrine neoplasias, neurofibromatosis and thyrotoxicosis.
- Diagnosis: involves 24-hour urinary assessment for metanephrines, creatinine, vanillylmandelic acid and catecholamines. Diagnostic imaging using magnetic resonance and computed tomography are safe in pregnancy. Ultrasound is often inadequate to assess the adrenals. If phaeochromocytoma is diagnosed, examine for multiple endocrine neoplasia.
- Management: use alpha-blockers, and then beta-blockers. Surgery can remove the tumour, but there may be difficulties with the large uterus.

Coarctation of aorta

This is an anatomical anomaly and a known independent cause of hypertension.

Cushing's syndrome

- rare in pregnancy
- clinical presentation: hypertension, pigmentation, striae, hyperglycaemia
- investigations: dexamethasone suppression test, computed tomography scan of the pituitary and adrenals

Conn's syndrome

- rare in pregnancy
- clinical presentation: hypokalaemia and hypertension (possibility of remission in pregnancy may be due to the antagonism of the action of aldosterone by progesterone)

Renal artery stenosis

AUTOIMMUNE CONNECTIVE TISSUE DISORDERS

Women with systemic lupus erythematosus may present with hypertension, renal complications or superimposed pre-eclampsia.

Long-term consequences

One cohort study (Skjaerven et al. 2012) has shown that women with preterm pre-eclampsia and no subsequent pregnancies had a 9.4-fold increase risk of cardiovascular death, and women with term pre-eclampsia and no subsequent pregnancies had a 3.4-fold increase risk of cardiovascular death. Women with term pre-eclampsia who went on to have further pregnancies only had a 1.5-fold increase in cardiovascular death, suggesting women who only had one pre-eclamptic pregnancy have health problems that discourage future pregnancies.

Table 44.5 Risk of developing subsequent disease after pre-eclampsia

MEDICAL CONDITION	RELATIVE RISK (95%)
chronic hypertension	3.7
ischemic heart disease	2.16
cerebrovascular disease	1.81
peripheral vascular disease	1.87
deep vein thrombosis	1.79
end-stage renal disease	4.3
type 2 diabetes	1.86
elevated thyroid stimulating hormone	1.7
all cancer	0.96

Source: SOMANZ. 2014. Guidelines for the management of hypertensive disorders of pregnancy. Sydney: Society of Obstetric Medicine of Australia and New Zealand. Available at: www.somanz.org

It is recommended all women with hypertensive disease in pregnancy have an annual review for blood pressure and other cardiovascular risk factors (Table 44.5).

References and further reading

Askie, L.M., Duley, L., Henderson-Smart, D.J., et al., 2007. Antiplatelet agents for the prevention of pre-eclampsia: a meta-analysis of individual patient data. Lancet 369 (9575), 1791–1798.

CLASP Collaborative Group, 1994. CLASP: a randomised trial of low dose aspirin for the prevention and treatment of pre-eclampsia among 9364 pregnant women. Lancet 343, 619–629.

Eclampsia Trial Collaborative Group, 1995. Which anticonvulsant for women with eclampsia? Evidence from the Collaborative Eclampsia Trial. Lancet 345, 1455–1463.

Magpie Collaborative Group, 2002. Do women with pre-eclampsia and their babies benefit from magnesium sulphate? The Magpie Trial: a randomised placebo-controlled trial. Lancet 359, 1877–1890.

Scott, J.S., 1958. Pregnancy toxaemia associated with hydrops foetalis, hydatidiform mole and hydramnios. J. Obstet. Gynaecol. Br. Emp. 65, 689–701.

Skjaerven, R., Wilcox, A.J., Klungsoyr, K., et al., 2012. Cardiovascular mortality after pre-eclampsia in one child mothers: prospective, population based cohort study. BMJ 345, e7677.

Society of Obstetric Medicine of Australia and New Zealand, 2014. Guidelines for the management of hypertensive disorders of pregnancy. SOMANZ, Sydney. Available at: <www.somanz.org>.

Chapter 45

Diabetes in pregnancy

Nikki Whelan

Diabetes in pregnancy is either preexisting/pregestational diabetes or newly diagnosed diabetes in pregnancy.

Physiology and pathophysiology

Maternal glucose homeostasis

- Normally, blood sugar levels are stable in all trimesters. This is achieved by doubling the insulin secretion from the end of the first trimester to the end of the third trimester.
- In early pregnancy, raised oestrogen and progesterone levels cause beta cell hyperplasia in the pancreas, which results in a rise in insulin secretion and an increase in fat stores.
- In the second and third trimesters, increases in the diabetogenic hormones human placental lactogen, prolactin and free cortisol cause insulin resistance and lipolysis. Therefore, the increased insulin concentration is counterbalanced by increasing insulin resistance, the mechanism of which is not clearly understood.
- Fasting blood glucose level (BGL) decreases, while postprandial BGL increases in pregnancy. The pregestational diabetic is at risk of hypoglycaemia in early pregnancy and ketoacidosis in later pregnancy, as the demand for insulin is increased.
- Fetal glucose homeostasis: maternal glucose crosses the placenta freely by facilitated diffusion. Therefore, the mother is responsible for regulating fetal blood sugar levels. Fetal insulin appears in the circulation at the end of the first trimester, but the exact role of fetal insulin is uncertain and it may act by promoting growth. It normally plays no role in blood glucose homeostasis. In response to fetal hyperglycaemia due to elevated maternal blood sugar, fetal pancreatic cells hypertrophy, leading to inappropriate release of insulin.

Pregestational diabetes

Effects on pregnancy

MATERNAL EFFECTS

Increased risks of:
- polyhydramnios
- pre-eclampsia
- placental abruption
- infection, including urinary tract and candidiasis
- diabetic ketoacidosis
- trauma during delivery
- caesarean section

FETAL EFFECTS

- Congenital malformation: pregestational diabetics (both type 1 and type 2) have an increased risk of fetal malformation with increasing levels of hyperglycaemia (see Table 45.1). Literature suggests only small increases in HbA1c are associated with increased risk.
- Type 1 diabetics with an HbA1c of 7.2% (normal range 6%) have double the risk of fetal malformation and type 2 diabetics may have twice the risk of fetal malformation of the non-pregnant population with a normal HbA1c. If their HbA1c rises to 7.3%, their risk of fetal malformation may be as high as 11%.
- Malformations include neural tube defects, cardiovascular and vertebral defects. The risk of malformation is proportional to imperfect metabolic control during organogenesis; improved blood sugar control decreases anomalies. Many malformations can be diagnosed by mid-trimester ultrasound.
- Abortion and perinatal mortality: diabetic women have higher abortion rates. An HbA1c of 6.5% increases the risk of spontaneous abortion by 3%. Perinatal mortality rates also rise in proportion to the rise in mean BGL. The exact mechanisms for the increased risk demise are uncertain.
- Abnormal fetal growth: there is an increase in the incidence of large-for-dates and small-for-dates fetuses, and consequently fetal morbidity. Macrosomia in all organs (except the brain) is due to an increase in cytoplasmic mass. Macrosomic babies are at risk of trauma during delivery, with definite risk of shoulder dystocia in the diabetic mother with a fetus > 4000 g. Intrauterine growth restriction (IUGR) may be a complication of placental vasculopathy and may be related to underlying renal disease or the development of pre-eclampsia.
- Preterm delivery is common.

Table 45.1 Maternal diabetes and risk of congenital malformation	
CONGENITAL MALFORMATION	**INCREASED RISK OVER NON-DIABETICS**
cardiac	4 times
neural tube defects	2–10 times
gastrointestinal atresia	3–10 times
caudal regression	200 times (though still rare)
urinary tract	10 times

NEONATAL EFFECTS

- Respiratory distress syndrome: carries six times the risk of non-diabetics. Fetal hyper-insulinaemia results in reduced pulmonary phospholipid production and a decrease in surfactant.
- Hypoglycaemia: 50% of babies of insulin-dependent diabetic mothers have blood sugar levels below 2 mmol/L due to fetal hyperinsulinaemia and discontinuation of the maternal glucose supply.
- Hypocalcaemia is present in 25%–50% of infants.
- Polycythaemia and jaundice: polycythaemia is due to an increase in erythropoietin caused by raised fetal insulin. Jaundice, which occurs in up to 50% of babies, is mainly due to elevated red cell destruction and immaturity of the liver.
- Macrosomia is common.
- Hypertrophic cardiomyopathy is usually reversible.
- Risk of diabetes: when one parent is diabetic, this is associated with a 3% risk of the offspring developing diabetes in 20 years. If both parents are diabetic, the risk is 20%.

Management

PREPREGNANCY COUNSELLING

General measures

- Stop smoking.
- Reduce alcohol intake.
- Review all medications, including complementary medications, for safety in pregnancy.
- Screen and vaccinate for infectious diseases, including rubella, varicella, *Bordetella pertussis* and cervical human papillomavirus (HPV).
- Provide weight management, nutrition and exercise advice.
- Provide contraceptive advice until conception is desired.

Diabetes-specific measures

- The multidisciplinary team should include an obstetrician, physician, diabetes educator and dietician (wherever possible).
- Achieve optimal glycaemic control: HbA1c should be maintained in the normal range wherever possible. This should be possible in most women with type 2 diabetes, but may not be possible in all women with type 1 diabetes.
- Preconception glucose levels significantly influence fertility and risk of congenital abnormalities, and probably impacts on developing embryo prior to organogenesis and that exposure can occur in fallopian tube and endometrium before implantation.
- The woman should take folic acid (5 mg daily).
- Medications include the use of the newer rapid-acting insulin analogues and insulin pump therapy. Oral agents should be reviewed and consideration given to switching over to insulin (e.g. basal bolus regimen). Oral agents such as metformin are not used routinely, but are becoming more commonly prescribed.
- Antihypertensive agents should be suitable for continued use in pregnancy.
- Statins should be ceased.
- Review diabetic complications, including retinopathy, nephropathy, macrovascular disease and autonomic neuropathy.
- Assess thyroid function and screen for other autoimmune diseases where appropriate.

ANTENATAL MANAGEMENT

Management should be by a multidisciplinary team wherever possible.

Medical

- Assess BGL control with HbA1c and reinforce the necessity for regular self-monitoring of BGLs.
- Aims: fasting BGL of 4.0–5.5 mmol/L, 1 hour postprandial < 8.0 mmol/L, and 2 hours postprandial < 7.0 mmol/L.
- Monitor with HbA1c every 4–8 weeks.
- Advise that hypoglycaemia is common, especially overnight from 6–18 weeks, and that insulin requirements may increase substantially in late second trimester with increasing insulin resistance.
- Basal and prandial insulin requirements may vary between ethnic groups; that is, South Asian and Middle Eastern women may have higher prandial insulin requirements than Caucasian women.
- Insulin requirements may reduce from 32 weeks gestation and should prompt assessment of fetal wellbeing if this is > 5%–10%.
- Assess diabetic complications if no prepregnancy counselling has been performed, especially retinopathy (regular formal eye examinations) and nephropathy (24-hour urine analysis, spot albumin : creatinine ratio, dip stick urine analysis and serum electrolytes, creatinine and urea).

OBSTETRIC MANAGEMENT

- First trimester dating scan.
- Offer nuchal translucency scan and serum screen at 12–13 weeks gestation for aneuploidy.
- Perform a fetal morphology scan at 18–20 weeks and in selected cases repeat a morphology scan at 24 weeks, especially targeting the heart.
- Assess fetal growth and wellbeing at 28–30 weeks and at 34–36 weeks, or more frequently in the presence of medical or obstetric complications.
- Aim for delivery at term unless obstetric or medical complications arise (e.g. fetal macrosomia, polyhydramnios, poor metabolic control, pre-eclampsia or IUGR).
- Vaginal delivery is preferable, unless obstetric or medical contraindications exist (e.g. risk of shoulder dystocia increases with birthweight > 4000 g).
- Anticipate the need for neonatal nursery admission if delivery is earlier than 36 weeks or poor metabolic control is present.

LABOUR

Monitor BGL 1–2 hourly, aiming for 4–7 mmol/L, which can be achieved with various regimens, including:
- insulin/dextrose infusion
- insulin/dextrose infusion if BGL is < 4 mmol/L or > 7 mmol/L
- subcutaneous insulin injections
- insulin pump therapy

POSTPARTUM

- Type 1 diabetes: insulin requirements fall rapidly post-delivery, and commonly require one third to one half of their pregnancy insulin dose.
- Avoid hypoglycaemia.
- Close monitoring is needed.

- Breastfeeding mothers need to be encouraged to test prefeeds and postfeeds to check for hypoglycaemia; commonly need two-thirds of their prepregnancy insulin dose.
- Type 2 diabetes: some women can be managed with diet alone; or in combination with oral agents. Some will need insulin therapy.

Contraception

There is no evidence that any present contraceptive methods are contraindicated in diabetes.

Gestational diabetes

Definition. This is the development of abnormal glucose tolerance during pregnancy in a woman who did not have diabetes before pregnancy.

Incidence. International criteria differ as to diagnosis, and so incidence varies considerably. Most Australian centres report a 15% incidence. These may include previously undiagnosed non-insulin-dependent diabetics. The Hyperglycaemia Adverse Pregnancy Outcome (HAPO) 2008 Study suggests there is a continuous, linear association between BGLs and major adverse pregnancy outcomes.

Diagnosis

- Diabetes mellitus in pregnancy should be diagnosed by the 2006 WHO criteria if one or more of following criteria are present:
  1. fasting plasma glucose > 7.0 mmol/l
  2. 2-hour plasma glucose > 11.1 following 75 g oral glucose load
  3. random plasma glucose > 11.1 in presence of diabetes symptoms
- Gestational diabetes mellitus (GDM) at any time in pregnancy:
  1. fasting plasma glucose 5.1–69 mmol/L
  2. 1 hr 75 g oral glucose load > 10 mmol/L
  3. 2 hrs 75 g oral glucose load > 8.5–11.0 mmol/L
- Diabetes in pregnancy may not necessarily be confirmed as diabetes in the postpartum period.
- Diabetes in pregnancy is more likely to be confirmed in the postpartum period when hyperglycaemia in pregnancy is diagnosed early and if the degree of hyperglycaemia is made.
- Incidence of 15% in Australia and higher in some ethnic groups (e.g. East Asia 23%).
- Gestational diabetes has increased perinatal morbidity, with characteristics for babies similar to preexisting diabetes. These include fetal macrosomia, neonatal hypoglycaemia, hyperbilirubinaemia and respiratory distress syndrome, with a probable long-term risk of obesity and diabetes.

RISK FACTORS FOR GDM

- previous hyperglycaemia in pregnancy
- previous elevated BGL
- family history of first-degree relative with diabetes or sister with GDM
- previous macrosomia, > 4500 g or > ninetieth percentile
- ethnicity: Asian Indian subcontinent, Aboriginal, Torres Strait islander, Pacific Islander, Maori, Middle Eastern
- body mass index (BMI) > 30
- maternal age > 40 years

- polycystic ovarian syndrome (PCOS)
- medications: corticosteroids, antipsychotics

SCREENING METHODS

Screening on a risk basis only or using a glucose challenge test have been shown to have a significant false-negative rate and have been largely abandoned.

TESTING

- All women not previously known to have prepregnancy diabetes or hyperglycaemia should undergo a 75 g oral glucose tolerance test (GTT) at 24–28 weeks.
- Women classified high risk may benefit from testing in early pregnancy.

DIAGNOSTIC CRITERIA

- Australian Diabetes in Pregnancy Society has accepted WHO recommendations.
- Hyperglycaemia first detected in pregnancy is either:
  - diabetes mellitus in pregnancy, or
  - gestational diabetes mellitus

Management

- a team approach with an obstetrician, endocrinologist, diabetic nurse educator and dietitian
- involves:
  - patient education
  - dietary management
  - increasing physical activity
  - limiting weight gain
- reduces risks of pre-eclampsia or caesarean section delivery/postpartum weight retention and long-term adverse metabolic outcomes in mothers and infants
- limit weight gain, especially in obese women (BMI > 30) to 5 kg
- additional treatments:
  - metformin (studies suggest it is a suitable treatment option)
  - insulin
- large gestational age infants are associated with excessive gestational weight gain, and fasting glucose levels > 5.5 mmol/L

OBSTETRIC MANAGEMENT

- Fetal growth and surveillance of fetal wellbeing: at 28–30 and 34–36 weeks gestation to monitor growth; more frequently if complications develop.
- Timing of delivery: if uncomplicated, await spontaneous labour, but avoid postdates.
- In labour: regular BGLs.

POSTPARTUM FOLLOW-UP

- 75 g 2-hour oral GTT at 6–12 weeks
- women diagnosed with hyperglycaemia in pregnancy have 30% risk recurrence in subsequent pregnancy
- 1%–10% risk 1 year of developing type 2 diabetes

FOLLOW-UP

- low-risk fasting plasma glucose or HbA1c 1–2 yearly
- high risk oral GTT 1–2 yearly

TREATMENT TARGETS
- fasting capillary blood glucose < 5.0
- hour BGL after commencing meal < 7.4
- hour BGL after commencing meal < 6.7
- risk of developing type 2 diabetes after GDM has significant ethnic variation; for example, the number of Indigenous women who had developed type 2 diabetes is as follows:
  - at 3 years   22%
  - at 5 years   25%
  - at 7 years   42%

Further reading

Australian Institute of Health and Welfare, Templeton, M., Pieris-Caldwell, I., 2008. Gestational diabetes mellitus in Australia, 2005–06. Diabetes Series No. 10. Cat. No. CVD44. AIHW, Canberra.

HAPO Study Cooperative Research Group, 2008. Hyperglycemia and adverse pregnancy outcomes. NEJM 358 (19), 1991–2002.

Nankervis, A., McIntyre, H.D., Moses, R., et al. for the Australasian Diabetes in Pregnancy Society, ADIPS Consensus Guidelines for the Testing and Diagnosis of Hyperglycaemia in Pregnancy in Australia and New Zealand (modified November 2014). Australian Diabetes in Pregnancy Society, Sydney.

Rowan, J.A., Hague, W.M., Wanzhen, G., et al. for the MiG Trial Investigators, 2008. Metformin versus insulin for the treatment of gestational diabetes. NEJM 358 (19), 2003–2015.

Chapter 46

Thromboembolism in pregnancy

Amy Mellor

- Venous thromboembolism (VTE) occurs in approximately 1 in 1600 pregnancies.
- Pregnancy is associated with a 10-fold increase in risk of VTE compared with the non-pregnant population.
- VTE is the leading cause of maternal mortality in developed countries. Pulmonary embolism (PE) accounts for 20%–30% of maternal deaths; approximately 1 death per 100 000.
- The prevalence of VTE is distributed equally between the trimesters. Although two-thirds of events occur antenatally, the daily risk is greatest in the postnatal period.
- The risk of VTE after caesarean section is double that of vaginal delivery.
- Deep venous thrombosis (DVT) is more common in the left leg. Pelvic vein DVT is also more common in the pregnant population.

Predisposing factors

All three components of Virchow's triad (venous stasis, endothelial injury and a hyper-coagulable state) are present in pregnancy.

Venous stasis
Compression of large veins by the gravid uterus, along with changes in venous capacitance, result in a reduction in venous return from the lower limbs.

Endothelial injury
Delivery results in vascular injury which contributes to the increased risk of VTE immediately postpartum. Instrumental and operative delivery heighten this risk.

Hypercoagulability
Pregnancy is associated with alterations in both thrombotic and fibrinolytic mechanisms. In the first trimester there is an increase in fibrinogen, prothrombin, and factors VII, VIII, IX and X. There is increased platelet aggregation and resistance to activated

protein C. There is a reduction in protein S, factor XI and factor XIII. A reduction in fibrinolytic activity occurs due to a decrease in antithrombin levels and an increase in function of fibrinolytic inhibitors PAI-1 and PAI-2. After delivery there is an elevation in factors V, VII and X, and antithrombin levels return to normal.

Risk factors
- previous VTE
- age > 35, parity > 4, obesity, multiple birth
- diabetes, hypertension, cardiac disease, irritable bowel diseases (IBD), varicose veins
- immobilisation, infection, surgery, smoking, dehydration
- thrombophilia
  - inherited: antithrombin deficiency, prothrombin gene mutation, factor V Leiden mutation, protein C deficiency, protein S deficiency
  - acquired: antiphospholipid antibodies
- nephrotic syndrome, pre-eclampsia
- preterm birth, intrauterine fetal death (IUFD)
- operative delivery, prolonged labour

Clinical assessment

The clinical diagnosis of VTE has low sensitivity and specificity. A high index of suspicion is required, as is a low threshold for initiating treatment despite a lack of objective evidence. Symptoms and signs of VTE include leg pain and swelling, erythema, warmth, tenderness, lower abdominal or back pain, low-grade pyrexia, dyspnoea, cough, pleuritic chest pain, haemoptysis and collapse.

Investigation

Deep vein thrombosis (DVT)
- Doppler ultrasound is the modality of choice for the diagnosis of DVT.
- Lack of compressibility is 95% sensitive and > 95% specific for a proximal leg vein thrombosis. It is less sensitive for calf and pelvic vein thromboses. If ultrasound is negative but clinical suspicion high, ultrasound should be repeated on days 3 and 7.
- Poor Doppler flow in the iliac vein has reasonable accuracy for diagnosis of pelvic vein DVT where compressive ultrasonography has been negative.
- Venography is considered the gold standard investigation for suspected DVT in the general population, but data in pregnancy are lacking. It is rarely used due to exposure of the fetus to ionising radiation and because Doppler ultrasound is almost as reliable.
- Magnetic resonance venography is a useful modality in the diagnosis of pelvic vein DVT, with a sensitivity approaching 100% in the non-pregnant population. Data in pregnancy are lacking.
- D-dimer level rise throughout normal pregnancy, making it a less useful test for the diagnosis of VTE. The negative predictive value remains high throughout.

Pulmonary embolism (PE)
- Arterial blood gas analysis is neither sensitive nor specific for the diagnosis of PE. A normal result is common in the presence of a PE, while respiratory alkalosis is a common feature of pregnancy.

- The two most common imaging modalities for the investigation of suspected PE are the ventilation/perfusion (V/Q) scan and computed tomographic pulmonary angiography (CTPA). V/Q scanning during pregnancy carries a slightly increased risk of childhood cancer but a lower risk of maternal breast cancer when compared with CTPA. The absolute risk of either is very small.
- A chest X-ray (CXR) and electrocardiogram (ECG) should be performed when PE is suspected clinically. A CXR may identify other pulmonary pathology (e.g. pneumonia), or may reveal features associated with PE (focal opacities, atelectasis, pulmonary oedema). However, in > 50% of cases of PE, the CXR will be normal.
- If the CXR is normal, a V/Q scan should be performed.
- V/Q scanning remains the investigation of choice for the diagnosis of PE in pregnancy. There is high diagnostic accuracy and a high negative predictive value for the exclusion of PE.
- CTPA is highly sensitive and specific for the diagnosis of PE in the non-pregnant population. It is useful where V/Q scanning is unavailable or inconclusive, or the CXR is abnormal.
- The value of magnetic resonance pulmonary angiography (MRPA) in pregnancy has not been established.

Management

- Before anticoagulant therapy is commenced, a full blood count, coagulation screen, urea and electrolytes, and liver function tests should be performed. A thrombophilia screen is not recommended acutely.
- In clinically suspected VTE, treatment with low-molecular-weight heparin (LMWH) should be given until the diagnosis is excluded by objective testing.
- In the initial management of DVT, the affected leg should be elevated and a compression stocking worn. Mobilisation should be encouraged. A temporary inferior vena caval filter may be considered in cases of iliac vein thrombosis.
- In massive PE associated with cardiovascular compromise, immediate administration of intravenous unfractionated heparin (UH) is required (e.g. loading dose of 80 units/kg should be followed by an infusion of 18 units/kg/hour). Thrombolysis or urgent thoracotomy may be considered in certain cases.
- LMWH is the treatment of choice for confirmed VTE. Administration is via subcutaneous injection once or twice daily, at a dose calculated from booking weight (e.g. enoxaparin 1 mg/kg twice daily). Anti-Xa monitoring and routine platelet count monitoring is not warranted in routine cases. Treatment with therapeutic doses should continue for the remainder of the pregnancy and for 6 weeks postpartum (for at least 3 months of treatment in total) due to the risk of recurrence in this period.

Labour and delivery

- Women should be advised to cease anticoagulant therapy once labour has commenced. Therapeutic LMWH should be ceased 24 hours before planned delivery. A prophylactic dose can be given the night before a planned induction of labour or caesarean section. Regional anaesthesia should not be employed until 24 hours after a therapeutic dose.
- For women at high risk of recurrence of VTE around the time of delivery, intravenous UH should replace LMWH 24 hours before intervention, and cease once labour is established or 6 hours prior to caesarean section. Protamine sulfate can be given to reverse the effect of heparin if the activated partial thromboplastin time (APTT) remains elevated at the time of delivery or abnormal bleeding occurs.

- The risk of haematoma at caesarean section in anticoagulated women is increased by about 2%. For this reason, wound drains and staples or interrupted sutures (to allow for drainage of haematoma) should be considered.

POSTPARTUM
- The third stage of labour should be actively managed. Prophylactic doses of anticoagulant can be given 2–6 hours after vaginal and caesarean deliveries. A dose should not be given for 4 hours after spinal anaesthetic or removal of an epidural catheter, and removal should be delayed until 12 hours after the last dose. Therapeutic doses of anticoagulant can be administered 24 hours after vaginal delivery and 36–48 hours after caesarean section. Warfarin should not be commenced until day 5 due to increased risk of postpartum haemorrhage. Heparin should be continued until the international normalised ratio (INR) is between 2 and 3 on two consecutive days.
- A thrombophilia screen should be performed once anticoagulation therapy has been ceased and follow-up arranged.

Anticoagulant agents

LOW-MOLECULAR-WEIGHT HEPARIN (LMWH)
- LMWH is the agent of choice for prophylaxis and treatment of VTE in pregnancy.
- It is as effective as UH, with improved bioavailability and a longer half-life. The safety profile is better, with less risk of haemorrhage, heparin-induced thrombocytopenia and osteoporosis.
- Monitoring is by anti-factor Xa assay if required (e.g. extremes of body mass index, renal disease).
- It does not cross the placenta, and is not contraindicated in breastfeeding.

UNFRACTIONATED HEPARIN (UH)
- UH combines with antithrombin to accelerate the inactivation of thrombin, factor Xa and other factors.
- It is the agent of choice in massive PE associated with cardiovascular collapse.
- It may be used subcutaneously for prophylaxis or treatment of VTE where LMWH is contraindicated (e.g. allergy, renal failure).
- Dosage is titrated to achieve an APTT 1.5–2.5 times the normal value, which is monitored regularly for the duration of treatment.
- The incidence of heparin-induced thrombocytopenia (HIT) in pregnancy is very low. Platelet count should be monitored with long-term use.
- It does not cross the placenta, and is not contraindicated in breastfeeding.

WARFARIN
- Warfarin interferes with the action of vitamin K on coagulation factors II, VII, IX and X, protein C and protein S, rendering them inactive.
- Warfarin crosses the placenta and has a 5% chance of teratogenesis and increased risk of miscarriage if used in the first trimester. It is associated with fetal and neonatal haemorrhage (especially intracranial), IUFD, and maternal haemorrhage when used later in pregnancy. Women anticipating pregnancy should be switched to LMWH.
- It is safe to use postpartum from 5 days after delivery with close INR monitoring. It is not contraindicated in breastfeeding.

OTHER AGENTS

- Newer agents, such as the direct thrombin inhibitor dabigatran, and direct factor Xa inhibitors rivaroxaban, apixaban and edoxaban, are not recommended in pregnancy or with breastfeeding due to a lack of clinical data. Fondaparinux and parenteral direct thrombin inhibitors should be used only in women with a history of severe allergic reaction to heparin.

PREVENTION

All women should be assessed for their risk of VTE early in pregnancy or pre-conceptually. Anticoagulant regimens are based on the degree of risk for the individual. Non-pharmacological methods of prevention include mobilisation, adequate hydration, compression stockings and pneumatic compression devices where indicated.

- A history of a single previous provoked VTE requires antenatal surveillance and 6 weeks of postpartum prophylaxis.
- Antenatal prophylaxis with 6 weeks of postpartum prophylaxis is recommended for the following groups:
  - single previous unprovoked, OCP-related or pregnancy-related VTE
  - recurrent VTE
  - single previous VTE and thrombophilia
  - long-term anticoagulation for any indication
- Therapeutic antenatal anticoagulation is required in women with antithrombin deficiency and a previous VTE, and in women with a history of recurrent unprovoked VTE.
- Women with no history of VTE and a thrombophilia are treated according to the level of risk associated with their thrombophilia. Prophylaxis throughout pregnancy and for 6 weeks postpartum is recommended in antithrombin deficiency and for homozygosity or compound heterozygosity for factor V Leiden and prothrombin gene mutations. Women with a lower risk thrombophilia may require prophylaxis in the postpartum period only.
- In women with antiphospholipid syndrome with a history of VTE, there is a 70% chance of recurrence in pregnancy. Prophylaxis is required antenatally and for 6 weeks postpartum. In women with antiphospholipid antibodies but no history of VTE, 5 days of postpartum prophylaxis only is required.

Further reading

Queensland Clinical Guidelines – Venous thromboembolism (VTE) prophylaxis in pregnancy and the puerperium. Queensland Health, Feb 2014.

Royal College of Obstetricians and Gynaecologists, 2015. Thrombosis and embolism during pregnancy and the puerperium; reducing the risk. Green-top Guideline No. 37a, April. RCOG, London.

Royal College of Obstetricians and Gynaecologists, 2015. Thromboembolic disease in pregnancy and the puerperium: acute management. Green-top Guideline No. 37b, April. RCOG, London.

Schwartz, D.R., Malhotra, A., Weinberger, S., 2014. Deep vein thrombosis and pulmonary embolism in pregnancy: epidemiology, pathogenesis and diagnosis. Up to Date, December.

Schwartz, D.R., Malhortra, A., Weinberger, S., 2015. Dee vein thrombosis and pulmonary embolism in pregnancy: treatment. Up to Date, July.

Schwartz, D.R., Malhotra, A., Weinberger, S., 2014. Deep vein thrombosis and pulmonary embolism in pregnancy: prevention. Up to Date, Nov.

Thrombosis Adviser – a Venous & Arterial Thrombosis Resource for Physicians. Available at: <www.thrombosisadviser.com/en/> (accessed July 2015).

Chapter 47

Cardiac disease in pregnancy

Will Parsonage
Karen Lust

Incidence. Approximately 1% of all pregnancies are affected by maternal cardiac disease.

Physiology of cardiovascular changes in pregnancy

Increase in intravascular volume

This increases from the first trimester and peaks at approximately 50% from baseline by 32–34 weeks gestation. In a woman with limited cardiac output secondary to cardiovascular disease, volume overload may be poorly tolerated and exacerbate congestive cardiac failure.

Decrease in peripheral resistance

This begins to fall in early pregnancy to a nadir of approximately −30% in mid pregnancy before slowly increasing towards term. A fall in peripheral resistance (after-load) may be advantageous in many cardiac conditions but can exacerbate shunting in the woman with right-to-left shunts (e.g. Eisenmenger's syndrome).

Cardiac output

Cardiac output rises early in pregnancy and is unrelated to rise in plasma volume, peaking at around 40% by mid pregnancy.

Labour leads to an additional increase in cardiac output. The cardiac output rises progressively from the first stage to an additional 50% in the late second stage, with an increase of up to 7 L/minute from resting, non-pregnant values. This demand, together with the dramatic shifts of fluid that occur at delivery, may be poorly tolerated in women whose cardiac output depends on adequate preload (pulmonary hypertension) or those with fixed cardiac output (mitral stenosis).

Epidural anaesthesia and general anaesthesia produce additional changes in cardiac output.

Maternal mortality risks in cardiovascular disease

Mortality is most likely in conditions where pulmonary blood flow cannot be raised secondary to obstruction. Maternal mortality risk from cardiac disease is best classified using a modification of the World Health Organization (WHO) criteria for the risk of pregnancy associated with medical conditions (Table 47.1).

Fetal risks in maternal cardiovascular disease

General considerations

Several maternal cardiac conditions are associated with adverse fetal outcomes.

Cohort studies of the outcome of pregnancy in women with cardiac disease show an increase in most adverse fetal outcomes including fetal loss, intra-uterine growth retardation, prematurity and low birth weight when compared to matched controls.

Table 47.1 Modified WHO criteria for maternal risk associated with cardiovascular disease		
WHO CLASS	**RISK OF PREGNANCY**	**ILLUSTRATIVE EXAMPLES (NOT AN EXHAUSTIVE LIST)**
1	No detectable increased risk of maternal mortality or morbidity	• Uncomplicated, small ventricular septal defect or patent ductus arteriosus • Mild pulmonary stenosis; mitral valve prolapse with no more than trivial mitral regurgitation • Successfully repaired simple lesions ostium secundum atrial septal defect, ventricular septal defect or patent ductus arteriosus • Isolated ventricular extrasystoles and atrial ectopic beats
2	Small increased risk of maternal mortality or morbidity	• Unoperated atrial septal defect • Repaired tetralogy of Fallot
2 or 3 depending on individual		• Mild left ventricle impairment • Hypertrophic cardiomyopathy • Native or tissue valvular heart disease not considered Class 4 • Marfan's syndrome without aortic dilation (with/ without a family history of aortic dissection) • Heart transplantation
3	Significantly increased risk of maternal mortality or severe morbidity. Expert counselling required. If pregnancy is decided upon, intensive specialist cardiac and obstetric monitoring needed throughout pregnancy, childbirth and the puerperium	• Mechanical valve • Systemic right ventricle (i.e. atrial 'repair' of transposition of the great arteries) • Post Fontan operation • Cyanotic heart disease • Other complex congenital heart disease
4	Extremely high risk of maternal mortality or severe morbidity: pregnancy contraindicated. If pregnancy occurs termination should be discussed. If pregnancy continues, care as for Class 3	• Pulmonary arterial hypertension of any cause • Severe systemic ventricular dysfunction • NYHA III-IV or ventricular ejection fraction < 30% • Previous peripartum cardiomyopathy with residual impairment of left ventricular function • Severe left heart obstruction • Marfan's syndrome with aorta dilated > 40 mm

Source: Adapted from Thorne S, Nelson-Piercy C, MacGregor A, Gibbs S, Crowhurst J, Pannay N et al. Pregnancy and contraception in heart disease and pulmonary arterial hypertension. J Fam Plann Reprod Health Care; 2006; 32: 75-81.

Family history

- The presence of a congenital cardiac anomaly in either parent or sibling increases the risk of cardiac anomaly in the offspring to about 2%–4%, or twice that of the normal population. The risk is substantially higher (5%–15%) when the mother is affected with certain congenital defects including atrial septal defect, ventricular septal defect and pulmonary stenosis. These have multivariant inheritance.
- Certain acquired conditions, such as hypertrophic cardiomyopathy exhibit autosomal dominant inheritance with variable expression.
- Environmental risk factors include rubella virus and alcohol consumption.

Management of cardiovascular disease in pregnancy

History

- The commonest symptom of heart disease is breathlessness on exertion but when mild, and unaccompanied by physical signs, may be difficult to distinguish from the effects of normal pregnancy.
- Syncope can also occur with normal pregnancy but is a critical symptom in the context of aortic stenosis, hypertrophic obstructive cardiomyopathy, tetralogy of Fallot and dysrhythmias.
- A history of rheumatic fever or previous investigation for a heart murmur are important and should be fully clarified as early as possible in pregnancy (and preferably preconception).

Physical examination

- In normal pregnancy, the following may all be normal findings: extrasystoles, peripheral oedema, a loud first heart sound and an added third heart sound.
- Flow murmurs with an ejection systolic character across the pulmonary and/or aortic valves may be present in up to 90% of women and reflect the increased stroke volume of pregnancy.

Investigations

- Chest X-ray in normal pregnancy is usually avoided but shows slight cardiomegaly and increased pulmonary vascular markings.
- Electrocardiograph in normal pregnancy shows inversion in T waves, Q wave in lead III.
- Echocardiography is safe in pregnancy and should be readily used to clarify clinical suspicions of structural abnormalities.

Counselling

Ideally, cardiovascular disease is identified and investigated before pregnancy, with the maternal risks evaluated, therapeutics discussed and appropriate contraception advised.

A number of commonly used cardiac medications are contraindicated (e.g. angiotensin-converting enzyme [ACE] inhibitors, angiotensin receptor blockers [ARB], statins) during pregnancy and may be better to be withdrawn prior to planned pregnancy.

Termination of pregnancy is rarely indicated due to cardiac disease but may be offered in certain circumstances. Termination is safer if performed in the first trimester and should always be performed in a hospital setting. Prostaglandins have significant systemic haemodynamic effects and should be used with caution. Some indications for termination include conditions associated with very high maternal risk (WHO class IV) including Eisenmenger's syndrome and primary pulmonary hypertension.

Endocarditis and pregnancy

- The efficacy of antibiotic prophylaxis against infective endocarditis in pregnancy has not been proven. In general, antibiotic prophylaxis is only recommended in patients at high risk during high-risk procedures (e.g. dental procedures). Antibiotic prophylaxis is not indicated for uncomplicated vaginal or caesarean delivery.
- Women at high risk include those with prosthetic heart valves, most unrepaired or palliated congenital lesions or past history of infective endocarditis.

Antenatal management

Patients with significant cardiac disease during pregnancy (i.e. WHO class II or above) should be managed by a multidisciplinary team with experience in the management of cardiac problems during pregnancy. Ideally, patients should be counselled preconception but failing that as early in pregnancy as possible.

Labour

- Spontaneous vaginal delivery at term is an appropriate and safe mode of delivery in most cardiac conditions. Induction of labour is associated with an increased risk of sepsis and caesarean section.
- Maintain strict fluid balance.
- Adequate analgesia is essential, although epidural should be used with caution, especially in conditions with left heat obstruction or right-to-left shunts where a reduction in peripheral vascular resistance may be detrimental (e.g. hypertrophic obstructive cardiomyopathy, aortic stenosis and Eisenmenger's syndrome).
- Manoeuvres to minimise aortocaval compression are recommended.
- The second stage of labour should be shortened.
- If possible, avoid delivery in the lithotomy position.
- Haemodynamic monitoring, continuous electrocardiogram (ECG) and pulse oximetry monitoring should be individualised but planned prior to labour if possible.
- Avoid ergometrine.
- Avoid sympathomimetic drugs.

Postpartum

- Maintain a strict fluid balance to predict cardiac failure associated with the major fluid shifts after delivery of the placenta.
- Significant haemodynamic and fluid shifts occur during the first 72 hours postpartum and can lead to cardiovascular instability. The need for further cardiac monitoring, or nursing in a cardiac care or intensive care setting, during this period should be individualised but planned prior to labour if possible.

Congenital heart disease

Atrial septal defect

This is a common congenital anomaly, usually asymptomatic but associated with left-to-right shunting, a risk of paradoxical embolus and arrhythmias (usually atrial). Hypervolaemia in pregnancy in the presence of a large defect can cause an increase in left-to-right shunting, an increased burden on the right ventricle, and may result in cardiac failure. Most patients tolerate pregnancy, labour and delivery well.

Ventricular septal defect

There is a risk of cardiac failure, arrhythmias and aortic regurgitation with large defects. If uncomplicated, the pregnancy, labour and delivery are tolerated well. The management is otherwise similar to atrial septal defect.

Patent ductus arteriosus

While usually asymptomatic and well-tolerated in pregnancy, labour and delivery, the possibility of high-pressure, high-flow left-to-right shunting with large lesions may worsen prognosis in some patients.

Eisenmenger's syndrome

This is a syndrome arising from conditions of congenital left-to-right shunt, in which progressive pulmonary hypertension leads to shunt reversal or bidirectional shunting. In the antepartum period, reduced vascular resistance causes an increase in right-to-left shunting. This leads to a reduction in pulmonary perfusion, with hypoxia and deterioration of the fetal/maternal condition.

Hypotension in the woman with Eisenmenger's syndrome reduces right ventricular filling pressure and lowers perfusion in pulmonary beds. Therefore, reduction in blood pressure with haemorrhage or anaesthesia can lead to sudden death.

MANAGEMENT

- Eisenmenger's syndrome is a very high-risk condition. Systemic vasodilatation and/or increased pulmonary vascular resistance during pregnancy may lead to increased right-to-left shunting, diminished pulmonary blood flow and deterioration.
- Maternal mortality as high as 20%–50% has been reported and pregnancy is generally considered contraindicated.
- Advise the patient about the risks of continuing pregnancy and offer termination.
- Antenatal care and delivery should *always* be undertaken in a tertiary centre.
- Anticoagulation should be carefully managed on an individual basis. There are competing risks of thromboembolism *and* bleeding in patients with Eisenmenger's syndrome.
- Early caesarean delivery may be required if maternal condition deteriorates.
- Regional anaesthesia should be performed with caution to avoid sudden changes in peripheral vascular resistance.

Coarctation of the aorta

The commonest site is at the origin of the left subclavian artery and can be associated with bicuspid aortic valve, other aortic abnormalities, ventricular septal defect, patent ductus arteriosus and intracranial aneurysms.

Pregnancy is generally well tolerated in patients with previously repaired coarctation. In patients with residual coarctation there is an increased risk of hypertensive disorders, aortic dissection and miscarriage. Maternal risk is otherwise usually dependent on whether there are associated vascular or cardiac lesions.

Hypertension should be actively treated but consideration given to the risk of reduced placental blood flow (distal to the coarctation) if treatment is overly aggressive.

Tetralogy of fallot

This cyanotic heart condition consists of ventricular septal defect, right ventricular outflow obstruction, overriding aorta and right ventricular hypertrophy. In uncorrected tetralogy, maternal mortality as high as 4%–15% has been reported.

Pregnancy is usually tolerated well in repaired tetralogy but there is an increased risk of arrhythmia and heart failure. The latter is usually due to right ventricular dysfunction secondary to residual or recurrent pulmonary valve dysfunction.

Consequently, tetralogy should be repaired or significant residual abnormalities revised, prior to pregnancy.

Patients should be advised by an experienced tertiary centre.

Vaginal delivery is safe and appropriate in most cases.

Pulmonary hypertension

Pulmonary hypertension is defined as a *mean* pulmonary artery pressure of ≥ 25 mmHg. Pulmonary artery *systolic* pressure of 36–50 mmHg indicates mild pulmonary hypertension. In practice, these measurements are usually derived from transthoracic Doppler echocardiography.

Pulmonary hypertension may be secondary to left-sided heart disease (e.g. mitral stenosis, lung disease) or primary pulmonary vascular conditions (e.g. primary pulmonary arterial hypertension, pulmonary thromboembolic disease). Pulmonary arterial hypertension may be idiopathic, familial or associated with congenital heart lesions.

The specific diagnosis and cause of pulmonary hypertension is of critical importance during pregnancy and any patient with documented pulmonary hypertension should be referred promptly for specialist obstetric medical/cardiac care (preferably preconception).

Primary pulmonary hypertension carries a particularly grave prognosis, a high risk of maternofetal complications, including substantial maternal mortality, and is generally considered incompatible with pregnancy (WHO class IV). Death typically occurs late in pregnancy or in the early weeks postpartum. Consequently, contraceptive advice is an important part of management of these patients and termination of pregnancy may need to be offered when appropriate.

In cases of established pregnancy in the presence of significant pulmonary hypertension, close monitoring, careful fluid balance, avoidance of hypoxia and judicious use of appropriate medical therapy are important. These decisions should all be undertaken in a tertiary facility and under the guidance of a team experienced in management of this group of patients.

Acquired cardiac lesions

Rheumatic heart disease

Rheumatic heart disease remains a significant cause of maternal heart disease in the developing world as well as in Australian and New Zealand indigenous communities.

ACUTE RHEUMATIC FEVER

- This is relatively uncommon in pregnancy but does occur.
- Presents with malaise, a rash, fleeting, migratory polyarthritis and heart murmurs due to valve regurgitation. Central nervous system involvement (chorea) and clinical evidence of heart failure and/or pericarditis are less common.
- Diagnosis is based on the typical clinical presentation in the presence of evidence of recent streptococcal infection. Evidence of carditis may be apparent on the electrocardiogram and echocardiogram. There is pathologic evidence of a systemic inflammatory response (elevated acute phase biomarkers).

CHRONIC RHEUMATIC HEART DISEASE

After episodes of acute rheumatic fever, there is accelerated degeneration of cardiac valves affected by valvulitis. This most commonly leads to clinically relevant lesions of the mitral and aortic valves but can affect any valve.

MITRAL STENOSIS

- This is the most common clinically relevant rheumatic valvular lesion in pregnancy. The main problem is that mitral stenosis leads to an increased resistance to left ventricular filling, elevated left atrial pressure, a relatively fixed cardiac output and a risk of pulmonary congestion and pulmonary oedema. These clinical features are exacerbated by the normal physiology of pregnancy. Atrial fibrillation may be established, or can occur during pregnancy, and is poorly tolerated due to the associated loss of atrial function. Atrial fibrillation is also associated with a risk of thromboembolism, and requires anticoagulation therapy.
- Clinical symptoms include increasing fatigue, shortness of breath and ankle swelling. These symptoms may be difficult to distinguish from those of normal pregnancy. Orthopnoea and paroxysmal nocturnal dyspnoea are ominous signs.
- On examination, there may be signs of cardiac failure in addition to the clinical features of mitral stenosis. Atrial fibrillation may be apparent clinically.

Management

- Cardiac output in mitral stenosis depends on adequate diastolic filling time and left ventricular preload. Therefore, the usual increase in heart rate with pregnancy is counterproductive and excessive tachycardia (from infection, iron deficiency or blood loss) and fluid overload must be carefully avoided. Similarly, onset of atrial fibrillation during pregnancy is likely to be poorly tolerated and requires careful therapy.
- Labour is a vulnerable time. Intrapartum fluctuations of cardiac output can be minimised with the use of epidural anaesthesia and a careful watch postpartum for fluid shifts.
- Antibiotic prophylaxis is indicated to avoid endocarditis.
- Immediately after delivery of the baby, there is a sharp rise in left atrial pressure, which may precipitate cardiac failure.

MITRAL INSUFFICIENCY

This may be secondary to acute rheumatic fever or chronic rheumatic valve disease. However, the more common cause in general is mitral valve prolapse. It is usually well tolerated in pregnancy if the degree of regurgitation is not severe, except for the risks of atrial fibrillation and endocarditis.

AORTIC STENOSIS

- There is a higher maternal mortality in rheumatic compared with congenital aortic stenosis.
- It is not considered haemodynamically significant, and is unlikely to become symptomatic during pregnancy, until the aortic valve area falls below 1.0 cm^2.
- In critical aortic stenosis, there is relatively fixed cardiac output, resulting in inadequate coronary artery and cerebral perfusion causing dyspnoea, angina, syncope and rarely sudden death. The times of greatest risk are delivery and pregnancy termination.
- It is very important to maintain adequate cardiac output. If hypotension occurs with blood loss, epidural or inferior vena caval occlusion then haemodynamic collapse can occur.

- Surgical correction of the disease before conception greatly improves prognosis in patients with severe and/or symptomatic aortic stenosis.

AORTIC INSUFFICIENCY

This is usually well tolerated in pregnancy, as tachycardia results in less time for regurgitation.

Cardiomyopathy

HYPERTROPHIC OBSTRUCTIVE CARDIOMYOPATHY

- There is abnormal left ventricular hypertrophy with histological abnormalities. Haemodynamic effects may include left ventricular outflow obstruction (usually dynamic) and mitral regurgitation but neither of these are essential to the diagnosis. Left ventricular systolic function is usually maintained. There is an increased risk of arrhythmias including life-threatening ventricular arrhythmias and sudden cardiac death in some patients.
- Symptoms are variable and may include dyspnoea, fatigue, chest pain, syncope and palpitations.
- Diagnosis is usually made on echocardiography or other non-invasive cardiac imaging demonstrating evidence of abnormal hypertrophy.
- Pregnancy is often well tolerated, and outcome is dependent on the severity of associated haemodynamic abnormalities (as mentioned earlier).
- Management includes beta-blocker if indicated, avoiding hypotension because of the risk of obstruction of left ventricular outflow tract, which may occur in volume depletion, aortocaval compression, and antepartum/postpartum haemorrhage.
- Hypertrophic cardiomyopathy may occur sporadically but is usually an inherited condition with an autosomal dominant pattern. Several causative mutations have been identified and genetic screening has an important role in the management of families affected by the disease. Referral to a clinical geneticist should be discussed with all pregnant women with hypertrophic cardiomyopathy.

PERIPARTUM CARDIOMYOPATHY

- This rare cardiomyopathy may develop in the last month of pregnancy or the first 5 months postpartum, with a peak incidence in the postpartum period.
- It is more common in older multiparous patients who breastfeed and have a history of hypertension, pre-eclampsia or multiple pregnancy with poor nutrition.
- Investigations include chest X-ray with non-specific cardiomegaly, electrocardiography, showing non-specific changes or widespread abnormalities or arrhythmias, and echocardiography with a grossly dilated heart.
- Management includes standard treatment for heart failure including fluid and sodium restriction, beta-blockade, vasodilators (recognising that ACE inhibitors and ARB are contraindicated during pregnancy) and judicious use of diuretics. Anticoagulation may be indicated. ACE inhibitors and ARBs can be reconsidered after delivery.
- Counsel the patient regarding the recurrence rate in future pregnancies. Peripartum cardiomyopathy has a high risk (20%–30%) of recurrence with any subsequent pregnancy even if cardiac function has returned to normal. In cases where cardiac function has not normalised, the risk of developing worsening heart failure is higher (40%–50%) and is associated with an increased risk of maternal death. Consensus, suggests that subsequent pregnancy should be avoided (and termination of pregnancy offered where appropriate) in this setting.

Aortic pathology and Marfan's syndrome

This is an autosomal dominant disorder characterised by a generalised weakness of connective tissue. It is associated with mitral or aortic regurgitation and aneurysmal dilatation of the aortic root and aorta with an associated risk of aortic dissection.

MATERNAL RISKS

- These include vascular aneurysms, including rupture or dissection of the aorta or splenic artery, and aortic valve regurgitation secondary to aortic root enlargement.
- Initial echocardiography evaluation includes the diameter of the aortic root. If the aortic root is < 40 mm the risk of aortic complications is low. If the aortic dimension is > 45 mm, pregnancy should be avoided. In this setting, preventive aortic repair is indicated. In patients with diameters 40–45 mm, management is individualised based on the rate of aortic enlargement, indexation of measurement for body surface area and historic features such as a family history of aortic dissection.

MANAGEMENT

- Treat hypertension aggressively.
- The benefit of beta-blocker medication in patients with aortic enlargement is contentious but is usually recommended during pregnancy.
- Perform a caesarean section if there is evidence of significant aortic disease, usually if the aortic dimensions are > 40 mm. Vaginal delivery with a shortened second stage and regional anaesthesia is appropriate for patient with aortic diameter <40 mm.

Bicuspid aortic valve

Bicuspid aortic valve can lead to significant valve stenosis or regurgitation although this usually does not occur in women of child bearing age. More importantly, bicuspid aortic valve can be associated with a similar (although usually less severe) aortopathy to Marfan's syndrome. Management principles are based on aortic dimensions, with a dimension of > 45 mm most clinically relevant in this setting.

Myocardial infarction

Acute coronary syndromes (ACS) during pregnancy are rare but carry a poor prognosis and management is complex. Although ACS can occur due to coronary atherosclerosis, there is also an over-representation of other mechanisms including spontaneous coronary dissection and coronary artery emboli when ACS occurs during pregnancy.

MANAGEMENT

- Management is similar to that for non-pregnant patients, although certain treatments are contraindicated (e.g. ACE inhibitors and HMG CoA reductase inhibitors) or problematic (e.g. dual antiplatelet therapy) during pregnancy and delivery.
- Delivery close to ACS (within 2 weeks) raises mortality.
- Labour/delivery must be in a monitored environment with onsite access for invasive management of unstable ischaemia or recurrent myocardial infarction if necessary.
- Management includes elective shortening of the second stage and regional anaesthesia.
- Ergometrine is contraindicated, as it may cause coronary artery spasm.

Chapter 48

Connective tissue disease in pregnancy

Karen Lust

Systemic lupus erythematosus (SLE)

- SLE is a multisystem autoimmune disease, involving direct attack by autoantibodies and deposition of immune complexes.
- SLE has a prevalence of 1.5/1000 population, peak incidence is between 15–40 years of age, and has a female-to-male ratio of 9:1.
- SLE is thought not to impair fertility.
- Pregnancy in women with SLE, especially in the presence of lupus nephritis, is associated with increased risks of pre-eclampsia, fetal growth restriction, fetal loss and preterm delivery. These increased risks are present even if the lupus nephritis is quiescent but are higher in the presence of hypertension or proteinuria.
- Risk factors for poor obstetric outcome include pulmonary hypertension, past adverse obstetric history, chronic kidney disease, active (especially renal) disease and recent stroke (< 6 months), hypertension and proteinuria.
- Lupus activity preconception and intrapartum is the best predictor of adverse pregnancy outcome.
- Pregnancy outcome for mother and offspring is best when the disease has been quiescent for at least 6 months prior to conception, and renal function is stable.
- There is conflicting information if pregnancy has an effect on rate of disease flares. Flares occur across the trimesters, and the immediate postpartum period.
- Flares present most commonly as fever, lymphadenopathy, skin and joint involvement, and renal impairment. Neurological, cardiovascular and respiratory manifestations may also occur. Flares are more common if disease is active 6–12 months pre conception, women with repeated flares preconception, in the presence of active glomerulonephritis at conception and if hydroxychloroquine is ceased preconception.
- Flares are associated with low complement, an active urine sediment and an increase in anti-double stranded DNA titres.

- Antiphospholipid antibodies (aPL) are present in 30%–40% of SLE patients, but only 10% have antiphospholipid syndrome and 30% have anti-Ro/SSA or anti-La/SSB antibodies.

Maternal effects
- pre-eclampsia: occurs in around 13% of patients with SLE, but up to 30% of patients with preexisting renal disease, and can be difficult to distinguish from lupus nephritis
- lupus nephritis: associated with an increased risk of pre-eclampsia, fetal growth restriction, fetal loss, worsening of renal and extra-renal manifestations
- venous thromboembolism
- postpartum haemorrhage

Fetal effects
- intrauterine growth restriction (IUGR)
- intrauterine fetal death: risk is higher in women with active disease at conception, hypertension, renal disease, aPL, low complement, elevated anti-DNA antibodies and thrombocytopenia
- preterm birth

Neonatal lupus
- results from passive transfer of anti-Ro/SSA or anti-La/SSB antibodies to cause congenital heart block and neonatal lupus
- risk of neonatal cutaneous lupus 5%, rash within 6 months of birth, usually non-scarring
- risk of congenital heart block 2%; risk of recurrence if a previously affected pregnancy 15%–20%
- no congenital anomalies associated with SLE

Management
- Pregnant women with SLE require high-risk multidisciplinary care.
- Medication should be reviewed and disease management optimised preconceptually.

INITIAL INVESTIGATIONS
- full blood count, renal function tests (including urinalysis, urine protein/creatinine ratio)
- aPL antibodies: anticardiolipin antibody, beta-2-glycoprotein and lupus anticoagulant
- anti-Ro/SSA and anti-La/SSB antibodies
- C3 and C4 titres
- anti-double stranded DNA antibody titres

ONGOING MANAGEMENT
- auscultation of fetal heart at each visit
- in presence of Ro or La antibodies: fetal echocardiogram around 20 weeks gestation, with repeat at 28 weeks if the initial 20-week scan was normal
- monthly platelet count
- repeat aPL, complement, anti-double stranded DNA antibodies and renal function tests each trimester

- surveillance for exacerbation of disease, pre-eclampsia and fetal complications
- regular surveillance of fetal wellbeing if complications arise
- delivery timed according to complications/fetal condition

DRUG THERAPY
- The potential for medication to cross the placenta and cause fetal harm must be weighed against the risks of active disease to the mother and fetus.
- Consider Low-dose aspirin.
- Prophylactic Heparin or low-molecular-weight heparin (LMWH) should be given in the presence of prior VTE, APLS.
- Non-steroidal anti-inflammatory drugs (NSAIDs) should be avoided after 32 weeks gestation because of the risk of premature closure of the ductus arteriosus and subsequent development of pulmonary hypertension in the neonate as well as fetal renal effects.
- Glucocorticoids are safe in pregnancy and breastfeeding. They increase the risk of gestational diabetes and adrenal suppression, necessitating hydrocortisone in labour.
- Hydroxychloroquine is not teratogenic and is safe to continue in pregnancy and breastfeeding.
- Azathioprine can be continued in pregnancy and breastfeeding.
- Cyclophosphamide, methotrexate and mycophenolate mofetil are teratogenic and are contraindicated in pregnancy. They should be ceased preconception and the patient changed to an alternative medication.
- No interventions have been shown to reverse established congenital heart block.
- Studies of pregnancies where hydroxychloroquine is started < 10 weeks gestation has been shown to reduce the occurrence of congenital heart block by 77%.
- Newer biological drug therapies used in SLE can cross the placenta and can be associated with neonatal B cell depletion. Consult treating rheumatologist to determine if needs adjustment preconception or in pregnancy.

Antiphospholipid syndrome (APS)

APS is characterised by arterial or venous thrombosis and specific pregnancy complications, in association with laboratory evidence of antiphospholipid antibodies (aPL.)

Antiphospholipid antibodies (aPL)
The diagnosis of APS requires the presence of anticardiolipin antibody (aCL) IgG and /or IgM, lupus anticoagulant (LA) or anti-beta-2-glycoprotein-1 on two occasions at least 12 weeks apart. aCL antibodies were found in 10% and lupus anticoagulant in 8% of healthy blood donors.

Pregnancy complications
- Complications are thought to arise due to:
  - antibody-induced thrombosis in the uteroplacental circulation
  - defective placentation: aPL antibodies have a direct effect on placental trophoblast
  - placental inflammation due to complement activation and deposition
- Pregnancy loss: early (recurrent miscarriage up to 17 % and late including intrauterine fetal death (IUFD) up to 6%.
- IUGR occurs in 15%–30%.

- Preterm births—up to 35%.
- Pre-eclampsia up to 35%; can be early and severe.
- Maternal thromboembolic disease: 5% risk.
- Lupus anticoagulant is the strongest predictor of adverse pregnancy outcome.

Management
- Women with known APS should be managed in a high-risk multidisciplinary setting.
- Additional surveillance includes baseline renal and liver function tests, and serial growth and wellbeing ultrasounds.
- Low-dose aspirin has been associated with an increase in successful pregnancy outcome. It should be commenced as soon as possible from conception, and can be ceased at 36 weeks gestation.
- Heparin should be given to women with a past history of thrombosis antenatally and postnatally. Recent studies have not supported a role for heparin to prevent recurrent miscarriage. It can be used to prevent IUGR, fetal loss, severe pre-eclampsia and neonatal death but there is limited evidence to support its use.
- Women with a history of early, severe pre-eclampsia or IUGR in a previous pregnancy should be commenced on low-dose aspirin ideally prior to 16 weeks gestation and continued throughout pregnancy.
- The addition of first-trimester low-dose prednisolone has resulted in a higher live-birth rate than conventional therapy alone.

Rheumatoid arthritis

Rheumatoid arthritis (RA) occurs predominantly in females, many of whom are in the reproductive age group.

Pregnancy
- Less than 25 % of women remain in remission throughout pregnancy.
- Reported improvement in RA in pregnancy by 40%–75% of women.
- If it improves, 90% experience exacerbation of disease postpartum.
- Pregnancy outcomes in women with RA are similar to the general population.
- Women with active RA or severe RA do have increased adverse outcomes in pregnancy.
- Medication may need to be continued, or reintroduced if flare occurs.
- NSAIDs should be avoided after 32 weeks gestation to avoid premature closure of the ductus arteriosus and renal effects.
- Prednisone can be safely used to treat disease flares and as maintenance therapy to control disease.
- Sulfasalazine, azathioprine and hydroxychloroquine are safe in pregnancy and breastfeeding.
- Leufonamide, methotrexate, mycophenolate mofetil and cyclophosphamide are teratogenic and should be ceased preconception.
- There is increasing evidence on the safety of anti-tumour necrosis factor (anti-TNF) and other biologics agents in pregnancy. These drugs all have different molecular structures, transplacental transport and half-lives. Recommendations regarding their use should be individualised. Expert advice should be sought on whether to continue these drugs and if and when they need to be ceased in pregnancy.
- Elective caesarean section may be necessary where joint disease precludes vaginal delivery.

Further reading

Lockshin, M.D., Salmon, J.E., Erkan, D., 2014. Chapter 64. Pregnancy and rheumatic diseases. In: Creasy, R.J., Resnik, R. (Eds.), Maternal–fetal Medicine: Principles and Practice, 7th ed. Saunders Elsevier, Philadelphia, pp. 1092–1099.

Østensen, M., Andreoli, L., Brucato, A., et al., 2015. State of the art: reproduction and pregnancy in rheumatic diseases. Autoimmun. Rev. 14 (5), 376–386.

Soh, M.C., Nelson-Piercy, C., 2015. High-risk pregnancy and the rheumatologist. Rheumatology (Oxford) 54 (4), 572–587.

Chapter 49

Haematology and pregnancy

Amy Mellor

Haematologic changes in pregnancy

Plasma volume increases during pregnancy by up to 50%, and is maximal at around 34 weeks gestation. In comparison, red blood cell mass increases by up to 30% at most by the end of pregnancy, resulting in relative fall in haemoglobin levels. Iron requirements increase throughout pregnancy, with 60 mg/day of elemental iron needed during the second and third trimesters. Folate requirements increase from 50 µg/day pre-pregnancy to around 400 µg/day. Pregnancy has minimal impact on vitamin B_{12} levels, as most adults have a 2–3-year store available.

Platelet count remains in the normal range for most pregnant women, though the average is slightly lower than in the non-pregnant population. Pregnancy is associated with a leucocytosis due to an increase in circulating neutrophils, while the lymphocyte count remains stable. The average white blood cell count in the second and third trimesters is between 9 and 15×10^9/L.

Anaemia in pregnancy

Anaemia is a reduction in red cell mass relative to plasma volume, measured as the amount of haemoglobin (Hb) per litre of blood volume. Anaemia in pregnancy is defined as an Hb < 110 g/L in the first and third trimesters, and < 105 g/L in the second trimester. Around 20% of women are anaemic in the third trimester of pregnancy. Anaemia should be investigated and treated, as severe anaemia has been associated with miscarriage, preterm birth, intrauterine growth restriction (IUGR) and fetal death.

Causes of anaemia
- microcytic: iron deficiency, haemoglobinopathies, chronic disease
- normocytic: haemolysis, haemorrhage
- macrocytic: vitamin B_{12} or folate deficiency

IRON DEFICIENCY

- Iron requirements average around 1000 mg over the course of a normal pregnancy. 300 mg is required for the fetus and placenta, 500 mg for the expansion of maternal Hb, and 200 mg is lost through the gut, urine and skin.
- Iron deficiency is responsible for 75% of cases of anaemia in pregnancy.
- Prevalence may approach 50%.
- Iron deficiency results in a microcytic, hypochromic anaemia, with low plasma iron, high iron-binding capacity and low serum ferritin.
- When used as a screening test for iron deficiency, serum ferritin is 90% sensitive and 85% specific.
- Treatment is with oral iron (e.g. 325 mg of ferrous sulfate) once to three times daily.
- Absorption is enhanced by administration of 500 mg of vitamin C.
- Side effects of iron include nausea, vomiting, abdominal pain, constipation or diarrhoea.
- Parenteral iron may be used where there has been intolerance or an inadequate response to oral therapy. Ferric carboxymaltose can be given as a single dose of 1000 mg of elemental iron over 15 minutes. Incidence of adverse reactions, including allergy and anaphylaxis, is < 1%.

FOLIC ACID DEFICIENCY

- Folate deficiency is much more common than vitamin B_{12} deficiency as a cause of megaloblastic anaemia. It occurs due to poor nutrition or decreased absorption.
- Findings include macrocytic (or normocytic), normochromic anaemia with hyper-segmentation of leucocytes. Reticulocyte count is normal or low. White blood cell and platelet counts are often reduced.
- Deficiency is defined as a red blood cell folate level < 165 ng/mL or serum folate < 2 μg/L. Vitamin B_{12} is within the normal range.
- Treatment is with oral folic acid, 1–5 mg/day.

VITAMIN B_{12} DEFICIENCY

- Deficiency is rare. It occurs in strict vegans or with intrinsic factor deficiency.
- Neurological deficits may result. It is critical that women with vitamin B_{12} deficiency not be treated with folic acid alone, as neuropathy may worsen.
- Treatment is with 1 mg of intramuscular vitamin B_{12} daily for 1 week, then weekly for 4 weeks.

Thalassaemia

Thalassaemia is an inherited defect in Hb, resulting from decreased globin chain production. Both alpha- and beta-thalassaemias result in defective synthesis of HbA. Alpha-chain synthesis is controlled by two pairs of genes on chromosome 16, and thalassaemia results from one or more gene deletions. Beta-chain synthesis is controlled by one pair of genes on chromosome 11, and thalassaemia results most commonly from a point mutation.

Alpha-thalassaemia

- Alpha-thalassaemia is most common in South-East Asian populations.
- A single gene deletion results in a 'silent carrier' state and is clinically undetectable.
- Two genes are deleted in alpha-thalassaemia minor, resulting in a mild hypochromic, microcytic anaemia.

- A deletion of three alpha genes results in HbH disease, the most severe form compatible with life. Abnormally high levels of HbH ($\beta 4$) and Hb Barts ($\gamma 4$) accumulate, resulting in severe haemolytic anaemia.
- In the homozygous state, all four genes are deleted. The fetus is unable to synthesise HbF or any form of adult Hb, resulting in high output cardiac failure, hydrops and fetal death. This is associated with significant maternal morbidity and mortality if pregnancy continues.

Beta-thalassaemia

- Beta-thalassaemia is autosomal-recessive and occurs most commonly in Mediterranean populations.
- Beta-thalassaemia minor or trait results in a variable clinical picture, depending on beta-chain production. If both parents are carriers, there is a 25% chance that offspring will be affected with beta-thalassaemia major.
- In homozygous beta-thalassaemia or beta-thalassaemia major, unimpeded beta-chain production results in severe haemolytic anaemia. The fetus is protected by the production of HbF. This protection disappears after birth, with the infant becoming anaemic by 3–6 months of age.

Screening and treatment

- All pregnant women should have a full blood count with red cell indices as screening for thalassaemia. A mean corpuscular volume (MCV) < 80 fL in the absence of iron deficiency necessitates further testing, as does a significant family history or high-risk ethnicity.
- Hb electrophoresis identifies the presence of excessive or deficient levels of globin chains. More than 3.5% of HbA_2 ($\alpha_2\delta_2$) suggests beta-thalassaemia, while a normal amount of HbA_2 with an MCV < 80 fL may suggest alpha-thalassaemia.
- The definitive diagnosis of alpha-thalassaemia requires DNA analysis.
- When an abnormality is identified, paternal testing should be performed to determine the risk of disease to the fetus. Diagnosis can be made by analysis of fetal DNA obtained through chorionic villus sampling, amniocentesis or fetal blood sampling. Genetic counselling to discuss treatment options should follow. Preimplantation genetic diagnosis is also an option for at-risk couples.
- Pregnant women with thalassaemia require adequate iron and folate intake. Severe disease may necessitate regular blood transfusions.

Thrombocytopenia in pregnancy

Gestational thrombocytopenia

- Gestational thrombocytopenia occurs in 5% of women and accounts for more than 70% of cases of maternal thrombocytopenia.
- The platelet count rarely falls below 70×10^9/L, and lies between 130 and 150×10^9/L in the majority of cases.
- It is defined by the following criteria:
  - mild, asymptomatic thrombocytopenia
  - no history of thrombocytopenia outside of pregnancy
  - onset late in pregnancy
  - no association with fetal thrombocytopenia
  - spontaneous resolution after delivery

- Gestational thrombocytopenia may represent a mild and transient form of idiopathic thrombocytopenic purpura (ITP).
- There is no associated increased risk to the mother or fetus/neonate, so routine obstetric management should be employed.
- The maternal platelet count should be checked postpartum to ensure resolution.

Idiopathic thrombocytopenic purpura (ITP)

ITP is a syndrome in which antibody-bound platelets are destroyed by the reticulo-endothelial system, predominantly in the spleen. The rate of destruction exceeds that of production in the bone marrow, resulting in thrombocytopenia. The diagnosis is one of exclusion, with no definitive clinical or laboratory parameters. The condition may be difficult to distinguish from gestational thrombocytopenia when first encountered in pregnancy.

ITP AND PREGNANCY

- The prevalence of ITP is 1–10 per 10,000 pregnancies.
- The platelet count nadir occurs most commonly in the third trimester. The platelet count should be checked monthly, with more frequent monitoring if the count falls below 30×10^9/L.
- The course of ITP is not changed by pregnancy, while ITP results in an increased risk of maternal haemorrhage. Immunoglobulin G (IgG) antibodies can cross the placenta resulting in thrombocytopenia in the fetus/neonate.

TREATMENT

- Acute bleeding in the setting of thrombocytopenia is treated with platelet transfusion, along with therapy to increase the platelet count rapidly.
- Treatment of the mother does not affect the fetal platelet count, so should be based on maternal need only.
- Asymptomatic women with platelets $> 30 \times 10^9$/L do not require treatment until delivery is imminent.
- For a platelet count $< 30 \times 10^9$/L, first-line treatment is with corticosteroids (prednisone 1 mg/kg/day). Once the platelet count is normal, the dose is tapered to maintain platelets at $> 50 \times 10^9$/L.
- Intravenous immunoglobulin (IVIG) can be used if response to steroids is inadequate, or if a faster response to therapy is required.
- Splenectomy is the most effective treatment for severe symptomatic ITP, but should be avoided in pregnancy if possible due to risk of mortality. Indications may include ongoing bleeding or a platelet count $< 10 \times 10^9$/L despite treatment with steroids or IVIG. When necessary, splenectomy is ideally performed in the second trimester. Rituximab and thrombopoietin receptor agonists should also be avoided in pregnancy where possible.

DELIVERY

- A platelet count of $> 50 \times 10^9$/L is considered safe for both vaginal delivery and caesarean section.
- If required, treatment with steroids or IVIG should be initiated one week before delivery is anticipated.
- Local protocols vary, but a platelet count $> 80 \times 10^9$/L is generally considered safe for regional anaesthesia.
- Labour and delivery is managed normally, with caesarean section reserved for routine obstetric indications. Fetal scalp electrodes, fetal blood sampling and vacuum extraction should be avoided in case of fetal thrombocytopenia.

NEONATAL ISSUES

- Around 10%–15% of neonates born to mothers with ITP have significant thrombocytopenia (platelets $< 50 \times 10^9$/L) at birth.
- The risk of neonatal intracranial haemorrhage during delivery is $< 1\%$.
- Because the risk of fetal haemorrhage with umbilical cord sampling is higher at 2%, determination of the fetal platelet count prior to delivery is not indicated.
- Cord blood should be tested for platelet count at delivery. If $< 20 \times 10^9$/L or abnormal bleeding occurs, treatment with IVIG is initiated.
- The neonatal platelet count reaches a nadir 2–5 days after delivery due to an increase in splenic activity, so daily platelet counts are required.

Thrombotic thrombocytopenic purpura (TTP)

- TTP is characterised by thrombocytopenia and microangiopathic haemolytic anaemia. Fever, neurological symptoms and renal dysfunction may also occur.
- Multiorgan ischaemia results from profound intravascular platelet aggregation.
- Congenital TTP is associated with absence of the plasma enzyme ADAMTS13; levels are typically $< 10\%$ of normal.
- The incidence of TTP in pregnancy is 1 in 25 000; it may present at any stage of pregnancy or in the postpartum period.
- TTP can be difficult to distinguish from severe pre-eclampsia/HELLP syndrome; the diagnosis is clinical.
- There is a 33% chance of perinatal mortality.
- Unlike pre-eclampsia, delivery does not result in resolution of disease. If there is response to treatment, the pregnancy can be continued to term.
- Congenital TTP is treated with plasma infusion every 1–2 weeks throughout pregnancy. Acquired TTP is treated with plasma exchange. If the distinction has not been established at the time of diagnosis, plasma exchange should be used.
- Congenital TTP is likely to recur in subsequent pregnancy, while recurrence of acquired TTP is uncommon.

Further reading

Bauer, K.A., 2014. Hematologic changes in pregnancy. Up to Date, January.

Bowden, D.K., 2001. Screening for thalassaemia. Aust. Prescr. 24, 120–123.

British Committee for Standards in Haematology, General Haematology Task Force, 2003. Guidelines for the investigation and management of idiopathic thrombocytopenic purpura in adults, children and in pregnancy. Br. J. Haematol. 120, 574–596.

George, J.N., Knudtson, E.J., 2015. Thrombocytopenia in pregnancy. Up to Date, January.

Kilpatrick, S.J., 2014. Anemia and pregnancy. In: Creasy, R., Resnik, R. (Eds.), Maternal–fetal Medicine: Principles and Practice, 7th ed. Saunders Elsevier, Philadelphia, pp. 869–884.

Lockwood, C.J., Silver, R.M., 2014. Coagulation disorders in pregnancy. In: Creasy, R., Resnik, R. (Eds.), Maternal–fetal Medicine: Principles and Practice, 7th ed. Saunders Elsevier, Philadelphia, pp. 825–854.

Yates, A.M., 2015. Prenatal screening and testing for hemoglobinopathy. Up to Date, January.

Chapter 50

Gastrointestinal disorders in pregnancy

Michael Flynn
Thea Bowler

Abdominal pain in pregnancy

Pain arises either from inside an organ or the covering visceral peritoneum or, later, involvement of parietal peritoneum. Visceral pain is poorly localised, as it is mediated by the autonomic nervous system. With parietal peritoneum, localisation is more specific.

Pain pathways of pelvic organs

- Sensory afferent pathways from the body of the uterus travel via sympathetic nerves to T10–L1.
- The cervix is supplied by sympathetic nerves to T10–L1 and parasympathetic nerves to S2–S4.
- Pain pathways from the ovary travel via sympathetic nerves to T10.

Causes of abdominal pain in pregnancy

PREGNANCY-RELATED

- miscarriage
- ectopic pregnancy
- impacted retroverted uterus at 10–14 weeks gestation, with the pain caused by urinary retention (management is by draining the urine and laying the woman prone or lateral)
- labour or contractions
- placental abruption, uterine rupture, intra-amniotic infection
- pregnancy related liver disease: acute fatty liver of pregnancy, severe pre-eclampsia, HELLP

- postpartum: endometritis, wound complications, necrotising fasciitis, urinary infection or retention, ovarian vein thrombophlebitis, intra-abdominal infection/organ injury

GYNAECOLOGICAL

- fibroids (torsion tends to occur in the puerperium; red degeneration is most common at 12–18 weeks gestation; presenting complaint is of tenderness over a mass, with mild fever and nausea/vomiting; management is with rest and analgesia)
- fallopian tube: torsion, salpingitis
- ovary: ovarian tumour/mass; complications: rupture, haemorrhage or torsion
- others: gastrointestinal (e.g. appendicitis) and urinary tract (e.g. infection, stone)

NON-PREGNANCY RELATED

- gastrointestinal tract: heartburn/reflux (occurs in 70%–80% of pregnant women), constipation, peptic ulcer disease, cholelithiasis (occurs in 3%–5% of pregnant women, but is mostly asymptomatic), pancreatitis, acute appendicitis (incidence of about 1 in 2500 pregnancies; has a significant association with premature labour), acute obstruction (from bands/adhesions, volvulus, hernia), inflammatory bowel disease
- other causes: renal (pyelonephritis, calculus), malignancy, pneumonia, sickle cell crisis

Gastro-oesophageal disorders

Gastro-oesophageal reflux

- This is due to a combination of changes in lower oesophageal pressure, raised intragastric pressure and failure of acid clearance. The incidence is up to 80% in the third trimester.
- Initial management of reflux is with dietary change, upright posture and antacids.
- In persistent gastro-oesophageal reflux despite conservative measures, the use of histamine 2 receptor antagonists (e.g. ranitidine, cimetidine) is first line, followed by proton pump inhibitors (e.g. omeprazole). Metoclopramide may speed gastric emptying and help relieve reflux.

Nausea and vomiting

- Some degree of nausea and vomiting is present in up to 90% of early normal pregnancies.
- It commonly occurs at 6–16 weeks gestation, but 20% persist beyond this time.
- Hyperemesis gravidarum (0.1%–1% pregnancies): persistent vomiting with weight loss > 5% pre-pregnancy weight and ketonuria. Onset in first trimester (usually week 6–8). Women with hyperemesis often have higher levels of serum human chorionic gonadotrophin (hCG).
- Women with severe hyperemesis requiring multiple hospitalisations have a slightly increased risk of small for gestational age infants.

MANAGEMENT OF HYPEREMESIS GRAVIDARUM

- investigations: mid-stream urine for urinary infection/ketones; pelvic ultrasound scan to exclude gestational trophoblastic disease and multiple pregnancy; full blood examination and electrolytes (hypochloraemic alkalosis, hyponatraemia, hypokalaemia);

liver function tests (LFT) (mildly elevated transaminases and hyperbilirubinaemia) and thyroid function tests
- fluid resuscitation and electrolyte restoration
- dietary modification with frequent, small meals and avoidance of trigger events/foods
- ginger and vitamin B_6 have some effect (both reduce nausea but do not affect vomiting)
- antiemetics, including metoclopramide and prochlorperazine, and antihistamines have been used as first-line management safely
- ondansetron: used successfully as second-line management
- glucocorticoids: used in severe hyperemesis
- vitamin and mineral replacement: with severe, persistent vomiting replace thiamine, B12, B6, magnesium, calcium
- differential diagnosis of persistent hyperemesis: includes hepatitis, pancreatitis, gastrointestinal obstruction, peptic ulcer disease, thyroid disease and adrenocortical insufficiency, consider pre-eclampsia if onset in second half of pregnancy

Gastrointestinal disorders

Peptic ulcer disease

Incidence. Incidence is 1 in 4000.

Peptic ulcer disease rarely occurs for the first time in pregnancy. If it is present before pregnancy, there is often a reduction in symptoms. Peptic ulceration can increase in severity with pre-eclampsia and during the puerperium.

Management of peptic ulcer disease is similar to that in non-pregnant patients, with proton pump inhibitors forming the mainstay of treatment. *H. Pylori* eradication is usually delayed until after delivery.

Coeliac disease

Autoimmune gluten-sensitive enteropathy affects 0.1%–1% population.

Clinical features include diarrhoea, abdominal pain, steatorrhoea, anaemia.

Severe untreated disease may be associated with preterm birth and intrauterine growth restriction (IUGR).

Management of coeliac disease in pregnancy includes dietitian referral, a gluten-free diet, iron, folate and B12 supplementation, and fetal growth surveillance.

Inflammatory bowel disease

Fertility correlates inversely with disease activity. Active disease during pregnancy increases risk of miscarriage and preterm birth. Ninety per cent of women with quiescent disease deliver at term.

Pregnancy itself does not increase the risk of relapse of inflammatory bowel disease.

Acute exacerbations are managed by admission to hospital, full blood count, serum albumin, stool cultures, corticosteroids and sulfasalazine.

Occasionally azathioprine or 6-mercaptopurine are required to achieve remission and should be continued in pregnancy. Anti-tumour necrosis factor (anti-TNF) agents (infliximab, etanercept) have been used safely in pregnancy.

Caesarean delivery is required only for obstetric indications or severe perianal Crohn's disease.

Hepatic disorders in pregnancy

Liver function tests in pregnancy
- There is no change in serum bilirubin and transaminase levels, although reduced total protein and albumin levels are normal.
- The increase in serum alkaline phosphatase is secondary to placental production.

Intrahepatic cholestasis of pregnancy
Incidence. Intrahepatic cholestasis affects up to 2% of pregnancies.

Presentation. Pruritus and mild jaundice present in the third trimester. Pruritus usually resolves within 48 hours of delivery. It starts at the soles and palms of the hands, and then spreads to the rest of the body.

RISK FACTORS
- There is a family history in 45% of cases.
- Previously affected pregnancy.
- It is often worse with multiple pregnancies. Pre-eclampsia must be excluded.

INVESTIGATIONS
- liver biochemistry (raised liver transaminase and bilirubin)
- raised fasting bile acids (this is the diagnostic feature of this disease)
- full blood count, urea/electrolytes and urate
- coagulation profile (raised prothrombin time may occur)
- hepatitis, Epstein–Barr virus (EBV), cytomegalovirus (CMV) serology
- autoantibody screen
- antimitochondrial and anti-SM antibodies (exclude primary biliary cirrhosis)
- liver ultrasound scan to exclude cholelithiasis

PATHOPHYSIOLOGY
- altered bile acids and progesterone metabolism
- effect on pregnancy
  - maternal vitamin K deficiency and increased risk of postpartum haemorrhage
  - meconium liquor
  - preterm delivery
  - intrapartum fetal distress
  - possible small increase in risk of intrauterine fetal death; this is difficult to predict

TREATMENT
- weekly LFT and bile acid monitoring
- coagulation monitoring prior to delivery if severe derangement of liver function
- vitamin K supplementation (especially for women with prolonged prothrombin time)
- symptomatic treatment: topical emollients, antihistamines, ursodeoxycholic acid (UDCA) 1000–1500 mg/day in 2–3 divided doses, dexamethasone
- close monitoring with consideration of early delivery (although there is limited evidence that either intervention improves outcome)
- postpartum: check return of LFT to normal 10–14 days postpartum, 90% recurrence rate, avoid oestrogen-containing contraceptives

Acute fatty liver of pregnancy
Incidence. Incidence is 1 in 12000 deliveries, with associated maternal and fetal mortality.

RISK FACTORS
- primiparity, obesity, pre-eclampsia, male fetus and multiple pregnancy
- association with long-chain 3-hydroxyacyl CoA dehydrogenase deficiency (LCHAD); this also increases risk of recurrence

PRESENTATION
- abdominal pain, especially epigastric 50%
- nausea and vomiting in 75% of cases
- jaundice in over 90% of cases, ascites
- hypertension in 50% of cases with oedema, proteinuria
- deranged liver function, coagulopathy, renal impairment, hypoglycaemia in 70%, diabetes insipidus
- progression to fulminant liver failure with hepatic encephalopathy

INVESTIGATION
- full blood examination (reveals a raised white cell count with neutrophilia, reduced platelets and haemolytic anaemia)
- coagulation profile (shows evidence of disseminated coagulopathy)
- electrolytes and renal function (elevated urea, creatinine and markedly raised urate)
- liver biochemistry (elevated bilirubin, but not markedly so; markedly elevated aspartate transaminase)
- hepatitis serology
- blood sugar levels (hypoglycaemia is common)
- imaging: liver ultrasound, computed tomography (CT) or magnetic resonance imaging (MRI) may demonstrate microvascular fat deposits (but may also appear normal); liver biopsy confirms steatosis but is not often performed due to coagulopathy

MANAGEMENT
- treatment in intensive care unit
- expedite delivery
- correct hypoglycaemia, coagulopathy and hypertension prior to delivery (50% glucose and fresh frozen plasma/cryoprecipitate/albumin may be considered)
- ventilation, dialysis, plasmapheresis, N-acetylcysteine or liver transplantation may be required
- maternal mortality is 2% with a perinatal mortality rate of 11%

Acute viral hepatitis

There does not appear to be an overall increase in congenital abnormalities if acute hepatitis occurs in pregnancy. Common causes are hepatitis A, B and C, herpes virus (simplex, varicella, cytomegalovirus) and Epstein-Barr virus.

Hepatitis A virus is usually self-limiting, with no increased fetal risks.

There is risk of vertical transmission with Hepatitis B and C.

CHRONIC HEPATITIS

Chronic active hepatitis may be due to autoimmune diseases. In pregnancy, there is a risk of IUGR, fetal death, prematurity and pre-eclampsia. There does not appear to be an increased risk of fetal malformation.

CIRRHOSIS

- There may be a decrease in fertility secondary to oligomenorrhoea.
- Pregnancy is complicated by an increased incidence of abortion and intrauterine fetal death.
- Other complications of cirrhosis may also occur, such as bleeding oesophageal varices.
- Management: avoid increasing portal pressure, cease alcohol, increase carbohydrate consumption, lower protein and supplement with vitamins. In labour, shorten the second stage. Take precautions against the risk of postpartum haemorrhage. Avoid caesarean section because of large collateral circulation and adhesions.
- Primary biliary cirrhosis: antimitochondrial antibodies are present in over 95% of cases.
- There are no prospective studies to assess the effects of disease in pregnancy.

Causes of fulminant hepatic failure in pregnancy
- viral hepatitis
- acute fatty liver of pregnancy
- severe pre-eclampsia
- haemolytic uraemic syndrome
- paracetamol overdose

Gallbladder and biliary tract

Dilatation of the gallbladder is found in pregnancy. However, anecdotal evidence of an increased risk of developing cholelithiasis in pregnancy has not been substantiated.

Acute cholelithiasis and cholecystitis in pregnancy requiring cholecystectomy occurs in about 1 in 1000 deliveries. The prevalence of asymptomatic gallstones in pregnancy is 2%–10%, which is similar to the rate in non-pregnant women.

Further reading

Royal College of Obstetricians and Gynaecologists, 2011. Obstetric cholestasis. Green-top guideline No. 43. RCOG, London.

Chapter 51

Neurological disease in pregnancy

Michael Flynn
Thea Bowler

Epilepsy and pregnancy

Incidence. Epilepsy occurs in 0.5%–1% of the population. Over 90% of women with epilepsy have a normal pregnancy.

Effects of epilepsy on pregnancy

- reports of fetal bradycardia after generalised seizure
- increased risk of childhood epilepsy of 3%–4% if one parent has epilepsy
- increased association with pre-eclampsia, preterm delivery, low birthweight, higher perinatal mortality and congenital malformations due to the epilepsy and the anticonvulsant drugs; fetal effects include cerebral palsy, seizures and mental deficit

Effect of pregnancy on epilepsy

- About 50% remain stable, with improvement in seizure frequency in 25% and deterioration in 25% of women.
- The deterioration is attributed to hormonal and metabolic changes and diminished compliance with drug therapy.
- In about 70% of patients, serum levels of anticonvulsants fall in early pregnancy and return to prepregnancy levels by 4 weeks postpartum; so if seizure activity increases, it is often in the first two trimesters.
- If epilepsy presents for the first time in pregnancy, rigorous investigation is required to exclude other neurological abnormalities.

Pharmacokinetics of anticonvulsants in pregnancy

- Drug absorption may be lowered with vomiting in early pregnancy.
- Volume of distribution is increased due to raised plasma volume and total body water, and results in a reduced steady state of plasma levels.
- Increased fat stores will lower lipid-soluble drug excretion.

- Phenytoin and valproate are highly protein-bound. With the reduction of albumin in pregnancy, there is a lower percentage of bound drug. Therefore, unbound levels in plasma remain constant, but total plasma levels are reduced.
- The glomerular filtration rate rises, raising the clearance of renally excreted drugs.
- Hepatic hydroxylation of phenytoin is increased, and this causes a reduction in free drug.
- Non-compliance due to maternal fears of teratogenicity often reduces plasma levels of drug.

Teratogenicity of anticonvulsants

- In a woman with epilepsy treated with a single anticonvulsant, the fetus has a risk of congenital malformation of 7%, compared with 3% in non-epileptics. There may be a higher incidence with polypharmacy.
- The major defects include orofacial clefts, cardiovascular anomalies, neural tube defects (which are commonly primary myelomeningocele and anencephaly, and especially if valproate is taken in the first trimester).
- Minor defects include microcephaly, dysmorphic features, hypertelorism and digital hypoplasia.
- Epilepsy pregnancy registries indicate valproate at doses > 1100 mg/day confer significant risk compared to other doses and other drugs.

Other maternal effects of anticonvulsants

- reduced folate levels
- increased vitamin D metabolism with phenytoin and phenobarbitone, and risk of hypocalcaemia

Fetal/neonatal effects of anticonvulsants

- reduced fetal thyroxine as phenytoin competes for thyroxine-binding sites
- increased risk of haemorrhagic phenomenon of the newborn (mostly internal bleeding, secondary to decreased levels of vitamin K-dependent clotting factors as a result of drug-induced liver enzyme induction)
- increased drowsiness, jitteriness, irritability and poor suckling in the neonate

Anticonvulsants and breastfeeding

- Although all anticonvulsants except valproate cross the placental barrier, breastfeeding is not contraindicated.
- Neonatal serum levels are 40%–80% of maternal levels, and drowsiness may be a problem.

Anticonvulsants and contraception

- There is an increased risk of pregnancy and contraception failure secondary to hepatic enzymatic induction from anticonvulsants (carbamazepine, phenytoin, phenobarbitone, primidone, oxcarbazepine and topiramate > 200 mg/day). There is no interference for gabapentin, lamotrigine, valproate and levetiracetam.
- The higher dose oestrogen (50 µg ethinyloestradiol) pill or long-acting reversible contraceptives are indicated.

Management of epilepsy in pregnancy

BEFORE CONCEPTION

- If seizure-free for 2 years, consider withdrawing therapy. When possible, this should be 6 months prior to pregnancy.

- Aim for monotherapy or at least lowest possible dose.
- With the exception of valproate, there is no agreement as to which anticonvulsant drug should be used. It is appropriate to avoid valproate, especially at doses > 1100 mg, if epilepsy is controlled by other medications.
- High-dose folate supplementation.

PREGNANCY

- Adopt a combined approach with the obstetrician and neurologist.
- Continue current anticonvulsant therapy and folate. Do not change therapy in established pregnancy solely to decrease teratogenicity.
- Plasma levels of free anticonvulsant drugs should be monitored in patients with frequent or recurrent seizures.
- At 18 weeks gestation, a detailed fetal morphology ultrasound scan is required to assess for neural tube defects and orofacial clefts.
- Vitamin K 20 mg/day orally in the last 2–3 weeks of pregnancy for women taking hepatic enzyme-inducing drugs, may help reduce the risk of haemorrhagic disease of the newborn.
- Intramuscular vitamin K injection for the neonate is indicated.

DELIVERY

- 1%–2% epileptic women will have intrapartum seizure and 1%–2% postpartum
- early epidural anaesthesia and shortened second stage may limit the chance of intra-partum seizure
- seizures during labour and delivery should be treated with intravenous benzo-diazepines; magnesium sulfate is not first-choice management, but may be used if eclampsia is suspected

POSTPARTUM

- Return to prepregnancy medication dose.
- Advise on the importance of sleep and rest.
- Breastfeeding is encouraged.
- To limit risk to infant should seizure occur: change baby on floor, bath with supervision.

Cerebral and spinal tumours

Prolactinoma

- Hyperprolactinaemia stimulates an increase in dopamine secretion, thereby inhibiting the release of gonadotrophin-releasing hormone (GnRH). Most women will be infertile unless treated.
- During normal pregnancy, the pituitary increases in size by 50%–70% secondary to lactotroph hyperplasia, and prolactin levels rise. Pituitary tumours are also likely to expand in pregnancy.

MANAGEMENT

- Institute combined obstetrician/neurologist management.
- Review regularly to assess growth of prolactinoma.
- Microadenoma causing hyperprolactinaemia: bromocriptine or cabergoline is withdrawn after pregnancy is confirmed and reinstated after delivery without significant risk of disease progression.

- Macroadenoma: the risk of expansion in pregnancy is < 10%. It is recommended that pregnancy only be attempted when the tumour has shrunk to at least the confines of the sella turcica.
- Combined management during pregnancy with endocrinologists and neurosurgeons is indicated. The common complaints of tumour expansion are visual field defects and headaches. There is no evidence of teratogenesis with bromocriptine. Surgical management in pregnancy may be required.
- In symptomatic women, induction of labour at 38 weeks is indicated with elective use of forceps to shorten the second stage.

Neurofibroma
An acoustic neuroma can expand in pregnancy, as can cutaneous neurofibromatosis. This condition is associated with hypertension.

Neuropathies

Carpal tunnel syndrome
This is a common condition in pregnancy due to fluid retention, and resolves mostly in the postpartum period. It is often symptomatic at night, and management is initially with splints and physiotherapy. If these bring no improvement, then orthopaedic review and hydrocortisone injections or surgery may be indicated.

Bell's palsy
This is more common in pregnancy, especially in the last trimester with increasing oedema. Management is with corticosteroids, optimally within 1 day of onset. It is possibly more common in patients with pre-eclampsia due to oedema.

Spinal cord injury

Increased risk of respiratory and urinary tract infections, decubitus ulcers and constipation.

Management in labour
- Management is dependent on the level of spinal cord lesion.
- If the spinal cord is divided above T10, labour will be painless.
- If the division is above T5–T6, there is a risk of autonomic hyperreflexia. This is an autonomic and somatic hyperreflexia in response to intense sensory stimulation. In labour, uterine contractions can overstimulate the splanchnic sympathetic bed and release catecholamines, which results in hypertension, arrhythmia, headache, facial flushing and sweating. This response can be prevented by epidural and spinal anaesthesia to the level of the umbilicus (T10).

Multiple sclerosis in pregnancy

Effects of pregnancy on multiple sclerosis
- Pregnancy is generally considered to provide a stabilising effect on multiple sclerosis. This is thought to be due to the altered immune state in pregnancy.

- Relapses are common in the first 3–6 months postpartum.
- There is no significant effect on fertility or fetal wellbeing.
- When combining both the protective effect of pregnancy and postpartum risk period, there seems no change to multiple sclerosis relapse rate or long-term disability from pregnancy.

Management
- General measures include rest, counselling, preventing urinary tract infections and treating anaemia.
- Epidural anaesthesia has no effect on the disease.
- No contraindications exist to breastfeeding.
- Acute exacerbations of the disease are treated with high dose glucocorticoids.
- The majority of disease-modifying drugs (used to prevent relapses) such as interferons and glatiramer should be ceased prior to pregnancy due to a lack of safety data.

Migraine headache

- Clinical features include unilateral, throbbing headache with or without prodromal symptoms, nausea and vomiting, photophobia, phonophobia.
- Common triggers include fatigue, stress, dietary factors (e.g. wine, cheese, chocolate) and the oral contraceptive pill.
- Most women experience a decrease in frequency and severity of attacks. Preexisting migraine has been associated with hypertensive disorders of pregnancy.
- Management of acute attack: paracetamol, opioids, antiemetics, sumatriptan (ergotamine is contraindicated in pregnancy).
- Prophylaxis: low dose aspirin, β-blockers (may cause mild fetal growth restriction), calcium channel blockers and tricyclic antidepressants.

Further reading
EURAP Study Group, 2006. Seizure control and treatment in pregnancy: observations from the EURAP epilepsy pregnancy registry. Neurology 66, 354–360.

Vukusic, S., Hutchinson, M., Hours, M., et al., 2004. Pregnancy and multiple sclerosis (the PRIMS study): clinical predictors of post-partum relapse. Brain 127, 1353–1360.

Chapter 52

Thyroid disease in pregnancy

Helen L Barrett
Karin Lust

Incidence. In developed countries, 5 in 1000 pregnancies are complicated by hyperthyroidism and 3–10 in 1000 pregnancies are complicated by hypothyroidism.

Thyroid physiology and pregnancy

* During normal pregnancy, the thyroid gland grows in size due to gland hyperplasia and increased vascularity. This goitre development is exaggerated in the setting of iodine deficiency.
* Circulating levels of iodine are reduced in pregnancy. This may be secondary to reduced renal tubular absorption (with renal iodine clearance increasing approximately 1.5-fold), maternal–fetal transfer and fetal storage. There is a daily requirement of inorganic iodine of 250 μg. This is increased from the non-pregnant state of 150 μg per day. Iodine is absorbed from foods such as salt, milk, dairy products, seafood and eggs. Miscarriage rates are increased in iodine-deficient women. Iodine supplementation is recommended for all women except those with Graves' disease or a past history of hyperthyroidism. During lactation, urinary iodine excretion is normal, but with iodine being concentrated by the mammary gland, the infant is supplied with approximately 100 μg/day of iodine. The breastfeeding mother is recommended to take 250 μg/day of iodine.
* Thyroid-binding globulin production rises throughout pregnancy as a result of increased oestrogen and remains raised postpartum. Because of this, more T3 and T4 are protein-bound, thus raising total T3 and T4 levels.
* There may be a reduction in free T3 and T4 as pregnancy progresses. In late pregnancy, this may be in the non-pregnant hypothyroid range. Therefore, when low free T3/T4 levels are present in pregnancy, thyroid-stimulating hormone (TSH) is required for a diagnosis of hypothyroidism. Free thyroxine concentrations correlate to thyroid function.
* TSH levels fall in the first trimester. Free thyroid hormones are raised in about 70%–75% of women with hyperemesis, suggesting a relationship between high

human chorionic gonadotrophin (hCG) levels and thyroid stimulation (hCG and TSH have the same alpha subunit with different beta subunits; hCG may be a TSH agonist).

- Fetal thyroid commences functioning at 10–12 weeks gestation; however, it is the maternal thyroxine mostly supplying fetal needs until the third trimester when the fetal thyroid is sufficiently mature to be independent. In this trimester, the placenta acts as a barrier to maternal TSH, T4 and T3 and the fetal axis acts independently of the mother. The placenta freely transports iodine and thyrotrophin-releasing hormone. Fetal blood sampling correlates to fetal status most reliably. After birth, fetal TSH levels rise markedly due to a thyrotrophin-releasing hormone surge and decrease to normal over 3 days. The fetal dependence on maternal iodine continues during breastfeeding.

Maternal–fetal interactions

- Thyroid antibodies: microsomal and thyroglobulin antibodies (TPO) cross the placenta, but are not cytotoxic to fetal thyroid cells.
- TSH receptor antibodies are immunoglobulin G-type antibodies and therefore cross the placenta with a risk of neonatal complications.
- Antithyroid antibodies, if present, are associated with an increased risk of miscarriage.

Overt hypothyroidism

- Autoimmune thyroid disease is diagnosed by destructive antibodies (antithyroid peroxidase antibodies and anti-TPO antibodies). The underlying thyroiditis is known as Hashimoto's disease. Prevalence is unknown, although antibodies may be present in 5% of women of childbearing age.
  - Raised TSH, decreased free T4 and positive thyroid autoantibodies are diagnostic of autoimmune hypothyroidism.
  - Mild elevation TSH and normal free T4 are diagnostic of subclinical hypothyroidism with an increased chance of becoming hypothyroid as pregnancy progresses.
  - The presence of antithyroid antibodies and normal TSH and free T4 is controversial, but requires frequent monitoring in pregnancy.
- Overt hypothyroidism is associated with increased risks of miscarriage, hypertensive disorders of pregnancy, placental abruption, anaemia, postpartum haemorrhage as well as prematurity, low birth weight, increased perinatal morbidity and mortality. If adequately treated, these adverse associations are ameliorated.
- Treat with thyroxine to maintain TSH in the low–normal range (< 2.5 mIU/L in the first trimester, < 3 thereafter).
- Women with hypothyroidism prepregnancy will usually need an increase in their prepregnancy thyroxine dose by 30%–50% in the early second trimester.
- Thyroid function should be monitored approximately every 6 weeks or 4 weeks after thyroxine dosage adjustments.
- In the postpartum, thyroxine requirements decrease. If the patient was on thyroxine prepregnancy, they should have their dosage reduced to the prepregnancy dose at which they were stable. The thyroid function tests should be followed up 4–6 weeks postpartum.

Subclinical hypothyroidism

- It is possible that women with normal thyroid function when not pregnant are at risk of developing hypothyroidism in early pregnancy if the thyroid gland cannot increase the required production of thyroxine for pregnancy. Subclinical hypothyroidism is associated with increased rates of pregnancy complications but is less clearly adversely associated with infant neurocognitive development.
- Women with subclinical hypothyroidism and positive TPO antibodies should be treated with thyroxine. This is based on some evidence of benefit. The evidence of benefit for those who have negative TPO antibodies is debated. Guidelines differ on whether to recommend thyroxine treatment for women who are TPO antibody negative. Research is continuing in this area and is recommended that institutions develop local policy.

Congenital hypothyroidism
Incidence. It occurs in 1 in 4000 live births.
   It constitutes part of the neonatal screening test.

Hyperthyroidism in pregnancy

Incidence. It affects 2 in 1000 pregnancies.
   As described earlier, TSH levels fall in the first trimester. Causes of low TSH can be physiological (e.g. related to hCG elevations), but pathological causes need to be considered and excluded.

Causes
- Graves' disease (the commonest cause in pregnancy)
- gestational thyrotoxicosis
- toxic nodular goitre
- Hashimoto's disease
- subacute thyroiditis
- rare: hyperemesis gravidarum, hydatidiform mole, struma ovarii

Gestational thyrotoxicosis
- Gestational thyrotoxicosis is transient hyperthyroidism in the first half of pregnancy with elevated fT4, and suppressed or undetectable TSH, without autoimmune thyroid antibodies.
- It is usually associated with syndromes related to high hCG levels (e.g. hyperemesis, molar pregnancy).
- Serum fT4 returns to normal by 14–18 weeks gestation.
- Treatment of gestational hyperthyroidism with antithyroid drugs does not improve obstetric outcome.
- Treatment with antithyroid drugs can be considered if the diagnosis is unclear, very severe or thought to be possibly Grave's disease. Symptom control can be undertaken with Beta blockers if necessary.
   To differentiate gestational thyrotoxicosis from Grave's disease, helpful features can be a personal or family history of thyroid disease; clinical features (e.g. goitre and eye signs, presence of TSH receptor antibodies).

Graves' disease

This is caused by thyroid hyperactivity due to TSH receptor-stimulating antibody. This antibody is IgG and can cross the placenta.

MATERNAL EFFECTS DURING PREGNANCY

- In 80% of cases, the woman remains euthyroid throughout pregnancy.
- Episodes of thyrotoxicosis more often occur in the first trimester and postpartum, and treatment is required during these times.
- In 20% of cases, thyrotoxicosis remains stable during pregnancy and requires treatment throughout.

FETAL/NEONATAL EFFECTS

- Fetal thyrotoxicosis may occur, as the antibody readily crosses the placenta.
- Goitre may be seen on ultrasound. Fetal blood sampling can be performed.
- Even after treatment of the mother with thyroidectomy, or radioactive iodine, there may be persisting antibodies. It is therefore important to determine the cause of the hyperthyroidism or the indication of the patient being on thyroxine replacement.
- Fetal risks include increased risk of intrauterine growth restriction (IUGR), premature labour, fetal or neonatal hyperthyroidism or hypothyroidism. The fetal risk of thyroid dysfunction depends on maternal thyroid control, use of antithyroid drugs and elevation of TSH receptor antibodies at 22–26 weeks gestation.
- Fetuses at risk can be evaluated by assessment of maternal antibody concentrations and fetal heart rate. Fetal tachycardia begins from about 25 weeks gestation.
- Neonatal Graves' disease is seen in 10%–20% of neonates of mothers with Graves' disease. These babies suffer from tachycardia, poor weight gain and accelerated bone ossification.

Management of thyrotoxicosis in pregnancy

Failure to treat is associated with an increased risk of pre-eclampsia, premature labour, thyroid storm, congestive cardiac failure and perinatal mortality. The aim is to achieve the euthyroid state as early as possible (i.e. preconception) to minimise risks. The symptomatic woman requires treatment throughout pregnancy.

INVESTIGATIONS

Investigations include increased serum free T4 and/or free T3 and decreased TSH and measurement of TSH receptor antibodies.

Radioactive iodine scanning should not be performed in pregnancy.

MEDICAL MANAGEMENT

- Propranolol is used in acute events for treatment of maternal tachycardia, tremor and anxiety. The small risk of IUGR is outweighed by control of maternal symptoms.
- Both propylthiouracil (PTU) and carbimazole cross the placenta. PTU is recommended as first line in the first trimester. This is due to carbimazole being associated with congenital abnormalities. Rarely PTU has been reported to be associated with severe liver toxicity, hence the recommendation to change from PTU to carbimazole after the first trimester. If changing drug, assess thyroid function after 2 weeks. The fetal risks of both drugs are fetal goitre and transient hypothyroidism. Both drugs can cause maternal agranulocytosis.
- Surgical management: if possible, delay this until the second trimester.

- Thyroid function should be monitored every 2–4 weeks depending on clinical situation.
- Adjust medication to keep serum T4 at upper limit of normal.
- As pregnancy progresses, the dose of antithyroid drugs may be reduced and often patients do not require treatment for the whole of pregnancy.
- Monitor liver function for those on PTU every 3–4 weeks (although hepatic dysfunction can occur unexpectedly and acutely at any time).
- Check TSH receptor antibodies at 20–26 weeks; if elevated > 3 times the upper limit of normal, careful fetal monitoring for thyroid dysfunction is indicated.
- Fetal monitoring is indicated in the third trimester for assessment of fetal growth and fetal hyperthyroidism.
- Antenatal management: includes combined management with endocrinology clinic or a doctor with experience in managing thyroid disease in pregnancy.
- If treated with antithyroid drugs, monitor thyroid function tests for neonatal status; however, the risk is low.
- Postpartum reassess thyroid function tests approximately 6 weeks postdelivery, especially in patients who have been able to go off their antithyroid drugs in pregnancy. There is an increased risk of recurrence of Graves postpartum.

LABOUR AND DELIVERY
Notify the paediatrician, as the neonate requires monitoring for hyperthyroidism.

Postpartum thyroiditis

Incidence. About 10% of women develop subclinical postpartum thyroiditis.

Clinical presentation
- Symptoms typically develop 1–3 months postpartum.
- It often commences with symptoms of mild hyperthyroidism and then mild hypothyroidism at about 3–6 months postpartum, which then resolves.
- Consider the diagnosis in women with depression or difficulty coping.
- If symptoms persist, Hashimoto's thyroiditis is likely.

Aetiology
- Thyroiditis is associated with microsomal antibodies in 50%–80% of cases.
- It is considered an autoimmune disorder, with 20%–25% of women having a first-degree relative with autoimmune disease.
- Type 1 diabetics have a three-fold risk.
- Women with known thyroid antibodies should have TSH measured at 6–12 weeks and at 6 months postpartum.

Recurrence
There is a 10% recurrence risk in future pregnancies. There is an increased long-term risk of overt hypothyroidism.

Further reading

De Groot, L., Abalovich, M., Alexander, E.K., et al., 2012. Management of thyroid dysfunction during pregnancy and postpartum: an Endocrine Society clinical practice guideline. J. Clin. Endocrinol. Metab. 97, 2543–2565.

Earl, R., Crowther, C.A., Middleton, P., 2013. Interventions for hyperthyroidism pre-pregnancy and during pregnancy. Cochrane Database Syst. Rev. (11), Cd008633.

Reid, S.M., Middleton, P., Cossich, M.C., et al., 2013. Interventions for clinical and subclinical hypothyroidism pre-pregnancy and during pregnancy. Cochrane Database Syst. Rev. (5), Cd007752.

Taylor, P.N., Vaidya, B., 2012. Side effects of anti-thyroid drugs and their impact on the choice of treatment for thyrotoxicosis in pregnancy. Eur. Thyroid J. 1, 176–185.

van den Boogaard, E., Vissenberg, R., Land, J.A., et al., 2011. Significance of (sub)clinical thyroid dysfunction and thyroid autoimmunity before conception and in early pregnancy: a systematic review. Hum. Reprod. Update 17, 605–619.

Velkeniers, B., Van Meerhaeghe, A., Poppe, K., et al., 2013. Levothyroxine treatment and pregnancy outcome in women with subclinical hypothyroidism undergoing assisted reproduction technologies: systematic review and meta-analysis of RCTs. Hum. Reprod. Update 19, 251–258.

Vissenberg, R., Manders, V.D., Mastenbroek, S., et al., 2015. Pathophysiological aspects of thyroid hormone disorders/thyroid peroxidase autoantibodies and reproduction. Hum. Reprod. Update 21, 378–387.

Chapter 53

Renal disease in pregnancy

Michael Flynn
Anne-Maree Craven

Physiology

In pregnancy there is a rise in renal blood flow and a subsequent rise in glomerular filtration rate (GFR) by up to 50%, which is present from the first trimester. There is a slight fall in GFR in the last 3 weeks of pregnancy. This increase in GFR causes a fall in serum creatinine and urea levels to lower than non-pregnant levels (creatinine level < 75 µmol/L). The estimated glomerular filtration rate (eGFR) has not been validated in pregnancy.

Changes in renal tubular function result in a fall in serum urate levels in early and mid-pregnancy, with levels rising again in the third trimester. Similarly, up to 50% of normal women will have glycosuria at some point in pregnancy, as the rise in GFR exceeds the tubular capacity to reabsorb glucose. Proteinuria up to 300 mg per day is normal in pregnancy and 24-hour urine collection remains the gold standard for assessing proteinuria.

Anatomically, in pregnancy the kidney enlarges and the renal pelves and ureters dilate. The right side enlarges more than the left due to the dextrorotation of the uterus. Pelvicalyceal dilatation up to 2 cm diameter can be considered normal.

Urinary tract infections
Acute pyelonephritis occurs in 1%–2% of all pregnancies (*see Ch 29*).

Chronic renal disease

Pregnancy outcome in chronic renal disease is related to level of renal impairment, function and severity of hypertension blood pressure and degree of proteinuria before pregnancy. Traditionally, renal disease has been defined by level of creatinine. However, this fails to recognise body mass and age as an important determinant of estimated glomerular filtration rate, and as such may underestimate the level of renal impairment in slimmer or older women.

Mild renal disease is defined as serum creatinine < 125 µmol/L preconception. In the absence of severe hypertension or proteinuria, pregnancy outcomes are usually successful with only moderately elevated rates of pre-eclampsia and growth restriction. There is usually a successful outcome. For most kidney diseases, pregnancy usually does not affect the long-term progress of the disease at this level of creatinine. Risk of flare of glomerulonephritis is estimated at 3%, although proteinuria is common. Hypertension is usually not a feature. Proteinuria and hypertension can be present or absent at this level depending on the disease process rather than the creatinine.

Moderate renal disease is preconception serum creatinine between 125 and 250 µmol/L. Approximately 40% of pregnancies are complicated by intrauterine growth restriction (IUGR) and pre-eclampsia hypertension. Close monitoring is required. A minority of women within this group will have suffer irreversible decline in renal function but progression to end-stage renal failure and dialysis is rare (< 2%). The risk is especially in uncontrolled hypertension. The major predictor of permanent decrease in renal function from pregnancy is hypertension and prepregnancy serum creatinine, rather than underlying aetiology. Risk of miscarriage and fetal demise due to uncontrolled hypertension, and prematurity, is higher. Prematurity preterm delivery is usually secondary to severe pre-eclampsia and IUGR. Women with underlying renal disease are at risk of earlier and more severe pre-eclampsia.

Severe renal disease is seen with serum creatinine > 250 µmol/L. Although pregnancy is possible, many women are subfertile due to chronic disease and amenorrhoea. Pregnancy poses a significant risk to mother and baby, and general advice is to avoid pregnancy before renal transplantation. Rates of perinatal mortality and intrauterine death are significantly higher at this level of renal impairment. Creatinine levels tend to rise in the second trimester and, combined with severe hypertension, often result in the need for preterm delivery. Renal function commonly does not return to prepregnancy level. Close monitoring of the mother's creatinine is required in the postpartum period due to the possibility of rapid deterioration of renal function. Overall, the risk of deteriorating renal function to end-stage renal disease requiring dialysis during the pregnancy is approximately 35%. There is a tendency to worsen more rapidly in the postpartum.

Pregnancy in dialysis patients, while still rare, has seen increasing rates of live infant births over the last few decades. This has been associated with extension of total haemodialysis hours (> 20 hours per week). Mean duration of gestation at delivery is 32–33 weeks and the main contributors to preterm delivery are maternal hypertension, polyhydramnios and acute shifts in maternal fluid volumes leading to impaired fetal perfusion and IUGR.

Management of chronic renal disease in pregnancy
There should be joint management with the renal and/or obstetric physicians.

PREPREGNANCY COUNSELLING
- Counselling includes general health advice.
- Pregnancy is contraindicated with recent flares of renal disease such as lupus nephritis. Pregnancy should be delayed until in remission for at least 1 year.
- The pregnant woman will be closely monitored by renal/obstetric physician in addition to the obstetrician. Community midwife care alone is not appropriate.
- Genetic counselling may be required if the cause of chronic kidney disease is heritable (e.g. polycystic kidney disease, reflux nephropathy).

- In mild impairment, pregnancy is unlikely to change the underlying disease (except scleroderma and polyarteritis nodosa).
- Control of hypertension is essential, aiming for systolic blood pressure of 120–135 mmHg and diastolic measures of 80–90 mmHg. With the normal lowering of blood pressure in the first trimester, sometimes reduction of antihypertensives is required during this period.
- Review medications and avoid those contraindicated in pregnancy (including angiotensin-converting enzyme inhibitors, angiotensin receptor blockers and some immunosuppressive drugs). Change to non-teratogenic antihypertensives and immunosuppressants with stabilisation of blood pressure and creatinine prior to conception.
- Advise on possible pregnancy outcomes, notably increased risk of pre-eclampsia, premature delivery and IUGR.
- Pregnancy is not common among long-term dialysis patients, and there is no advantage to any dialysis route.

ANTENATAL MANAGEMENT
- Baseline assessment of serum creatinine, urea, electrolytes, creatinine clearance and 24-hour urinary protein, vitamin D status, disease markers if appropriate (e.g. dsDNA in lupus).
- Consider prophylaxis of preterm pre-eclampsia with aspirin and calcium. Check vitamin D levels and replace as required.
- Ultrasound scan: 18–20-week fetal morphology assessment with Doppler assessment of uterine artery blood flow to help predict pre-eclampsia.
- Mid-stream urine specimen to exclude infection.
- Prophylactic antibiotics and monthly urine analysis in patients with recurrent urinary tract infections (UTIs).
- Serial assessment of renal function and close monitoring of blood pressure, specifically hypertension and superimposed pre-eclampsia.
- Fetal surveillance and placental function in the third trimester.
- Admission for stabilisation if hypertension severe.
- Aim: delivery at 38–40 weeks (although preterm delivery is often indicated for fetal reasons, substantial deterioration of renal function, uncontrollable hypertension or pre-eclampsia). Caesarean section is only required for obstetric reasons.
- Differentiating between worsening of chronic kidney disease and pre-eclampsia can be difficult as both can cause increases in creatinine, blood pressure and proteinuria. Expert advice from renal/obstetric doctors should be sought.
- Most of the maternal risks of pregnancy are associated with hypertension and superimposed pre-eclampsia. (Fetal risks are around IUGR, preterm delivery which is not necessarily related to blood pressure.)

Nephrotic syndrome in pregnancy

The commonest cause of nephrotic syndrome in pregnancy is pre-eclampsia. Greater than 5 g/day proteinuria is associated with earlier onset of pre-eclampsia, preterm delivery and its associated neonatal complications. Maternal complication rates are similar to those with lower levels of proteinuria (significantly higher perinatal mortality and morbidity not seen in any data to support higher mortality apart from case study). If the nephrotic syndrome is not due to pre-eclampsia, the pregnancy may continue to

38–39 weeks gestation if blood pressure and renal function are near normal before pregnancy and the fetus seems well.

Management includes thromboprophylaxis with low-molecular-weight heparin (LMWH) (if creatinine is near normal) due to increased risk of deep vein thrombosis. Vitamin D, calcium and iron replacement are required as these are often depleted as a consequence of high-protein losses. Regular fetal monitoring of growth and wellbeing is indicated due to the risk of reduced utero-placental blood flow. (A high-protein diet is controversial as kidneys just excrete more protein which can damage the tubules and fetal monitoring.) Diuretics are contraindicated, as they may exacerbate the decreased intravascular volume.

Pregnancy and renal transplant

Incidence. About 2% of women of child-bearing age with a renal transplant become pregnant. Most studies report a live birth rate of 60%–80% in renal transplant recipients. The success rate of an ongoing pregnancy may be higher than 90%. Some studies show the miscarriage rate as approximately 20%.

There is a 30% chance of developing hypertension and/or pre-eclampsia, and risk of preterm delivery is high. Successful pregnancy outcome is markedly improved if pre-pregnancy creatinine is < 125 μmol/L. It is likely that pregnancy will not have any long-term effect on survival of allograft.

Prepregnancy advice
Advise to use contraception for at least 1–2 years after a transplantation, after which time risk of acute rejection will be lower and immunosuppressive therapy should be reduced to maintenance levels. In women with a stable renal transplant who are at low risk of complications, pregnancy could be considered at 12 months posttransplantation.

While mycophenolate is teratogenic, cyclosporine, tacrolimus, prednisone and aza-thioprine are considered safe in pregnancy. Cyclosporine use has been associated with low birthweight infants. Women need to be changed to appropriate immunosuppression well before conception with no evidence of rejection on the new regimen before stopping contraception. Bisphosphonates are contraindicated for 6 months prior to conception.

Risk of infection is higher in immunosuppressed patients, and special consideration should be given to the risk (to mother and fetus) of reactivation of certain viruses such as CMV.

Bone health should be maximised, especially in women on prednisone. Vitamin D levels should be checked and supplemented where necessary.

With good graft function post transplantation (creatinine < 150 μmol/L), women can be assured that pregnancy is not likely to have a significant adverse effect on long-term kidney function. This is also applicable to repeated pregnancies.

Consideration should be given to counselling in regard to maternal life expectancy following renal transplantation. These patients have a higher cardiovascular risk and 10-year mortality is markedly higher compared to women with no history of renal disease.

Neither prednisone nor azathioprine is likely to affect pregnancy and pregnancy is then not contraindicated, provided there is stable renal function and normotension.

Pregnancy

- Immunosuppressive medication should be maintained at current doses, unless there is a significant change in drug levels.
- Rejection rates are no higher than in the non-pregnant state.
- Aspirin is indicated for prophylaxis of preterm pre-eclampsia.
- A 2-hour glucose tolerance test is indicated, especially for those women on prednisone or tacrolimus.
- Increases in preexisting proteinuria is seen commonly, especially in the third trimester, and does not necessarily indicate pre-eclampsia or deteriorating renal function.
- There are increased risks of IUGR (20%–40%) and preterm delivery (40%–60%), especially in women with preexisting hypertension.
- The transplanted pelvic kidney is not injured during vaginal delivery.

Further reading

Davidson, J.M., et al. (Eds.), 2008. Renal disease in pregnancy. RCOG Press, London.

de Sweit, M., 1995. Medical Disorders in Obstetric Practice, 3rd ed. Blackwell Science, Oxford.

McKay, D.B., Josephson, M.A., Armenti, V.T., et al., 2005. Reproduction and transplantation: report on the AST Consensus Conference on Reproductive Issues and Transplantation. Am. J. Transplant. 5, 1592–1599.

Chapter 54

The puerperium

Michael Flynn

Definition. The puerperium is the period from the completion of the third stage of labour to the return of the prepregnant physiological state. It is said to last 6 weeks.

Physiology. Involution of the uterus is due to catabolism of the uterine muscle bulk, with the fundal height decreasing from the level of the umbilicus on day 1 postpartum to not being palpable abdominally on days 10–14. It returns to a non-pregnant size within 4 weeks. The cervix involutes with the uterus and the os is closed by 2–3 weeks. The endometrium starts to regenerate 2–3 days postpartum.

The lochia or vaginal discharge is usually red (lochia rubra) for 2–14 days, then serous (lochia serosa) for up to 20 days, and gradually ceases by 4–8 weeks (lochia alba). Ovulation is often inhibited in breastfeeding before 10 weeks; if lactation is suppressed, it may occur at 7–10 weeks.

Afterbirth pains are tonic contractions of the uterus. They are increased in multiparas and with breastfeeding. Diuresis occurs 2 days after birth, and there is a return of plasma volume and other blood parameters to normal within 2 weeks.

Abnormal postpartum bleeding

Normal duration of blood loss is a mean of 24 days, with approximately 10% of women still bleeding at 8 weeks. Treatment is investigation with ultrasound to exclude retained pregnancy tissue prior to antibiotic treatment and, if required, surgical management with curettage.

Puerperal infections

Incidence. Puerperal infections occur in 2% of women after delivery.

Sites
- The genital tract is the commonest site of infection.
- Other sites include respiratory, wound and breast.

- Milk fever can occur with engorgement on days 3–4 but does not imply infection.
- A urinary tract infection is uncommon unless catheterisation has been performed.
- On days 2–5 postpartum, the infection is commonly genital or urinary tract (*Escherichia coli* or haemolytic *Streptococcus*).
- During week 2 postpartum, sites are more likely wound, breast or complicated pelvic infections.
- Deep venous thrombosis and pulmonary embolism are possible.

Postpartum endometritis

RISK FACTORS

- prolonged rupture of membranes
- emergency caesarean section
- excessive blood loss
- prolonged surgery
- multiple vaginal examinations
- preterm delivery

MICROBIOLOGICAL CAUSES (MOSTLY POLYMICROBIAL)

- 60% anaerobic endometritis: *Peptostreptococcus, Bacteroides, Clostridium*
- 40% aerobic causes: *Streptococcus, Enterococcus, E. coli, Staphylococcus aureus*
- *Bacteroides fragilis*, which may cause invasive anaerobic endometritis, often with adnexal involvement
- *Mycoplasma* common although pathogenesis unsure

MANAGEMENT

- General examination should specifically assess the patient for infections of the breast, uterus, genital tract, chest, abdomen/wound and urinary tract. Deep venous thrombosis may present as a febrile illness.
- Microbiological assessment includes urine and blood for culture. Microbiological cultures of the genital tract are often not helpful, as the infective organisms are usually vaginal commensals.
- In the woman who is febrile with no other clinical symptoms and signs, empirical therapy of amoxycillin/potassium clavulanate 500/125 mg orally every 8 hours may be tried.
- If fever persists for more than 48 hours, add erythromycin 500 mg orally every 8 hours, as *Mycoplasma* may be involved.
- In the clinically unwell woman, intravenous therapy is indicated. A combination of (amoxy)ampicillin, gentamicin and metronidazole is used.

Breast infection

Incidence. Breast infection occurs in 1%–5% of postpartum infections.

CAUSES

- mostly *S. aureus*
- *Streptococcus*
- *E. coli*
- usually nosocomial, with transfer from infant to nipple (the causative organism can often be isolated from milk or pus)

TREATMENT
- The aim of early treatment with antibiotics is to avoid abscess formation.
- Breastfeeding should be continued or the breast manually emptied to avoid milk stasis and further abscess risks.
- Oral antibiotic treatment consists of flucloxacillin 500 mg to 1 g every 6 hours, dicloxacillin or cephalexin 500 mg to 1 g every 6 hours.
- Failure of antibiotic therapy may represent the presence of an abscess.

Breastfeeding

Physiology of lactation

During pregnancy, breast tissue is stimulated and hypertrophy of alveolar lobular structures occurs. Oestrogen, progesterone and prolactin are required for growth of the milk-collecting ducts. The milk production is inhibited in pregnancy by high levels of oestrogen and progesterone.

Milk production is regulated by prolactin, which causes glandular cells to secrete milk in response to a suckling reflex. Oxytocin is also released by suckling, although by different neuroendocrine pathways. Oxytocin acts on myoepithelial cells to induce milk ejection. The 600 mL breast milk made per day contains all vitamins except for vitamin K.

Establishing and maintaining lactation is complex, but several studies demonstrate beneficial effects of early contact of mother with baby. There appears to be no critical period for the first feed in the establishment of lactation. Colostrum, a yellow fluid, is made in the first 2 days. It differs from breast milk due to its increased fat globules and higher mineral and protein content. Immunoglobulin A can also be found.

Correct positioning of the baby on the breast is crucial to the avoidance of sore nipples and the successful establishment of feeding. In the correct position, the nipple forms the distal third of a teat and the baby's lower jaw and tongue are opposed to breast tissue, which makes the milk flow.

Frequency and duration of feeds
- Babies who are allowed to regulate their own feeds tend to gain weight more quickly and maintain breastfeeding longer than those on feeding schedules.
- There is no reason to restrict feeding duration, as small-volume high-caloric milk is present at the end of the feed.
- There is no evidence to support the use of routine supplemental formula or fluids.
- The combined oral contraceptive pill increases breastfeeding failure, and the progesterone-only pill is indicated in the postpartum period.

Common breastfeeding problems
- Nipple trauma: this is usually due to incorrect positioning, and education is required.
- Breast engorgement: this occurs when the volume of milk exceeds the capacity of alveoli to store it. Management involves correct positioning of the baby and the use of firm breast support.
- Insufficient milk: although a common reason for ceasing breastfeeding, objective evidence suggests that only 1%–5% of lactating mothers have inadequate milk supply. The treatment includes unrestricted feeding and dopamine antagonists (metoclopramide).

Lactational amenorrhoea

- This is due to a suckling-induced change in hypothalamic sensitivity to the negative feedback of ovarian steroids.
- Inhibition of lactation occurs with the combined oral contraceptive pill and smoking.
- Bromocriptine may suppress lactation if required.

Common postpartum problems

- Anaemia: postpartum anaemia occurs in 25%–30% of women, and sustained iron intake is recommended.
- Perineal trauma.
- Urinary problems include voiding difficulty and urinary tract infections.
- Constipation and haemorrhoids are also potential problems.

Chapter 55

Perinatal mental health

Susan Roberts

Definitions

Perinatal mental health refers to mental health in pregnancy and the first year postpartum. Depression and anxiety are the most common psychiatric illnesses in pregnancy and the postpartum.

Pregnancy and the postpartum can be a time of increased risk for mental health problems either occurring for the first time or as a relapse of prior problems. Detection and management is important for the following reasons.

Significant morbidity

Perinatal mood disorders
- Antenatal depression occurs as commonly as postnatal depression and begins antepartum in up to 40% of women.
- Postnatal depression occurs in 6.5%–12.9%.
- The 'baby blues' occurs in up to 80% of women. It is characterised by emotional lability, tearfulness and vague somatic complaints, and usually resolves within 2 weeks. More severe and long-lasting symptoms may evolve into postnatal depression.

Perinatal anxiety disorder
- Anxiety disorders are diagnosed in 4%–39% of pregnant women and up to 16% of women postpartum.
- Pregnancy-related anxiety.
- Preexisting anxiety disorder in women who have never received treatment or relapsed secondary to cessation of treatment.
- Adjustment disorder with anxiety.
- Anxiety symptoms are comorbid with depression in 66% of women with postnatal depression.

- Perinatal posttraumatic stress disorder (PTSD) occurs in 1%–2% of pregnant women and may be related to a history of childhood sexual abuse or prior traumatic birth. It may be associated with increased request for termination of pregnancy, requests for caesarean section, impaired mother–infant bonding and commonly associated with antenatal and postnatal depression.
- Obsessive compulsive disorder: 33%–46% of women with obsessive compulsive disorder report worsening in pregnancy and postpartum.

Severe mental illness and pregnancy
- Women with severe mental illness have been reported to have lower fertility rates; however, rates have increased with increasing use of non-prolactin raising antipsychotics and many women with schizophrenia and bipolar disorder have children.

Significant consequences

- Adverse pregnancy outcomes include low birth weight, hypertension and pre-eclampsia.
- Associated with increased body mass index (BMI); postnatal depression is associated with greater weight retention.
- Increased risk of negative health behaviours including smoking, alcohol and substance misuse, greater use of prescription drugs, inadequate nutrition, weight gain and poorer antenatal attendance.
- Antenatal depression and anxiety is associated with an increased fear of childbirth and increased requests for an elective caesarean section in some women.
- Decreased initiation and duration of breastfeeding.
- Suicide is a rare but a major cause of maternal mortality associated with a previous history of self-harm, early onset and more severe symptoms and comorbid substance misuse. It is in the top three causes of indirect mortality in Australia.
- Long-term mental health problems.
- Association between maternal stress and depression and fetal neurological development possibly via the mechanism of increased maternal levels of cortisol which cross the placenta affecting the developing fetus.
- Associated with poorer maternal attachment in some instances and poor emotional and behavioural outcomes for children.
- Increased feeding and settling difficulties in infants.
- Postnatal depression is associated with an increased risk of parenting stress and difficulties in the mother–infant relationship.
- Increased risk of paternal depression, marital discord and impact on other children.

The structure exists for detection and intervention by screening

- The Edinburgh Depression Scale is a widely used scale for screening women in pregnancy and the postpartum. It is a 10-item questionnaire that enquires about mood and anxiety symptoms in the last 7 days.
- Screening should ideally occur at the first prenatal contact, 4–6 weeks postpartum and 3–4 months postpartum and ideally it should be repeated in 2 weeks if there is a high score.

- It should be used in conjunction with a psychosocial screen to determine other risk factors for poor perinatal mental health.
- A score ≥13 indicates a need for further mental health assessment. A positive on Q10 regarding thoughts of self-harm always warrants further evaluation and referral for acute mental health assessment if it is determined there is an acute risk to the woman's safety.
- Screening should only occur if there are established referral pathways to care.

Risk factors for perinatal depression and anxiety

- a history of psychiatric illness
- depression and/or anxiety in pregnancy is a risk factor for postnatal depression and anxiety
- recent negative life events (death of a loved one, relationship break up, moving house)
- lack of social support
- poor marital relationship
- history of abuse or of domestic violence
- unplanned or unwanted pregnancy
- present/past pregnancy complications
- pregnancy loss
- anxious personality style
- lower socioeconomic status

Assessment

Perinatal depression

Biological symptoms of depression such as low energy, sleep and appetite disturbance can overlap with the somatic symptoms of pregnancy; however, women who have a high number of somatic complaints have an increased risk for antenatal depression and subsequent postnatal depression. The core features of pervasive depression including lack of reactivity of mood, lack of interest in things and negative thoughts are more reliable symptoms of depression.

Risk to self and baby should always be assessed by asking the following questions:
- Have you had thoughts of harming yourself/your baby?
- Have you made plans to harm yourself/your baby?
- What would stop you from harming yourself/your baby (protective factors)?

If the answers to these questions are affirmative and there is a lack of protective factors, an immediate safety plan and organising a support person to be with the woman should be discussed and a referral for urgent psychiatric review arranged.

An understanding of local regulations regarding mandatory notification of child safety is required if there are concerns regarding the safety of an infant or other children.

Perinatal anxiety

Anxiety symptoms regarding birth and safety of the baby may be normal in pregnancy, particularly if there is a past history of obstetric complications. The frequency and intensity of anxiety symptoms and the degree to which they interfere with sleep, appetite and daily activities or result in risky health and lifestyle behaviours determine 'normal' versus a potential anxiety disorder warranting further investigation.

Physical assessment and investigations

An appreciation that depressive and anxiety symptoms can result in adverse obstetric and fetal outcomes and be a result of poor physical health is integral to management. It requires a thorough assessment of physical wellbeing and exclusion of potential biological contributions such as thyroid disorders, anaemia, vitamin deficiency B12, folate and D, and infection (e.g. mastitis).

- A baseline organic screen should include full blood count, urea and electrolytes test, liver function test, thyroid stimulating hormone test, iron studies, B12, folate and Vitamin D.
- Assessment of comorbidities should also be performed:
  - drugs, alcohol and nicotine
  - other psychiatric disorders
  - an assessment of available psychosocial support, both emotional and practical.

Management of depression and anxiety in pregnancy and postpartum

- A comprehensive diagnostic assessment and biopsychosocial formulation considering risk factors will determine appropriate management.
- Address lifestyle factors such as exercise, diet, sleep and rest, smoking, alcohol and substance abuse, and support.
- Consider non-pharmacological options:
  - referral for social interventions such as home-visiting programs (e.g. continuity of midwifery care in pregnancy, child health postpartum)
  - psychological therapies which include non-directive counselling, cognitive behaviour therapy, interpersonal therapy and mindfulness-based psychological therapy should be considered for mild to moderate depression and couple therapy where indicated
  - psychoeducation for women and their significant others
  - internet-based support and therapy options are becoming increasingly available.

Pharmacological management of depression and anxiety in pregnancy

- Medication should be reserved for moderate to severe conditions.
- All medications cross the placenta.
- In decision-making about the use of medications in pregnancy, consideration should be given to the potential risks and benefits to the pregnant woman and the fetus of treatment and non-treatment. This should take into account past response, placental transfer, obstetric and neonatal outcomes of particular medication considered and breast milk transfer using up-to-date, established data.
- Awareness of clinical guidelines and prescribing within the guidelines from beyondblue.
- Consideration of risk of medication in pregnancy can be summarised under the following headings:
  - teratogenesis (being aware of the baseline risk of 2%–3%)
  - risk for the neonate: postnatal adaptation syndrome (PNAS)
  - risk of pregnancy complications such as hypertension and premature delivery
  - long-term neurodevelopmental outcomes for the infant.

- The following websites provide up-to-date information of psychotropic medications in pregnancy:
  - Motherisk: www.motherisk.org
  - MotherToBaby (OTIS Teratology Information Service): www.mothertobaby.org
  - Reprotox
  - Medications in Mother's Milk: www.medsmilk.com
  - Lactmed: www.toxnet.nlm.nih.gov
- Monotherapy should be used where possible and the lowest possible dose, being aware not to undertreat and keeping in mind altered pharmacodynamics in pregnancy.
- Informed consent to prescribe medications in pregnancy should be obtained from the woman and preferably their partner, and documentation regarding the risk–benefit discussion should be in the notes.

Pharmacological treatment of depression in pregnancy and postpartum

- If a decision is made to commence or continue antidepressant medication in pregnancy, the use of selective serotonin re-uptake inhibitors (SSRIs) can be considered, as this is the category about which most is known. The current evidence on SSRIs shows no consistent pattern of additional risk of birth defects. While the safety of tricyclic antidepressants (TCAs) is supported by a lesser body of evidence, they can also be considered, especially if they have been effective previously. If a decision is made to discontinue or decrease antidepressant medication, it is important to gradually taper the dose, closely monitor and have a plan to identify relapse early.
- No support can be given to discontinue antidepressants in the third trimester as this does not influence the risk of postnatal neonatal adaptation syndrome and exposes the woman to a higher risk of relapse.
- Women with healthy full-term infants and who plan to breastfeed can be advised that SSRIs are not contraindicated.

Pharmacological treatment of anxiety disorders in pregnancy and the postpartum

- Use of benzodiazepines can be considered for short-term treatment of severe anxiety in pregnant women while waiting the onset of action of an SSRI. Long-acting benzodiazepines should be avoided as much as possible. Prescribing benzodiazepines close to term is associated with withdrawal symptoms in the neonate.
- The use of benzodiazepines can be considered for short-term treatment of severe anxiety in breastfeeding women while awaiting the onset of action of an SSRI or TCA.

Postpartum psychosis

- acute onset of manic or affective psychosis in the immediate postpartum period
- occurs in 1–2/1000 deliveries

Risk factors

- women with a prior history of postpartum psychosis carry a risk of 1:2 for future deliveries

- women with bipolar disorder have a 1 in 5 risk of severe recurrence postpartum and 1 in 2 risk of recurrence of any mood disorder
- 97% of women relapse within 2 weeks postpartum
- women with a family history of postpartum psychosis
- BUT 50 % of women have no psychiatric history
- primiparity

Aetiology
- genetic vulnerability
- specific puerperal trigger
- abnormal response to normal hormonal fluctuations
- role of stress hormones
- possible role of immunological factors
- sleep disturbance
- psychosocial stressors ARE NOT associated (unlike postnatal depression)

Symptoms
- sudden onset and rapid deterioration with wide fluctuations in intensity of symptoms
- lability of mood with elation and euphoria
- thought disorder
- distractibility
- overactivity
- delirium-like symptoms such as confusion, perplexity, disorientation, visual, tactile and olfactory hallucinations, misrecognition may be common

Differential diagnosis
- eclamptic psychosis
- acute confusional state
  - infection
  - endocrine and metabolic disorders
- drug-induced psychosis

Assessment and management
- psychiatric emergency
- comprehensive physical and neurological examination
  - full blood count, urea and electrolytes test, liver function test, thyroid stimulating hormone test, calcium, glucose, computerised tomography (CT) of head, urine drug screen
  - safety assessment of woman and baby, being aware of rapidly changing mental state
- admission preferably to a mother and baby unit to maintain mother–infant relationship
- management of physical status
- medications
  - antipsychotics
  - lithium carbonate
  - electroconvulsive therapy (ECT)
- support for partner and family
- assessment and consideration of child protection

Prevention of postpartum psychosis

- pregnancy planning and preconception planning for all women with a history of psychotic disorder and bipolar affective disorder
- referral to specialist perinatal mental health service of all pregnant women with previous history of psychotic disorder, bipolar affective disorder, family history of postpartum psychosis
- plan timing of delivery to minimise sleep disruption
- management of comorbidities
- medication prophylaxis immediately postpartum with research evidence supporting the use of lithium carbonate
- high-level monitoring in pregnancy and postpartum with communication of the management plan to all involved in women's care

Management of women with preexisting bipolar disorder, affective psychosis and schizophrenia in pregnancy and the postpartum

- All women with a history of schizophrenia, bipolar disorder and other psychoses should be referred for monitoring and optimisation of care in pregnancy and the postpartum period preferably to a perinatal mental health service.
- Relapse rates are significantly increased after discontinuation of medication and pregnancy does not appear to confer any protection.
- Liaison with maternity care staff and other support improves outcomes.
- Guidelines recommend a perinatal care plan that is documented and communicated to the woman, her family and all health professionals involved in her care in the peripartum.
- While it appears that antipsychotics have not been implicated as a major teratogen adverse outcomes such as gestational diabetes, low birth weight and developmental outcomes have been reported.
- These pregnancies should be considered high risk and a higher level of monitoring for fetal size and gestational diabetes is recommended.
- Particular medications such as sodium valproate are associated with a three-fold risk of major malformations and subsequent cognitive impairment and are contraindicated in pregnancy.
- The safety of lithium in pregnancy is controversial, with recent studies showing a weaker link as a cardiac teratogen; however, frequent monitoring is required in pregnancy due to changes in blood volume with careful management intrapartum.

PRECONCEPTION COUNSELLING

- Referral to specialist perinatal mental health services for women with a prior history of significant mental illness.
- Childbirth is a powerful trigger for mania and psychosis.
- Educate regarding modifying risks for relapse in pregnancy and breastfeeding.
- Discuss medication management to minimise risk of sudden cessation of medications and subsequent relapse.
- Individualised risk–benefit analyses are needed when psychotropic drugs are used in the perinatal period.
- Considerations for continuing current regime, coming off some or all medications, or switching to drugs with greater evidence for safety in pregnancy.
- Address psychosocial issues related to parenthood.
- Consideration of genetic counselling.

- Address issues related to other risk factors for fetal health such as smoking, nutritional factors, obesity, drug and alcohol use and domestic violence.

References

Austin, M.-P., Kildea, S., Sullivan, E., 2007. Maternal mortality and psychiatric morbidity in the perinatal period: challenges and opportunities for prevention in the Australian setting. Med. J. Aust. 186, 364–367.

Ayers, S., 2004. Delivery as a traumatic event: prevalence, risk factors and treatment for postnatal posttraumatic stress disorder. Clin. Obstet. Gynecol. 47, 552–567.

beyondblue, 2011. Clinical practice guidelines for depression and related disorders- anxiety, bipolar disorder and puerperal psychosis - in the perinatal period. A guideline for primary care health professionals. beyondblue: the national depression initiative, Melbourne.

beyondblue, 2009. Emotional Health and Wellbeing in pregnancy and Early parenthood, 3rd ed. beyondblue: the national depression initiative, Melbourne.

Cox, J., Holden, J.M., Sagovsky, R., 1987. Detection of postnatal depression: development of the 10 item Edinburg postnatal depression scale. Br. J. Psychiatry 150, 782–786.

Deligiamidis, K., Freeman, M., 2014. Complementary and alternative medicine therapies for perinatal depression. Best practice and research. Clin. Obstet. Gynecol. 28, 85–95.

Galbally, M., Snellen, M., Lewis, A., 2011. The use of psychotropic medications in pregnancy. Curr. Opin. Obstet. Gynecol. 23, 1–7.

Gavin, N.I., Gaynes, B.N., 2005. Perinatal depression: a systematic review of prevalence and incidence. Obstet. Gynecol. 106 (5–1), 1071–1083.

Gentile, S., 2010. Antipsychotic therapy during early and late pregnancy. A systematic review. Schizophr. Bull. 36, 518–544.

Glover, V., O'Connor, T.G., O'Donnell, K., 2010. Prenatal stress and the programming of the HPA axis. Neurosci. Biobehav. Rev. 35, 17–22.

Grigoriades, S., VanderPorten, E.H., Mamisashvili, L., et al., 2013. The impact of maternal depression in pregnancy on perinatal outcomes: a systematic review and meta-analysis. J. Clin. Psychiatry 74, e321–e341.

Jones, I., Chandra, P., Dazzan, P., et al., 2014. Bipolar disorder, affective psychosis, and schizophrenia in pregnancy and the post-partum period. Lancet 384, 1789–1799.

Marchesi, C., Ossala, P.e., 2015. Clinical management of perinatal anxiety disorders: A systemic review. J. Affect. Disord. 190 (4), 543–550.

Mum Mood Booster, (n.d.). (P. I. Institute, & Oregon Research Unit, Producers). Available at: <mummoodbooster.com>.

Murray, L., Cooper, P., 1997. Effects of postnatal depression on infant development. Arch. Dis. Child. 77 (2), 99–101.

Russell, E.J., Fawcett, J.M., Mazmanian, D., 2013. Risk of obsessive compulsive disorder in pregnant and postpartum women: a meta-analysis. J. Clin. Psychiatry 74, 377–385.

Yonkers, K., Wisner, K.L., Stewart, D.E., et al., 2009. The management of depression during pregnancy: a report from the American Psychiatric Association and the American College of Obstetrics and Gynecology. Gen. Hosp. Psychiatry 31, 403–413.

Chapter 56

Perineal trauma

Peta Higgs
Judith Goh

Perineal trauma occurs commonly during vaginal delivery. Episiotomy is the commonest surgical procedure in obstetrics. Careful examination after vaginal birth is essential to detect the degree of perineal trauma. Rectal examination should be performed as part of the assessment of perineal injury to identify a 'button-hole' injury where the rectal mucosa is torn through the vagina above an intact anal sphincter complex.

Classification

- **first-degree tear**: injury to the skin of the perineum and vaginal mucosa
- **second-degree tear**: injury to the skin and musculature of the perineum, not involving the anal sphincter
- **third-degree tear**: injury to the perineum involving the anal sphincter
  - *grade 3a tear:* < 50% external anal sphincter torn
  - *grade 3b tear:* > 50% external sphincter torn
  - *grade 3c tear:* both external and internal sphincters torn
- **fourth-degree tear**: injury involving the anal sphincter and anorectal mucosa

Obstetric anal sphincter injury (OASIS)

This has a higher risk of morbidity including:
- anal incontinence (25%)
- perineal discomfort and dyspareunia (10%)
- abscess formation and wound breakdown (10%)
- rectovaginal fistula (0.4%–3%)

Risk factors for OASIS
- large baby (≥ 4 kg)
- primiparous
- instrumental delivery

- occipito-posterior position
- second stage of labour longer than 1 hour
- epidural
- shoulder dystocia
- midline episiotomy

Prevention of OASIS

- Perineal protection at crowning.
- Warm compression during second stage of labour.
- Mediolateral episiotomy (with an angle of 60 degrees from the midline) has a lower risk (1%–9%) of OASIS compared to midline episiotomy (up to 17%).
- Mediolateral episiotomy should be considered in instrumental delivery.
- Restrictive use of episiotomy (rate of approximately 27%) reduces the risk of OASIS compared to routine episiotomy.

Repair of OASIS

- experienced or supervised surgeon to repair
- repair in operating theatre
- good lighting
- adequate analgesia (regional or general)
- antibiotic cover

Method of repair of OASIS

- Anal mucosa repaired with 3-0 polyglactin using interrupted or continuous suture.
- Internal anal sphincter (IAS) identified and repaired separately, with delayed absorbable interrupted or mattress sutures.
- External anal sphincter (EAS) repair by overlap or end-to-end method using either 3-0 PDS or 2-0 delayed absorbable suture.
- For a partial thickness tear of the EAS, end-to-end technique should be used.
- Perineum repaired in two layers to superficial perineal muscles and perineal skin with polyglactin suture.
- Rectal examination to ensure suture has not passed through rectal mucosa (and removed if present).
- Careful documentation of classification of tear and repair technique.

Immediate post partum care

- Insert an indwelling catheter.
- Broad spectrum antibiotics to reduce postoperative infection and wound complications.
- Postoperative laxatives (without bulking agents) to reduce the risk of wound dehiscence.
- Analgesics.
- Ice to perineum.
- Supportive underwear.
- Plan for follow-up.

Follow-up

Follow-up after OASIS should be performed by a specialist obstetrician gynaecologist or colorectal surgeon at 6–12 weeks. Women should be referred to a perineal clinic if available.

History
- perineal pain
- dyspareunia and sexual dysfunction
- flatus incontinence
- faecal incontinence
  - type (urgency, passive)
  - how often
  - type of protection required
  - stool consistency
- discussion of events and debriefing if difficult and traumatic labour
- other pelvic floor symptoms (e.g. urinary incontinence)

Examination
- vulvar skin and irritation
- wound healing and scar of repair
- introital width for intercourse
- pain over scar or perineum/pelvic floor muscles or pelvic organ
- anal sphincter tone and squeeze
- recto vaginal fistula on ano-rectal examination

Investigation
This would depend on the history and examination.
- endo anal ultrasound
- ano-rectal physiology
  - resting pressure
  - squeeze pressure
- functional canal length
- pudendal nerve terminal motor latency (PTNML)
- colonoscopy
- defecating proctogram

Treatment of faecal incontinence
The extent and interpretation of evaluation must be tailored to the individual. A multi-disciplinary team approach optimises outcomes. Surgical treatment is usually only considered after childbearing is completed.

In Australia, resources available to women include government-funded or subsidised schemes such as home assessments and continence products. The Continence Foundation of Australia provides a 24-hour helpline for men and women with urinary and faecal incontinence.
- conservative
  - pelvic floor physiotherapy
  - dietary advice to soften and bulk stools
  - voiding and defecatory dynamics
- pharmaceutical
  - stool softeners and bulking agents
  - loperamide to avoid loose stools and increase internal anal sphincter tone
- surgical
  - secondary anal sphincter repair
  - sacral nerve stimulator implant

- internal anal sphincter bulking
- diverting colostomy

Treatment of perineal pain and dyspareunia

This depends on the findings on history and examination.

- discussion on normal sexual function postdelivery
- sexual counselling for couple
- physiotherapy for massage of scar tissue, pelvic floor relaxation and trigger point release
- perineal revision
- excision of perineal scar

Advice for future pregnancy

- Planned size of family and the subsequent risks of vaginal delivery versus elective caesarean section should be discussed.
- Women who have had symptoms of faecal incontinence (even if transient) are at risk of worsening symptoms after another vaginal delivery.
- Women with abnormal endoanal ultrasound and/or manometry should be counselled regarding the option of an elective caesarean section.
- Episiotomy in a subsequent vaginal delivery has not been shown to decrease the risk of further OASIS and should only be performed if clinically indicated.

References

Continence Foundation of Australia. Available at: <www.continence.org.au>.

Fernando, R.J., Sultan, A.H., Kettle, C., et al., 2013. Methods of repair for obstetric anal sphincter injury. Cochrane Database Syst. Rev. (12), Art. No.: CD002866, doi:10.1002/14651858.CD002866.pub3.

Royal College of Obstetrician and Gynaecologist, 2015. Management of third and fourth-degree perineal tears following vaginal delivery. Green-top Guideline 29. RCOG, London.

Chapter 57

Membership exam tips and tricks

Thea Bowler

The curriculum including breadth and depth of required knowledge is outlined on the RANZCOG website.

Written examination

- 3-hour short-answer question examination: 12 questions
- 3-hour multiple-choice question examination: 120 questions

Preparation
- Most registrars study for a duration of 6–12 months.
- Study plan: it is useful to have a timeline for topics to be covered.
- Study group: a study group may be of great value for motivation and consolidation of learning.
- Content: a comprehensive outline of required knowledge can be found on the RANZCOG website.
- Important resources:
  - online learning resources (www.ranzcog.edu.au): CLIMATE, StratOG
  - guidelines (especially those that are new/recently updated and topical): RANZCOG, Green-top, NICE, Management of Perinatal Infections (ASID)
  - landmark papers.
- Practice: it is important to do as many past examination questions as possible.
  - Past short-answer and multiple-choice questions can be found on the RANZCOG website.
  - Some use practice questions as a guide to the depth of knowledge to cover.
  - It is worth practising short-answer questions under exam conditions and timing (15 minutes per question).
  - Many short-answer and multiple-choice questions are repeated; therefore, it is advantageous to know past questions well.

Exam strategy

- Make sure your writing is legible.
- Consider using bullet points (avoid long-winded answers).
- Allow 15 minutes per question and then move on.
- If unsure of the answer, it is best to write something.
- If a list is requested in a question's stem (e.g. differential diagnoses), use the marks allocated as a guide to the number of answers to provide. If there are many possible answers, there may be half a mark allocated per point.
- Aim to finish the entire exam without leaving questions blank.

Oral examination

The oral examination consists of 10 stations: 4 minutes reading time and 12 minutes examination time.

There are 20 marks allocated per station, with 5 of these marks comprised of the Global Competency Score (overall impression of the candidate's performance).

There are eight clinical stations where information regarding a scenario is provided during reading time. The candidate is then required to obtain any further necessary information from the examiner and proceed to discuss their management of the case, responding to the examiner's questions.

There are two communication stations (with an actor playing the part of the patient) in which the candidate is assessed on their ability to establish rapport, communicate effectively, use appropriate body language, provide honest and realistic answers and demonstrate respect and consideration towards the patient.

Preparation

- Preparation for the oral examination requires practice. A study partner is useful to undertake as many practice cases with as possible, although it is helpful to do cases with a wide range of colleagues and consultants to obtain as much feedback as possible.
- Past questions can be found on the RANZCOG website and there are many books available with practice objective structured clinical examination (OSCE) questions and answers.
- Attend as many practice examinations as possible (these are held at various hospitals).
- Note-taking: establish a systematic note-taking technique that allows gaps in the history to be filled and pertinent information to be highlighted.
- History and examination: it is important to establish a systematic technique for obtaining all necessary information in the shortest amount of time, without missing pertinent points.
- Management: it is worth developing short spiels for common topics that give a summary of the condition and proposed management in a succinct and confident manner.

Exam strategy

- Speak clearly, confidently and succinctly. A confident approach contributes to global competency. Ensure that your dress mirrors your behaviour/attitude: professional and tidy.

- Reading time: read the question carefully, make notes regarding further information to be elicited and anticipate what further questions/scenarios may follow.
- Answer the question: any questions asked are associated with allocated marks. Straying from the question wastes time without gaining marks. If the candidate is unsure whether to discuss something in greater detail, it is reasonable to ask the examiner, 'Would you like me to discuss this further?'
- Investigations: only order investigations that are relevant to the clinical scenario. Over-investigation may negatively impact your score.
- Ask for clarification: if an element of a question is unclear, ask for further explanation before giving an answer.
- Answer in as much detail as possible (e.g. drug doses, investigations, clinical manoeuvers).
- Encounters: points can be gained in each encounter; don't allow perceived performance in one encounter to impact on the remainder of the station/exam.

Self-care

Studying for membership examinations is a stressful experience. Despite the time constraints imposed by the work/study schedule, it is important to make time to exercise, eat well, get adequate sleep and even occasionally socialise. Making time for these things is important for mental health and will actually improve the quality of study rather than detract from it.

Appendix

MRANZCOG oral examination (sample questions)

Case 1

Encounter 1

The candidate will be given 4 minutes to read the letter provided below, outside the examination room. It is a referral letter from a general practitioner in your city. The candidate will play the role of the consultant obstetrician gynaecologist and the examiner will play the role of the patient.

River Lakes Medical Centre
16 Fountain St
Brighton Heights

Dear Dr

Thank you for seeing Elizabeth Tate who is a 17-year-old girl with primary amenorrhoea. She has no significant past medical history or allergies. She lives at home with her parents, one younger sister and one younger brother. She attends the local high school and is in Year 12.

Regards
Thomas Bell

After 4 minutes, the candidate then comes in to meet the examiner and the station begins.

Encounter 2

Elizabeth has presented with her mother Margaret for a review of her results. Our roles will remain the same.

Encounter 3

Elizabeth has presented to you 3 years later. She is now 20 years of age, has a boyfriend and is now in a long-term relationship. Menarche occurred at the age of 18. She wants to discuss fertility issues. Our roles will remain the same.

This is the end of the case.

Model answer for case 1

Encounter 1

- Take adequate history and examination. Information given to the candidate when asked: height 150 cm; weight 60 kg; vital signs normal; breast development at Tanner stage 4; pubic and axillary hair present; cardiovascular and abdominal examination normal.
- Candidate should ask for pelvic ultrasound, hormone profile including luteinising hormone (LH), follicle stimulating hormone (FSH), oestradiol, progesterone, testosterone, sex hormone binding globulin, prolactin, thyroid-stimulating hormone (TSH), free thyroxine and karyotyping.

Encounter 2

The candidate receives the results of the requested investigation.
- Pelvic ultrasound: normal but small ovaries with few follicles, uterus 6 cm in length and the endometrium is thin

- Luteinizing hormone	< 2 IU/L	
- Follicle stimulating hormone	9 IU/L	
- Oestradiol	< 43 pmol/L	
- Progesterone	3 nmol/L	
- Testosterone	1.0 nmol/L	(0.3–2.8)
- free testosterone (calc)	7 pmol/L	(4–46)
- Sex hormone binding globulin	99 nmol/L	(18–114)
- Prolactin	19 ug/L	(< 20)
- Thyroid stimulating hormone	1.4 mU/L	(0.40–4.00)
- Free thyroxine (fT4)	14 pmol/L	(10–20)

- G-banding studies:
  - Maximum band resolution: 550 bands per haploid set
    — 15 cells counted
    — 5 cells analysed
- Karyotype: 46,X,i(X)(q10), with 45,X; consistent with Turner's mosaicism

Candidates are expected to:
- explain results to patient, in particular advise about Turner's syndrome
- list screenings test at the time of diagnosis of Turner's syndrome including cardiovascular evaluation, renal ultrasound, audiology assessment, lipid profile, thyroid function test and fasting glucose
- provide educational and psychosocial evaluations
- ongoing monitoring including blood pressure, lipid profile, renal function, fasting glucose, thyroid function, liver function, coeliac screening and ovarian function.

Encounter 3

Candidates are expected to:
- provide educational and psychosocial evaluations
- advise patient that chance of conception, although reduced, is still present and therefore discuss options of contraception
- advise patient of increased risks of chromosomal abnormalities with conceptus and increased risks of spontaneous abortion
- advise option of in vitro fertilisation (IVF) with donor oocyte.

Case 2

Encounter 1

The candidate will be given 4 minutes to read the letter provided below, outside the examination room. It is a referral letter from a general practitioner in your city. The candidate will play the role of the consultant obstetrician gynaecologist and the examiner will play the role of the patient.

Mountainview Family Practice
14 Montana Avenue
Heathridge

Dear Dr

Lisa Nguyen is now 10 weeks pregnant in her first progressive pregnancy. She is wanting to book to confine at your hospital. Her pregnancy has been uneventful so far but the only concern is her anaemia. She has been on iron for all of her pregnancy and no improvements have occurred. Enclosed are her results.

Thanks for seeing her.

Regards
Lynda Paine

Haemoglobin		100	g/L	(115–165)
Haematocrit		0.29		(0.35–0.47)
RCC		4.5	10 × 12/L	(3.9–5.6)
Reticulocytes		28	10 × 9/L	(10–100)
MCV		65 L	fL	(80–100)
WCC		3.5	10 × 9/L	(3.5–12.0)
Platelets		29	10 × 9/L	(150–400)
Blood group		AB Rh(D) positive		
Antibody screen		negative		
Varicella zoster IgG (EIA):		positive		
Hepatitis B virus surface antigen:		negative		
Hepatitis C virus antibody:		negative		
HIV 1/O/2 antibodies:		negative		
Syphilis screen:	RPR test:	negative		
	TP-PA test:	negative		
Rubella virus IgG antibody:		59 IU/ml		
	< 10 IU/ml	No evidence of immunity		

Encounter 2

Lisa returns with her results and a diagnosis of alpha thalassemia-1 trait. Our roles will remain the same.

Encounter 3

Lisa returns with her results and ultrasound scan performed today. Our roles will remain the same.

Review at 28 weeks
GTT normal
Ultrasound fetal measurement: 28 weeks, 40th percentile
Placenta is fundal and clear os.
Heart activity present and fetal movement seen.
Amniotic fluid is normal.
There is mild ascites.
There is also pleural effusion.
Skin oedema of more than 6 mm.

Model answer for case 2

Encounter 1

- Take adequate history and examination. Information given to the candidate when asked: height 166 cm; weight 54 kg; vital signs normal; breast examination normal; cardiovascular and abdominal examination normal. The patient has separated from her partner; therefore, other testing should be performed on her ex-partner.
- Candidate should discuss the findings on the results, in particular advising further investigation to include review of peripheral blood smear, reticulocyte count, serum iron studies, haemoglobin electrophoresis and genotyping patterns.

Encounter 2

- Candidate needs to discuss the findings of the results below:
  - homozygosity for alpha (+) thalassemia (a–/a–)
    — summary alpha thalassemia-1 trait.
- Candidate needs to discuss the management of alpha thalassemia trait in pregnancy.
- Candidate needs to explain to the patient that there is still a possible risk of fetal hydrops development for her unborn baby as her partner's genotype is not known.

Encounter 3

- Candidate needs to diagnose non-immune hydrops fetalis from the ultrasound report.
- Candidate needs to discuss management of non-immune hydrops fetalis and explain the prognostic outcome of the condition.

Credit

Box 28.1 Australian Categorisation of drugs in pregnancy
© Commonwealth of Australia

Disclaimer:

The Australian categorisation system and database for prescribing medicines in pregnancy have been developed by medical and scientific experts based on available evidence of risks associated with taking particular medicines while pregnant. This information is presented for the use of health professionals prescribing medicines to pregnant women, rather than for the general public to use. It is general in nature and is not presented as medical advice to health professionals or the public. It is not intended to be used as a substitute for a health professional's advice.

Index

Page numbers followed by '*f*' indicate figures, '*t*' indicate tables, and '*b*' indicate boxes.